Psychological Basis of Psychiatry

To Radha
'I have too little to give you, my dear…'

Commissioning Editor: Michael Parkinson
Project Development Manager: Barbara Simmons
Project Manager: Nancy Arnott
Designer: Erik Bigland
Illustrator: Chartwell Illustrators

Psychological Basis of Psychiatry

M S Thambirajah MB BS, FRCPsych

Consultant Child and Adolescent Psychiatrist, Ablewell House, Walsall NHS Teaching Primary Care Trust

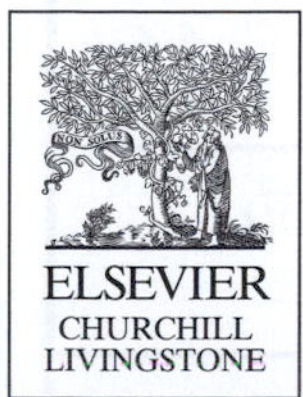

EDINBURGH LONDON NEW YORK OXFORD PHILADELPHIA ST LOUIS SYDNEY TORONTO 2005

ELSEVIER
CHURCHILL
LIVINGSTONE

First published 2005

ISBN 0443 100993

British Library Cataloguing in Publication Data
A catalogue record for this book is available from the British Library

Library of Congress Cataloging in Publication Data
A catalog record for this book is available from the Library of Congress

Notice
Medical knowledge is constantly changing. Standard safety precautions must be followed, but as new research and clinical experience broaden our knowledge, changes in treatment and drug therapy may become necessary or appropriate. Readers are advised to check the most current product information provided by the manufacturer of each drug to be administered to verify the recommended dose, the method and duration of administration, and contraindications. It is the responsibility of the practitioner, relying on experience and knowledge of the patient, to determine dosages and the best treatment for each individual patient. Neither the Publisher nor the author assumes any liability for any injury and/or damage to persons or property arising from this publication.
The Publisher

Printed in China

PREFACE

'We shall never have a science of medicine as long as we separate the explanation of the pathological from the explanation of the normal, vital phenomena'
Claude Bernard (1865)

In all sciences a sound grasp of the normal is considered to be a prerequisite for understanding the abnormal. In medicine, for example, physiology is considered to form the basis for understanding organ dysfunction and disease, as the above quote from Claude Bernard, the founder of experimental medicine, asserts. Psychiatry has grown up as a study of pathology, a specialisation in the abnormal without investing much effort in the understanding of normal mental phenomena. The latter has been left mostly to psychologists. Yet we have consistently undervalued the study of normal functioning. As Gregory Bateson (1987) has pointed out, although there is a reasonably comprehensive terminology in psychiatry to describe abnormality, no such vocabulary exists for describing normality. Nonetheless we accept that even in the most disturbed psychotic patients, apart from the pathology, large parts of their mental functioning such as cognitions, emotions and personality are normal, but our science is rather inarticulate about the operations of the normal aspects of the person. Instead psychiatry's theoretical focus is concentrated on the diagnosis of abnormality and normal processes, so important for therapeutic progress, are little studied.

This book aspires to gather together most of the 'knowns' in normal psychological functioning that are relevant to psychiatry. The second aim of the book is to extend our understanding of normal psychological processes to the realms of abnormal psychology, abnormal functioning and psychopathology. In our present state of knowledge the gap between the two areas is huge. For example, we know little about how normal emotions (e.g. sadness) are related to pathological emotional states (e.g. depression). Nor do we have even a rudimentary understanding of how normal thinking processes are related to thought disorders in psychotic states. The chasm between normal and abnormal psychological functioning is also mirrored by the gulf between the two professions – psychology and psychiatry – and their subcultures and worldviews.

But this has not always been the case. Sigmund Freud, the psychologist par excellence, was a physician. The contributions to psychology of later day psychiatrists like John Bowlby and Aron Beck have been monumental. William James, considered to be the father of American psychology, trained initially as a medical physiologist. After a long period of professional rivalry and mutual recriminations there are now signs that the two groups are coming together. More recently there had been a certain degree of rapprochement between the two professions. Although in the US this has come about partly because of the necessities of managed care, the recent advances in cognitive behaviour therapy, especially CBT for psychoses, appear to be bringing the two disciplines closer together than ever before.

It is my hope that this book will go some way in encouraging psychiatrists, especially psychiatric trainees, to develop an interest in the theoretical, clinical and research aspects of psychology. The discipline of psychology is fortunate in having many fine textbooks. In general, psychologists have been excellent teachers and produced some of the best texts in any field, but most of these books approach the subject matter from a discipline specific point of view. These texts cater for students and trainees in psychology and have little appeal for the psychiatrist or nurse in training. Medically-trained practitioners prefer to read precise and compacted texts rather than the more loquacious and longwinded psychology textbooks. I have attempted to keep the material in the book as brief and succinct as possible. Like a bee collecting honey from different flowers, I have gathered together the essentials in psychology and present it to the busy reader in a condensed form. In trying to keep the book within reasonable proportions some topics have been sacrificed and others abridged. For example, topics such as consciousness and thinking have been omitted and the chapter on psychoanalytic concepts is very brief (and, in my view, does an injustice to Freud!).

This book arose out of my experience in teaching in the various courses for psychiatric trainees and others. I am deeply indebted to Professor C. Mohan and Professor George Mohan for inviting me to teach in the MRCPsych revision courses they have organised. I owe a special word of thanks to the staff at Walsall Central Library for their untiring efforts in acquiring reference books and journal articles for me. Without their help this book would not have seen the light of day. I am grateful to Dr Thilak Ratnayake for his useful comments on the first draft of this book. Finally I must express my gratitude to Susan Burns and Carole Wright for typing the manuscript.

M S Thambirajah Walsall 2004

References

Bateson G (1987) Psychiatry and society, In Ruesch J & Bateson G Communication: the social matrix of psychiatry, New York: W.W. Norton.

Bernard C (1885) An Introduction to the Study of Experimental Medicine, p. 146, New York: Dover.

CONTENTS

Learning theories and their applications

1

'What we have learned is [comparable to] a handful of soil; what we have not learned is as large as the World.'
Thiruvalluvar, Tamil poet

In simple terms learning is defined as *'a relatively permanent change (or potential for change) in behaviour which occurs as a result of experience'*. Several aspects of this definition are worthy of note. The phrase 'relatively permanent' serves to exclude changes that may be due to temporary states such as fatigue, hunger or illness. In learning, the 'change in behaviour', may not necessarily be revealed in immediate behaviour and refers also to a capacity for behavioural change. Difference between learning and performance of the learned behaviour deserves emphasis. Learning may not manifest itself in performance until a later time. This has been referred to as latent learning. By emphasising 'experience', the definition draws attention to a salient fact: learning theorists assign overwhelming pre-eminence to environmental influences. Although this does not rule out genetic predisposition and biological influences, learning theories hold that environmental factors, by and large, determine behaviour.

Types of learning

Learning, be it a simple exercise such as learning to read a new word or a complicated set of procedures to be mastered like driving a car or understanding a story or an abstract principle, is a complex procedure, which involves numerous biological and psychological systems. Several types of learning have been described. One way of ordering them from simple learning to complex forms of learning is as follows:

1. Classical conditioning (respondent learning).
2. Operant conditioning (instrumental learning).
3. Observational learning (vicarious learning or modelling).
4. Cognitive learning.
5. Complex learning – abstraction, problem solving, learning rules and strategies, hypothesis testing and concept formation.

CLASSICAL CONDITIONING

Ivan Pavlov, the Russian physiologist, while studying the digestive system, discovered that dogs salivated not only when food was introduced into the mouth but also whenever the experimenter entered the room with the food. Pavlov called this stimulus–response relationship *conditioned reflex*. Systematic study of the phenomenon led him to develop a general law of conditioning: when a previously neutral stimulus is repeatedly paired with a stimulus that normally causes salivary secretion, the neutral stimulus alone eventually comes to elicit the response. In a typical Pavlovian experiment, first a tone is sounded (for about five seconds) and two or three seconds later, food is presented. The procedure is repeated several times. After a number of such trials or pairings only the tone is presented without the presentation of food and the number of drops of saliva and the time interval between presentation and initiation of salivation is measured. The results have been unequivocal: after about 30 pairings a neutral stimulus such as a tone or the sounding of a bell produces salivation. Pavlov investigated this process in detail by changing each of the variables.

Simply stated, the Pavlovian paradigm holds that if a conditioned stimulus (CS), such as a bell, tone or flash of light, is repeatedly and consistently followed by an unconditional stimulus (UCS) like food, over time the CS comes to elicit the conditioned response (CR). The acquisition of a conditioned response may be represented as in Figure 1.1.

Key features of classical conditioning

The phenomenon of classical conditioning has been the subject of intense study, especially during the period when 'behaviourism' dominated the field in the 1950s and 1960s (see later). As a result, a number of robust features about classical conditioning have been described:

1. Extinction. Once a conditioning response has been established, presentation of the CS (e.g. bell) alone without the UCS (e.g. food) leads to gradual disappearance of the CR. This phenomenon, when CS no longer produces CR, is known as extinction.

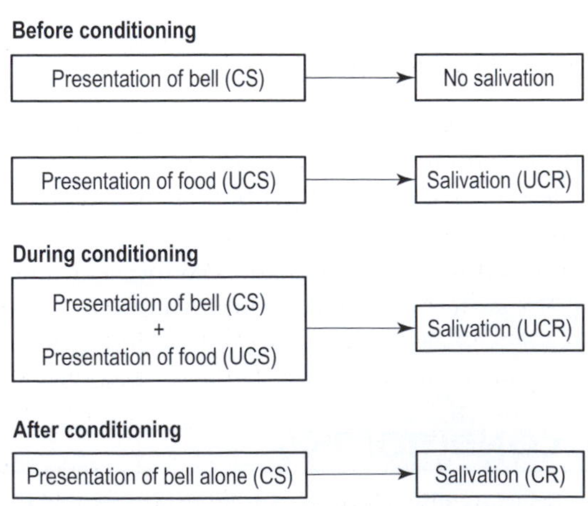

Fig. 1.1 The classical conditioning paradigm

2. Spontaneous recovery. If CS is reintroduced after extinction has been produced, the CR reappears but the response is rather weak and fragile.

3. Generalisation. This refers to the tendency to respond to stimuli that are roughly similar to the original CS. Dogs conditioned to a tone of say 2000 Hz salivate to tones of increasing and decreasing in frequency. However, the response is maximal when the 2000 Hz tone is presented. The pattern of responding is roughly an inverted U centred around the actual CS.

4. Discrimination. If two widely different CSs are used and one is paired with the UCS (CS+) and the other one is not (CS–) then the organism will discriminate between the two stimuli provided they are not too similar.

5. Higher-order conditioning. After classical conditioning has taken place, the CS can be successfully paired with a second CS (CS2). After a series of trials in which CS2 precedes CS1, the CS2 acquires the conditioning properties of the US. This is called second-order conditioning. The experiment can be repeated with a CS3 to produce third-order conditioning. Such higher-order conditioning produces weaker conditioning and it is almost impossible to go beyond third-order conditioning before extinction sets in.

6. Counter-conditioning. If an established CS (CS1) is paired with a new CS (CS2), which elicits a new response that is incompatible with the old one so that only one of them can occur at a time, it leads to suppression of the original CR. For example, fear conditioning induced in dogs following mild electric shocks is abolished by repeated presentation of food with the shocks.

Shock → Escape (fear)

Shock + Food → Salivation (not escape)

Counter-conditioning is another method (in addition to extinction) for abolishing conditioned responses and bringing about extinction. It is the basis of *reciprocal inhibition*, a behavioural technique used in anxiety states (see later).

Factors affecting classical conditioning

1. Contiguity. Pavlov found that pairing the CS with the US was essential for conditioning to occur. Contiguity refers to the temporal relationship between the CS and US. In standard experiments on classical conditioning the CS occurs before the onset of the US and remains on until the CS is presented, i.e. the CS and US are contiguous. This basic pairing condition is called *delayed* or *forward conditioning*. In animal experiments optimal conditioning occurs under these conditions; the strongest conditioning takes place when the time interval between the onset of the CS and US is 0.5 seconds. Three other variations in the sequencing of the two stimuli have been carried out (Figure 1.2):

1. *Trace conditioning*. The CS is presented before the US as in the standard condition, but it is terminated before the UCS begins. The UR is usually weak and gets weaker as the time interval between the two is increased. It is

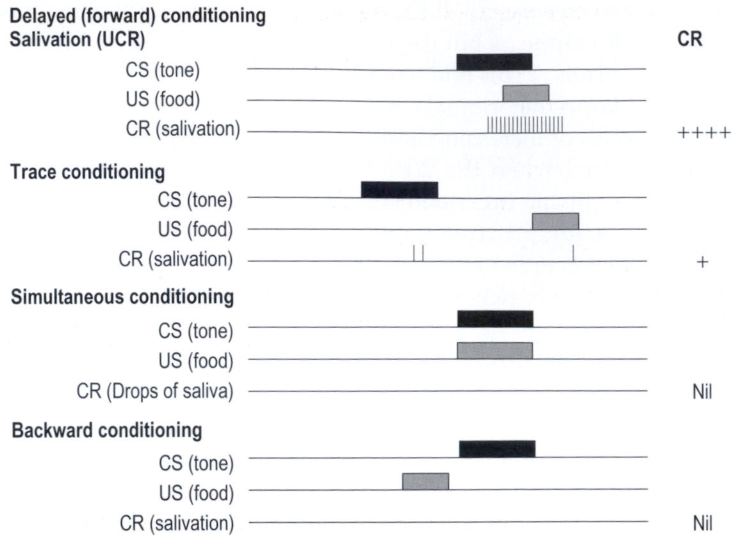

Fig. 1.2 Classical conditioning and the four temporal sequences

called trace conditioning because 'traces' of the CS are thought to remain in memory.

2. *Simultaneous conditioning*. Here the CS and US are presented and terminated simultaneously. It produces virtually no conditioning.
3. *Backward conditioning*. In this the US comes on before the CS. There is hardly any conditioning.

Thus, for strong conditioning CS should precede the US and remain on until the US occurs. In animal experiments the optimal CS–US interval is 0.5 seconds.

2. *Contingency.* For a long time it was held that contiguity was both a necessary and sufficient conditioning for classical conditioning to occur. This understanding was powerfully challenged by the work of Rescorla (1968). He produced experimental evidence to show that the traditional view of pairing of the CS and US embodied two different characteristics: contiguity and contingency. In contiguity the critical factor is the timing: the CS is contiguous with the US if the two stimuli occurred close together in time. Contingency refers to the probability or likelihood of the one event following the other. Applied to classical conditioning, UCS is contingent upon CS when the probability or chances that the UCS will occur when the CS has been presented is high. In the later condition of contingency, the UCS acts as an accurate predictor of the occurrence of the US. Rescorla devised a series of experiments in which the two conditions of contiguity and contingency could be separated out. This is shown in the Figure 1.3

Rescorla carried out his experiments with rats using a tone as the CS and a mild shock as the US. His main finding was that conditioning only occurred in the contingency group. In the contiguity group there was little or no evidence of conditioning. These findings led him to conclude that it was

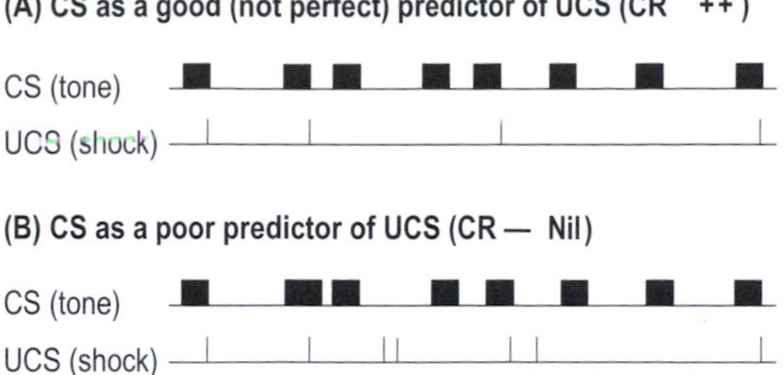

Fig. 1.3 Contiguity and contingency. In condition (**A**) CS is a good predictor that a UCS will follow. In condition (**B**) the CS is of no value in predicting the UCS. A CR developed readily in condition (**A**) but not in (**B**). Note that the number of CS–UCS pairings are identical for both groups

not sufficient for two stimuli to be just associated in time but the neutral stimulus, the CS, should reliably predict the occurrence of the UCS for strong classical conditioning to take place (Rescorla's *predictive hypothesis*). The same conclusion has been reached by others studying classical conditioning. The current understanding of classical conditioning is that simple contiguity of two events is insufficient to explain Pavlovian conditioning. Rather, conditioning depends on the information that the CS provides about the US; if the CS is a good predictor of the US then conditioning occurs. (Rescorla, 1988). The situation is complicated by the fact that in some instances simple contiguity alone does produce conditioning.

3. ***Nature of the conditioned stimulus.*** Not all CS–US relationships result in conditioning to the same extent. Pavlov held that any natural stimulus, such as sound, smell or sight, could be converted into a conditioned stimulus. This idea, known as the *equipotentiality assumption*, has been shown not to be true. Research has established that not all conditioned stimuli are equally effective. The most convincing evidence for this assertion comes from *taste aversion experiments* in rats. In a series of conditioning studies Garcia demonstrated that rats could not be conditioned to noise or light but that they conditioned to taste quite readily. Rats that developed nausea (through experimental radiation) after exposure to light or sound while drinking plain water showed no suppression of drinking whereas rats that were given flavoured water followed by nausea induction stopped drinking it almost immediately afterwards (Garcia & Koelling, 1966). Thus rats appear to develop aversion more readily to taste than to other stimuli. Aversive taste conditioning, also known as the *Garcia effect*, is common in both animals and humans and this has obvious survival advantages. It helps the rats avoid poisoned food and human beings are 'disgusted' by spoilt food.

These findings are important because the selectivity shown by animals and man to stimuli for conditioning shows that conditioning is constrained by biology. There appears to be an inborn predisposition to learn certain associations and not others. The tendency to form certain CS–US associations has been termed *preparedness* by Seligman (1970). Further evidence for the concept of preparedness comes from conditioning experiments carried out by Ohman. He showed that human beings could be conditioned to fear-relevant stimuli, such as snakes and spiders, with just one pairing with electric shock (US) whereas it took numerous trials before fear conditioning developed to neutral stimuli like flowers or mushrooms. Moreover, conditioned fear induced by fear-relevant stimuli was more persistent and lasted longer. Evolution appears to have prepared the human race to fear some stimuli rather than others (Ohman, 1993).

4. Number of 'trials'. In conditioning experiments, typically, the conditioned response increases in strength with repeated trials until it reaches a maximum, known as the asymptote, after which no further increase occurs. This relationship has been termed the 'learning curve'. But this is not always the case, the Garcia effect, conditioned aversion to taste and smell of food, and fear conditioning to snakes and spiders are acquired after a single trial. One-trial learning is important in conditions where survival is crucial. The rat might not live to avoid the bait if it took the standard 30 trials to learn the association!

Conditioned responses

Classical conditioning was originally demonstrated for autonomic reflexes such as salivation and secretion of gastric juice. As has been noted above, it was later shown that another autonomic reflex, nausea induced by taste aversion, was readily conditionable. What is the scope of classical conditioning? It is obvious that it applies to a limited rage of responses. More importantly, unlike other forms of learning, it does not produce any new responses that are not in the repertoire of the organism. Classical conditioning has been shown to be demonstrably relevant in the following responses:

- *Autonomic responses*. The range of autonomic responses that can be conditioned are numerous. Most studies have involved responses such as salivation, heart rate, vasoconstriction, nausea and eye blinking. There is also some evidence of conditioning of blood glucose levels, sensitivity to pain and changes in immune systems.
- *Emotional responses.* Conditioned emotional reactions are common. Conditioning plays an important role in the acquisition of fears and phobias (see later).
- *Motivational states*. Hunger and sexual arousal are subject to the rules of classical conditioning to some degree. Stimuli associated with food have been shown to induce hunger in both humans and animals (see Chapter 5). Classical conditioning may play a part in human sexual arousal. In one study, when previously paired with slides of nude women, pictures of long fur boots were shown to produce conditioned penile erection in male volunteers. This has led to the postulation that conditioning may be a feature in fetish formation. (Rachman & Hodgson, 1968).

Another question that has been raised is: Is the conditioned response identical to the unconditioned response for a particular pair of CS and US? Pavlov postulated that CRs were no different from URs. Subsequent research has demonstrated that all CRs are not identical to their corresponding UCRs. In some instances the associated CRs are weak or, even, the opposite of the original UCRs. For example, injection of adrenaline normally increased the heart rate and blood sugar. But when conditioned to CSs such as flashes of light or a buzzer, the conditioned response is a *decrease* in heart rate and blood sugar.

Nature of learning in classical conditioning: what is learned?

What is the mechanism underlying classical conditioning? The theories that attempt to explain the process fall into two groups, associative theories and cognitive theories

1. ***Associative theories.*** Pavlov argued that, at a basic level, dogs were learning about the association or the relationship between the tone (CS) and the appearance of food (US). According to him the CS becomes a substitute for the US, so that after conditioning it (the CS) turns into the US. This is known as the stimulus–stimulus theory (S–S theory). There is some evidence to support this proposition.

2. ***Cognitive theories.*** Other groups of workers have argued that it involves complex cognitive processes, such as attention, thinking and expectation. Several experiments have demonstrated that the critical factor in classical conditioning is that the animal learns to expect the CS and that it is the predictive power of the CS that determines conditioning. Conditioning, they assert, involves predicting the occurrence of one stimulus from the presence of the other. Prediction is inevitably dependent on cognitive processes such as attention and memory

As research into Pavlovian conditioning has progressed it has become abundantly clear that classical conditioning, once considered a simple form of learning, has turned out to be a complex phenomenon. The best conclusion that one can come to is that, in humans, conditioning involves at least two systems: (1) A relatively primitive system that is outside awareness and operates in the automatic processing mode underpinned by associative processes and stimulus substitution; and (2) a cognitive system in which conscious awareness leads to rapid learning, this involves prediction, expectation and memory.

Classical conditioning and human behaviour

Classical conditioning can be seen in most aspects of our day-to-day behaviour although we may not be aware of it. Aversion and attraction to certain types of food (and people!), the aura of tranquillity that people experience in places of worship, the garrulousness and excessive drinking in bars and the way we feel about and use various parts of our homes (the study, bedroom) are examples of conditioning seen in everyday life. The advertising industry has attempted to exploit conditioning by pairing highly desirable stimuli with the products that they want to sell. An image of an attractive (and, often scantily clad) young female model often accompanied by pleasant music followed by the image of a car, for example, is a common advertising technique to induce people to buy the product.

Conditioning and psychopathology

The classical conditioning paradigm has been used to explain and understand abnormal and maladaptive behaviours. The best-known application has been to the acquisition of fears and phobias.

Acquisition of fears and phobias

One of the earliest demonstrations of conditioning in human beings was by J. B. Watson, the founder of radical behaviourism. Watson induced phobia for white rats in an 11-month-old infant called Albert. 'Little Albert' was a well-adjusted child with no fear of white rats – in fact, when presented with the rat he tended to play with it. Like most infants he was afraid of loud noises. Watson subjected him to conditioning trials in which a loud noise was produced out of his sight by striking a steel bar with a hammer every time Little Albert saw the rat and tried to reach for it. Little Albert would jump violently and start crying at the loud sound. After several pairings of exposure to the rat and the sound, Albert developed an intense fear of the white rat. Thus, Watson was able to convincingly demonstrate that classical conditioning could be applied to human beings. He also showed that the fear response generalised to other white objects such as cotton, fur coats, a rabbit and a dog (Watson & Rayner, 1920).

The acquisition of the phobia could be summarised as follows:
Before conditioning:

Loud noise (US) → Fear (UR)

Conditioning trials:

White rat (CS) + Loud noise (US) → Fear

After conditioning:

White rat (CS) → Fear (CR)

Generalisation:

White furry objects → Fear (CR)

Watson and Rayner's experiment has been replicated several times. An interesting finding was that the CS had to be a live animal; when the CS was an inanimate object such as a bottle, a piece of wood, or a toy animal, no conditioning took place. This finding emphasises the biological limits of conditioning and is consistent with Seligman's concept of 'preparedness', that is, human beings and animals are biologically predisposed or 'prepared' to form certain associations rather than others.

Habit formation and addictions

It had been suggested that some habits are cue dependent. Sights and smells are particularly potent cues for eating and drinking. As mentioned above conditioning may play a part in sexual behaviour.

Clinical applications of classical conditioning

The discovery of the principles of classical conditioning inspired many workers to attempt to apply it to clinical problems. As a result several clinical interventions have been devised to treat emotional and behavioural problems. The most well-known applications of classical conditioning are:

Systemic desensitisation

One of the best-known applications of the principles of classical conditioning is systemic desensitisation developed by Joseph Wolpe (1958) for the treatment of phobias. It involves gradual exposure of the subject to the feared stimulus or situation by one step at a time while getting him or her to undergo relaxation during each stage. The mechanism thought to underlie the procedure is *counterconditioning*. In counterconditioning the conditioned response is eliminated by pairing the CS with another US that produces a new response that is incompatible with the old CR. Since only one response is possible the new one replaces the old. The first human experiment that demonstrated desensitisation most powerfully was carried out on a boy named Peter. Peter had a phobia for rabbits but, like all children, liked eating. In the desensitisation procedure Peter was shown the rabbit at a distance while he was also given food. The pairing was repeated in several trials and at each trial the rabbit was moved a little closer. At the end of the experiment Peter was completely free of the phobia and even started playing with the rabbit (Jones, 1924).

Systemic desensitisation involves three phases. The first phase entails the *construction of a fear hierarchy*, this consists of drawing up a list of conditions under which the identified phobia occurs and ordering them in sequence from the most feared situation to the least feared. For example, in the case of spider phobia a (shortened) hierarchy may consist of:

1. Drawing spiders.
2. Showing pictures of spiders.
3. Touching photographs of spiders.
4. Seeing spiders at a distance.
5. Watching a spider at closer quarters.
6. Touching the spider.

The second element in systemic desensitisation is learning progressive relaxation. In this the subjects learns to relax the muscles and regulate their breathing. Wolpe called this process of inducing incompatible responses *reciprocal inhibition*. The third and most important component of the procedure is *exposure*. In this the subject is exposed to the least threatening stimulus in the hierarchy while inducing relaxation. When exposure to the first item in the hierarchy is successfully completed the subject moves to the next item in the list and the processes is repeated until the phobia is overcome.

During exposure to the target stimulus the subject's level of anxiety increases until it reaches a plateau and then begins to diminish. It is essential that each exposure session be prolonged long enough for the anxiety

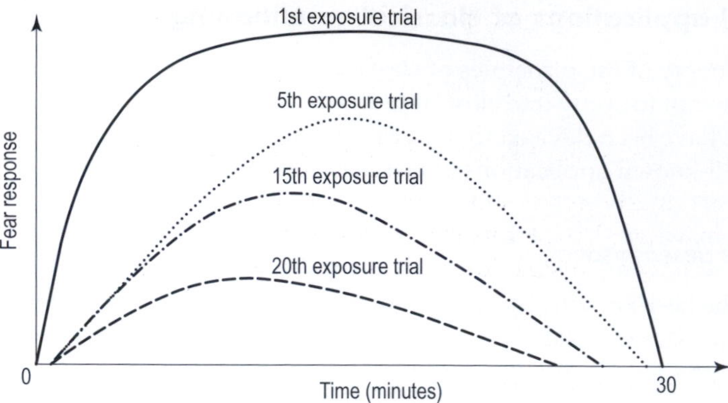

Fig. 1.4 Successive exposure to a feared stimulus produces habituation and eventually extinction of the fear response, provided each exposure is long enough for the fear response to subside

experienced by the subject to return to the base line. This usually takes about 20 to 30 minutes (Figure 1.4). The aim is to produce *habituation* so that on subsequent exposures the amount of anxiety induced gets progressively less and less, until eventually it leads to extinction of the fear response.

If for any reason the session is prematurely aborted before anxiety levels return to normal it leads to *sensitisation* rather than habituation, resulting in heightened fear responses. This is common if the procedure is not well planned. When desensitisation is carried out in imagination it is known as *covert desensitisation*

Flooding

Flooding is based on the principle that presentation of the feared stimulus for sufficiently long periods of time (provided the subject can tolerate the anxiety) leads to dissipation of the anxiety, thus bringing about the extinction of the fear response. It is a forced exposure procedure that has been shown to be highly clinically effective but often not acceptable to patients. Flooding may be carried out with objects and situations in real life (*in vivo*) or in imagination.

Aversion therapy

Aversion therapy involves the pairing of an unpleasant or painful stimulus with the target behaviour. This technique has been employed mainly with drug addiction and alcohol misuse. The unconditional stimulus is a painful or unpleasant stimulus such as electric shock, or induction of nausea and vomiting. For example, smoking may be paired with an injection of apomorphine that produces nausea and vomiting. Extinction is thought to be brought about by the subject's avoidance of the unpleasant CR, nausea.

Apomorphine (US) → Nausea (CR)

Apomorphine + Smoking → Nausea (CR)

Smoking → Nausea (CR) → Avoidance of smoking

In the past, mild electric shocks have been used as aversive unconditioned stimuli to treat alcohol misuse. Aversion therapy has not been popular because of patients dislike for the treatment methods and their limited effectiveness.

The use of the enuresis alarm

Nocturnal bed-wetting (enuresis) in childhood is a developmental disorder that occurs in 10% of five year olds and 5% of 10 year olds. The usual form of treatment is the use of an enuresis alarm. The device consists of a small pad (containing the electrodes) that is placed in the child's nightclothes, with the alarm being placed in a waistband. The first drop of urine completes the circuit and activates the alarm, which wakes the child. When the alarm goes off the child is expected to get up, go to the toilet and change the pyjamas and sheets usually with parental help. The alarm is thought to act as the US that is paired with the sensation from the distended bladder (CS). After several pairings the child learns to wake up in response to a full bladder.

Alarm (US) → Waking

Distended bladder (CS) + alarm (US) → Waking

Distended bladder (CS) → Waking

The predictions made by the classical conditioning theory have indeed been shown to be correct. In general, enuresis alarms are a safe and effective way of treating nocturnal bed-wetting. Studies have shown that about 80% of the children become dry after using the alarm for two to three months.

OPERANT CONDITIONING

Two features of classical conditioning are worth repeating. First, it applies largely, but not exclusively, to somatic and emotional reflexes and some motivational phenomena. This limitation of the classical conditioning paradigm has important implications. Much of human behaviour is voluntary, purposeful and wilful and, therefore, the applicability of the rules of classical conditioning to human behaviour is rather restricted. Second, its focus is on stimuli. One of the remarkable discoveries of early learning theorists was that the response to a stimulus depends not only on the stimulus but, more importantly, on what happens as a result of the response, i.e. on the consequence.

It is common knowledge that if a response is followed by a reward, or pleasurable experience, it tends to be repeated. In short, positive consequences of an act or behaviour increase the probability of that behaviour being increased. This was scientifically demonstrated by Edward Thorndike (1898). A hungry cat was placed in a box (called Thorndike's puzzle box) that had a door, which could be opened by a latch inside the box. When food was placed outside the box the cat randomly ran around the box until by accident it managed to open the door by pushing on the latch. In a short time, by a process of trial and error, the cat learned to open the door every time food was placed outside it. From these experiments Thorndike postulated the *Law of Effect* which states that 'the positive consequences of an act or behaviour increases the chances of that behaviour being repeated'. He called the learning resulting from such consequences *instrumental learning*.

B. F. Skinner (1953) took this line of work further. He devised a piece of apparatus (called the Skinner box) that was equipped with an inside lever. Pressing the lever resulted in the delivery of pellets of food through a food dispenser. A hungry rat or pigeon is placed inside the box and its bar pressing behaviour is recorded. Typically, as the animal learns that its bar pressing behaviour produces the consequence of delivering food, the bar pressing behaviour increases. Skinner called the responses, in this case the bar pressing response, *operants* because they operate on the environment to change it. *Operant conditioning* refers to learning in which a voluntary response is increased or decreased, depending on positive or negative consequences. Learning theorists use the term *reinforcer* to describe any event that increases the probability of a response when presented after it. The process by which an act, event or response increases the probability that the preceding behaviour is repeated is known as *reinforcement.*

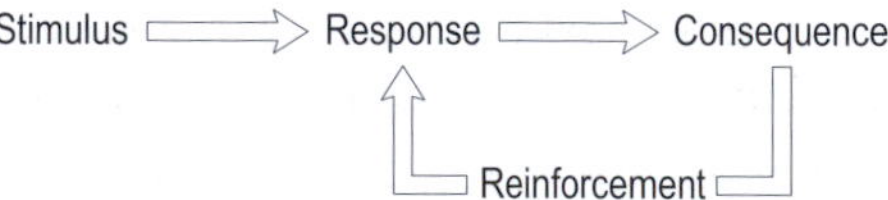

The relationship between the behaviour and its consequence is called a *contingency*. Thus, another way of describing the process is to say that the increase in responses is the result of *contingency* between the lever-pressing response and the delivery of food. Two events are said to be contingent with each other if the occurrence of the second event is dependant on the first and does not happen in the absence of it. Therefore, it could be said that reinforcement is contingent upon the consequence that follows the response. Thus, unlike classical conditioning, in operant conditioning, it is the consequences of behaviour that are all-important. The stimulus acts as a cue for the behaviour or sets the context for the behaviour. The relationship between the stimulus or antecedent, behaviour and consequence can be written as:

Stimulus → Response → Behaviour +

or

Antecedent → **B**ehaviour → **C**onsequence +

The acronym 'ABC' is an important relationship in analysis of behaviour. We will return to it later.

Positive and negative reinforcement

There are two types of reinforcement contingencies: positive reinforcement and negative reinforcement. *Positive reinforcement* is said to take place when the behaviour is maintained or increased by producing consequences that the person or animal finds rewarding. In Skinner's experiments with rats the delivery of food positively reinforced bar-pressing behaviour. In childhood sleep problems, the repeated attention (consequence) the child receives from the parents positively reinforces the child's crying at bedtime and the sleeping difficulties. *Negative reinforcement*, on the other hand, is the increase in probability of a response or behaviour through the *removal* of an aversive consequence. Taking a hypnotic to relieve insomnia, an aversive experience, negatively reinforces the behaviour and increases the likelihood of the act being repeated.

In real life, positive and negative reinforcements may act together to maintain behaviour patterns. In the above example of the child who cries at bed times, while parental attention positively reinforces the child's behaviour, the cessation of crying upon receiving attention results in the removal of the aversive response for the parents and produces negative reinforcement of the parent's behaviour.

Negative reinforcement can occur through either postponement of the aversive consequence or by removal of the unpleasant event. The former reinforcement contingency is known as avoidance conditioning and the latter as escape conditioning. In *avoidance conditioning* the response or act *prevents* the aversive stimulus from occurring. For example, taking a different road to work after a previous accident avoids cues associated with the accident and therefore the anxiety that may be induced by it. Avoidance conditioning is relatively resistant to extinction. In *escape conditioning* the behaviour *terminates* or removes the unpleasant event. People learn to escape from fires and animals take shelter from the rain. In both these situations learning occurs by the process of escape conditioning. Experimentally, lever pressing in the Skinner box could be arranged to terminate a shock delivered through the floor. As the intensity of the shock increases so does escape behaviour.

Negative reinforcement should not be confused with punishment. *Punishment* is the *reduction* of the probability of the response or behaviour by the application of an aversive consequence. If fines imposed for a traffic offence reduce such transgressions in the future, they could be deemed a punishment. In lay usage, punishment implies the application of an unpleasant consequence, such as smacking a child or passing a death sentence for murder. In learning theory, punishment is said to have occurred only if the procedure had brought about a reduction or abolition of the target behaviour.

The four reinforcement contingencies are summarised in Table 1.1.

Reinforcers

A reinforcer is an event or stimulus that increases the probability of the behaviour that precedes it. *Primary reinforcers* satisfy biological needs and are,

Table 1.1 The four reinforcement contingencies

Contingency	*Pleasant consequence*	*Aversive consequence*
Presentation of consequence	Positive reinforcement (resulting in increased response)	Punishment (resulting in decreased response)
Removal of consequence	Negative punishment (resulting in decreased response)	Negative reinforcement (resulting in increased response)

therefore, inherently rewarding. Food and water are examples of primary reinforcers. They are effective from birth and need no special training. A *secondary reinforcer* is a previously neutral stimulus that, if paired with the stimulus that is already reinforcing, will itself take on reinforcing properties. Hence their reinforcing properties are acquired through experience. Money is the most obvious secondary reinforcer. In social situations praise, affection and attention are important secondary reinforcers (social reinforcers).

Timing the delivery of reinforcers has been found to be crucial in bringing about reinforcement. Operant conditioning is strongest when there is little delay in delivering a reinforcer. In animal experiments, it has been shown that delaying a positive reinforcer, even for a few seconds, impairs learning. Hence, for maximal effect positive and negative reinforcements need to be delivered without much delay. For example, to increase desirable and prosocial behaviours in children, rewards need to be provided as soon as possible. The other factor that affects the effectiveness of reinforcers is their salience. The receiver needs to feel that the reinforcer is important or worthwhile. Most often experiments conducted in operant conditioning have dealt with hungry rats where the reinforcement has been food.

It is sometimes possible for reinforcement contingencies to occur accidentally. In experimental situations, animals have been shown to develop strange ritualistic responses such as turning in a circle, ending up on their back legs, or producing odd head movements because, by accident, these movements had been reinforced by delivery of food at the time of their occurrence. Such accidental reinforcement results in strengthening the actions that precede it. This has been termed *superstitious behaviour*. Superstitious behaviour is common in human beings. Thus, someone who passes an examination while wearing a particular shirt may begin wearing the 'lucky' shirt for every examination.

Schedules of reinforcement

Thus far, the above discussion of reinforcement has assumed that reinforcers were delivered every time a particular response occurred. This condition of reinforcement, where every time a behaviour is performed it is reinforced, is known as continuous reinforcement. Oddly enough, continuous reinforcement does not lead to the strongest learning. Using laboratory animals, a number of different schedules of reinforcement and their effect on behaviour have been observed. These partial or intermittent reinforcement schedules can be classified as follows:

- Fixed ratio (FR) schedules provide reinforcement following a fixed number of responses. For example, rats may be given food after every 10th lever press (FR10). Here the response requirement is fixed at 10 responses. With FR schedules the response rate is very high indeed but it also has low resistance to extinction.
- Variable ratio (VR) schedules where reinforcement is provided after a given number of responses but the number varies from one reinforcement to the next. For example, on a VR-15 schedule, a rat might sometimes be reinforced after 10 lever presses, sometimes after 25 presses but an average of 15 responses would occur before reinforcement was given. Most gambling machines offer a variable ratio schedule. With VR schedules response rates are very high and extinction cannot be achieved easily.
- Fixed interval (FI) schedules provide reinforcement for the first response that occurs after some fixed time has passed since the last reward, regardless of the number of responses made during that interval. For example, on a FI-20 schedule, the first response to every 20 seconds will be rewarded and the first response that occurs once a further 20 seconds has elapsed will be reinforced and so on. FI schedules produce a slow but steady rate of response and extinction occurs quickly.
- Variable interval (VI) schedules reinforce the first response after some period of time but the amount of time varies. In a VI60 schedule, for example, first response to occur after an average of one minute is reinforced but the actual time between reinforcements may vary from 1 to 120 seconds. VI schedules produce a slow but steady increase in response that cannot be extinguished easily.

Generally speaking, behaviours learned under partial reinforcement schedules are far more difficult to extinguish than those learned on continuous reinforcement schedules. The partial reinforcement schedules and fixed ratio schedules provide the highest response rates while the variable ratio schedules are the most resistant to extinction.

Features of operant conditioning

Like classical conditioning, instrumental learning appears to conform to certain 'rules':

- *Extinction*. As with classical conditioning, if the reinforcer is removed from the operant conditioning situation, the operant behaviour declines and eventually undergoes extinction. Thus, if the feeder mechanism in the Skinner box is suddenly disconnected, thereby preventing lever pressing from producing pellets of food, the rat's lever-pressing behaviour gradually becomes less and less until it reaches the basal level.
- *Spontaneous recovery*. After extinction, if an animal is returned to the experimental situation where lever pressing produces delivery of food, it learns to press the lever quickly without any additional training.
- *Generalisation*. Reinforcement in one situation may not necessarily generalise to other situations. For example, a boy rewarded with praise for being helpful in class may not 'learn' to be helpful at home. Lack of generalisa-

tion of operant learning in day-to-day situations is a consistent feature and is overcome by providing training in a variety of situations.

Operant conditioning and psychopathology

The operant conditioning paradigm has been applied to explain the development and/or maintenance of a number of clinical phenomena. Two explanatory models that have been influential are the learned helplessness model of depression and the two-factor aetiological model of phobia.

Learned helplessness

In 1975, Martin Seligman published his laboratory studies on dogs, which formed the basis of his paradigm of depression called 'learned helplessness' (Seligman, 1975). Seligman was studying avoidance conditioning in dogs. He set up an avoidance conditioning situation with three conditions:

1. In the first condition a group of dogs were given electric shocks from which they could not escape.
2. In the second condition another group of dogs were also given electric shocks but they were able to jump a fence to avoid them.
3. In the third condition a further group of dogs were not given any shocks (control group).

After 24 hours all dogs were given shocks that they could escape from (i.e. the same as condition two).

Seligman found that dogs in condition two quickly jumped the fence to avoid the shock as they had learned this the day before. Dogs in condition three also jumped the fence but took a few trials to learn this behaviour. Dogs in condition one did not try to jump the fence and just lay down and accepted the shocks. It seems that the helplessness that these dogs had learned on day one had shaped their future behaviour. Seligman postulated that when exposed to repeated adversities over which they had little or no control individuals learned to be helpless and so feel depressed.

The theory was revised in 1978 (Abrahamson, Metalsky & Alloy, 1978) to include explanations for the feelings of pessimism, hopelessness and low self-esteem that are prominent in depression. The reformulated theory holds that the helplessness and uncontrollability by themselves do not sufficiently explain the cognitive and emotional components of depression. Rather the *attributional styles* that are adopted to explain the causal events are thought to be more important. They argued that people respond to failure in a variety of ways but characterised these as lying along three dimensions:

1. *Internal–External*. Failure is attributed to an internal cause, namely themselves, or to some external cause, such as other people or the circumstances – 'I am no good at passing examinations' versus 'A particular exam was difficult'.
2. *Stable–Unstable*. Failure is attributed to a cause that is likely to continue in the future (stable) or to a cause that might easily change in the future

(unstable) – 'I always fail examinations' versus 'This was a particularly difficult examination'.

3. *Global–Specific.* Failure is attributed to a cause that applies to a range of situations that influence all or most of one's life (global) or to a cause that is specific to only one situation (specific) – 'I am no good in anything' versus 'I may be no good at performing in examinations, but I am a good clinician'.

Vulnerability to depression is said to be derived from a tendency to attribute negative events to internal, stable, global causes. Such a *'depressogenic attributional style'* is viewed as a stable trait with its origin in early childhood experiences. It has been found that people who are currently depressed do indeed show these negative attributional styles. But there is little evidence to date to show that these negative cognitive styles are present before the onset of depression, and they have not been demonstrated in patients who have recovered from depression. It is worth noting that the original theory was based on the S–R paradigm of behaviourism. The reformulated theory, on the other hand, had taken cognisance of the cognitive revolution that swept through psychology and placed cognitive factors at the centre of the model. The revised model may be summarised as:

Negative events + perceived uncontrollability → Learned helplessness → Depressogenic attributional style (internal, stable, global) → Depression

The conditioning model of phobia

The learning theory holds that fears and phobias are acquired by pairing of a potentially phobic stimulus (e.g. white rat in the case of Little Albert, the CS) with an unconditioned stimulus (e.g. a loud noise caused by striking an iron bar, the UCS). In these situations, fear is thought to be a learned response to danger signals (conditioned stimuli) that are indicative of situations of injury or pain (unconditioned stimuli). Neutral stimuli, which are associated with the fear or pain producing state of affairs, develop fearful qualities, i.e. they become fear CS.

The second factor involved is thought to be the avoidance of the phobic stimulus (in Little Albert's case, the white rat) bringing about a reduction of fear and anxiety, thus maintaining the phobia. This has been called the *two factor theory* of Mowrer (1939). According to the theory there are two stages in the formation of phobias: (1) an initial acquisition phase in which an aversive or traumatic event becomes associated with a neural event resulting in an intense emotional reaction of fear through the process of classical conditioning; and (2) maintenance and intensification of the phobic reaction by avoidance of the feared situation. This involves the operant conditioning process, negative reinforcement and avoidance learning.

For example, an accidental fall or experiencing a fainting attack in a public place may condition a subject to associate going out to public places with fear. Subsequently, the person finds that attempting to go out results in severe anxiety or fear. Avoiding going out results in evasion of the negative feelings. This results in continuation of the phobia (Figure 1.5). The theory has also been applied to obsessive-compulsive behaviours. In obsessive hand washing, classically acquired anxiety about contamination (because of past experience) makes the

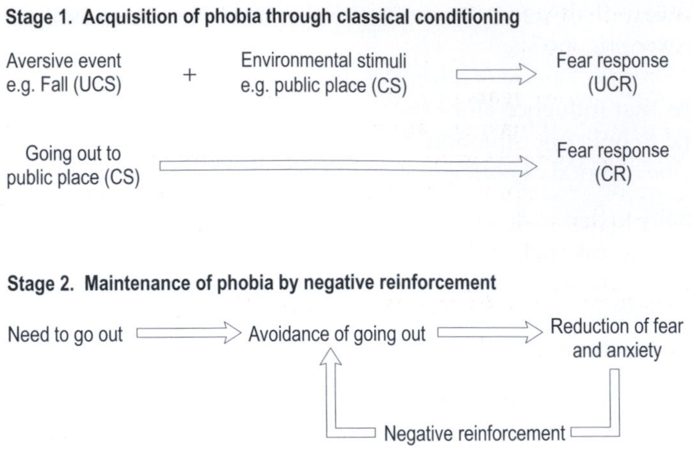

Stage 1. Acquisition of phobia through classical conditioning

Aversive event e.g. Fall (UCS) + Environmental stimuli e.g. public place (CS) ⇒ Fear response (UCR)

Going out to public place (CS) ⇒ Fear response (CR)

Stage 2. Maintenance of phobia by negative reinforcement

Need to go out ⇒ Avoidance of going out ⇒ Reduction of fear and anxiety

Negative reinforcement

Fig. 1.5 The two factor model of phobia

person wash the hands continually and repeatedly after touching things believed to be contaminated. The hand-washing behaviour reduces anxiety. Alleviation of anxiety negatively reinforces and maintains the hand washing.

Several criticisms have been directed at the two factor model, the most important of which are:

1. Most patients with phobic disorders do not give a history of traumatic events or fearful experiences relevant to the phobic stimulus. The converse also seems to be true – not everyone who has had a traumatic experience develops a phobia for stimuli associated with it. For example, very few people who have been bitten by a dog develop dog phobia and few who have been involved in a traffic accident show phobia for driving.
2. In some instances, after initial conditioning, presentation of the CS without the UCS increases the degree of fear, a phenomenon known as *incubation.* Contrary to the assertion by the two factor theory, rather than bringing about its extinction, (short) exposures to a threatening or phobic situation increase conditioned fear.
3. The conditioning model fails to explain why people develop some phobias more readily than others. For example, human beings are more likely to develop phobias about snakes and spiders but not about guns, knives or electrical items, which could be equally dangerous.

It is thought that the two-factor theory of fear acquisition and maintenance accounts only for part of the available information about phobias. It has been proposed that other mechanisms might be responsible for acquisition of fears. Rachman (1977) proposed three overlapping phenomena that may underlie the formation of phobias:

1. Conditioning, both classical and operant, as described in the two factor theory.
2. Observational or vicarious learning.

3. Dissemination of information about the stimuli that cause fear, including cultural transmission.

It is likely that intense fears of biological significance, such as snake phobias and blood injury phobias, are more likely to be acquired by a conditioning process, whereas common everyday fears are thought to be acquired by indirect and socially transmitted processes of information-giving type and by vicarious exposure.

Clinical applications of operant conditioning

Token economy and star charts

Token economy was introduced by Ayllon and Azrin (1968) as a way of modifying patients' behaviour in psychiatric wards. It utilises the principle of positive reinforcement by providing secondary reinforcers to encourage desired behaviours. Patients are required to perform the target behaviours, such as making the bed, getting ready in time and exercising, in order to receive a particular number of tokens. Tokens usually consist of coins or cards, which can be exchanged for privileges like going out, cigarettes or listening to music. Token economy systems have been successfully employed in a variety of settings (classrooms, prisons, homes for people with learning disabilities) to increase appropriate behaviour.

Another method of providing positive reinforcement to encourage positive behaviour, especially in the case of children, is the system of star charts or 'smiley faces'. In children with encopresis (soiling) or nocturnal enuresis (bedwetting), a star is given for a symptom-free or 'good' day and pre-agreed privileges are provided for achieving a given number of stars.

Biofeedback

In biofeedback continuous feedback is provided regarding one's physiological state, such as skin conductance, blood pressure or heart rate, in the form of visual or auditory signals. The individual attempts to control the signals voluntarily using methods that they have been taught. Biofeedback has been used in relaxation training, especially in patients with anxiety. An electrode attached to a machine 'reads' the level of subclinical sweating (skin conductance) and converts it into a continuous tone or red light. The subject's task is to extinguish the signal by relaxation. Biofeedback techniques have been successfully employed in the control of tension headache, migraine, and epilepsy.

Use of punishment

In theory, and under experimental conditions, punishment procedures are effective in bringing about extinction of undesirable behaviours. Unpleasant consequences, when made contingent upon performance of an undesirable behaviour, can quickly reduce that behaviour. However, there are both practical and ethical considerations concerning the application of punishment contingencies. Punishment is most effective in reducing maladaptive behaviour when it is immediate (inflicted without much delay), severe and consistent

Application of aversive consequences to overcome maladaptive behaviours, i.e. positive punishment procedures are associated with a number of 'side effects':

1. The use of physical punishment in children, for example, could result in modelling of aggressive behaviour. Children subjected to physical punishment learn to use coercive methods to achieve their ends.
2. Punishment may produce avoidance behaviour such as lying or aggression in order to evade the unpleasant consequence. In keeping with the theory of negative reinforcement, such negative behaviours get reinforced and, eventually, become difficult to eliminate.
3. Punishment provokes intense feelings of anger and resentment directed at the person providing the punishment, especially if it is perceived to be unfair, resulting in a variety of retaliatory responses and damage to relationships.

Given that punishment procedures carry with them the above disadvantages, it is often a better option to reinforce desirable behaviours than attempt to punish maladaptive behaviours in applied settings.

Operant conditioning and behaviour therapy

Reinforcement strategies have been employed in clinical and educational settings to: (1) reduce maladaptive or unwanted behaviour; and (2) to increase prosocial or desired behaviours

Establishing new behaviours

1. *Differential reinforcement of other behaviour (DRO).* This involves the reinforcement of positive behaviours rather than focusing on undesirable ones. Thus, a child who steals occasionally may be praised and rewarded on the days he is *not* stealing. A child who has a phobia of adult dogs may be rewarded for looking after a puppy. DRO is often more effective than mere withdrawal of reinforcement or punishment and may be used in combination with these procedures.

2. *Shaping.* In shaping, the desired response is achieved by reinforcing those responses that become increasingly similar to the one the experimenter wants. The target behaviour that may not be in the repertoire of the individual is first identified. As responses that are more similar to the desired final response occur, these are reinforced. Shaping, therefore, involves two components:

1. Differential reinforcement, that is, reinforcement of some responses and not others.
2. Successive approximations, which refers to the reinforcement of those responses that become increasingly similar to the final desired target response.

Shaping represents a practical approach to teaching new behaviours. Shaping has been used in teaching children with learning disabilities to feed themselves. First, the client is reinforced for touching the spoon. When this step is achieved, holding the spoon is reinforced. Next raising the spoon to the mouth is reinforced, while the first two steps are taken for granted and not reinforced. Thus each successive step is reinforced until the final goal, eating using the spoon, is achieved.

3. ***Chaining.*** This refers to a specific sequence of responses in which each response serves as a stimulus for the next response. Reinforcement is delivered after the performance of the entire sequence of actions according to a predetermined criterion. It differs from shaping in that it is not successive approximation but the specific S–R links that are reinforced. In *forward chaining* behaviours are linked together, beginning with the first behaviour in the sequence (Figure 1.6). In *backward chaining* the behaviours are linked together, beginning with the last behaviour in the sequence.

For example, in preparing a person with learning disabilities to go out, the therapist may say, 'Please put on your coat'. This serves as a discriminant stimulus, which brings about the first response of obtaining the coat from the closet. It serves as a conditioned reinforcement for putting one arm through the sleeve. The second response uses the onset of the actions of placing the arm through the next sleeve and so on, until the coat is put on and zipped. After zipping the coat, the therapist praises the subject thus reinforcing the entire forward chain.

Reducing unwanted or undesirable behaviours

1. ***Non-reinforcement of undesired behaviour.*** Withdrawal of reinforcement of the undesirable target behaviour is by far the commonest method employed to overcome or unlearn maladaptive behaviours. This invariably involves careful analysis of the behaviour that is to be corrected.

2. ***Time out.*** This is a form of negative punishment in which the person is removed from all positive reinforcing events for a brief period of time. It is, therefore, best termed 'time out from reinforcement'. Typically time out procedures are employed with disruptive or maladaptive behaviours. For example, a child with a temper tantrum is removed from the situation and made to sit in a chair in the corner of the room for a short period of time during which he is not provided with reinforcement in the form of attention or other activities. Once his tantrum stops and he has been silently seated in the chair for a few minutes, usually less than 5 minutes, he is allowed to resume activities. Such measures have been shown to be remarkably effective in reducing temper tantrums and other disruptive activities in children.

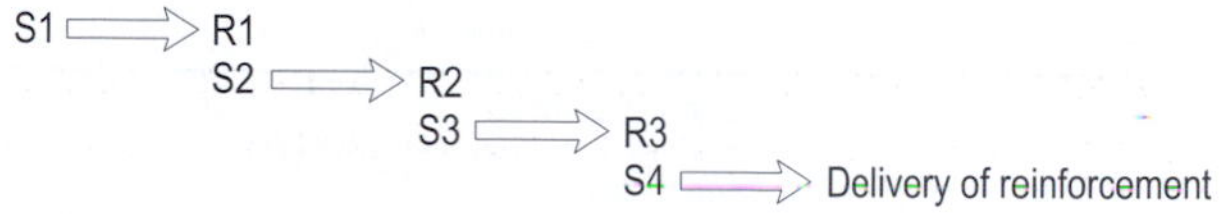

S1 ⇒ R1
S2 ⇒ R2
S3 ⇒ R3
S4 ⇒ Delivery of reinforcement

Fig.1.6 Chaining procedure. The previous response (R1) acts as a discriminant stimulus (S2) for the next response (R2), and so on

3. Response cost. This is a punishment technique that involves removal of a positive event as a response to certain forms of undesirable behaviour. Typically these involve enforcing penalties for undesirable behaviours. For example, in the case of a teenager a contract might be agreed such that making their bed in the morning means going out with a friend in the evening. Failure to make the bed in the morning entails the response cost of the loss of the evening reinforcer. The technique may also include restitution, as when an adolescent is made to clean up the place after throwing things in anger.

Table 1.2 summarises the common applications of classical and operant conditioning procedures.

Behaviour analysis

As a general paradigm, behaviour analysis views current behaviour (B) as a function of two sets of variables: antecedent events (A) and consequences (C). The basis of the ABC paradigm may be represented as follows:

Antecedent (A) → Behaviour (B) → Consequence (C)

Thus, in order to understand any piece of behaviour it is important to specify both the antecedent events (A) that determine the occurrence of behaviour (B) and, more importantly, its consequences (C), which reinforce and maintain the behaviour.

Behaviour analysis is underpinned by the belief that deviant behaviour is due to inappropriate learning and that the presenting behaviour is the focus for assessment and not some underlying cause. Behaviour analysis involves several important steps:

1. Identification of target behaviour. The target behaviour(s) should be operationally defined and objectively described (behavioural description). For this purpose the behaviour is defined as any change in the organism's activities that is observable and measurable.
2. Observation, measurement and recording of target behaviour(s).
3. Identification of antecedents and consequences affecting the behaviour.

ABC analysis is the key to any form of intervention. It involves the collection of baseline data regarding the frequency, intensity and duration of target behaviour, together with the context in which the behaviours occur,

Table 1.2 Summary of some of the applications of classical and operant conditioning principles

Classical conditioning	*Operant conditioning*
Systemic desensitisation	Token economy
Flooding	Star charts
Aversion therapy	Biofeedback
Use of enuresis alarm	Aversion therapy, punishment techniques

implying that the antecedents set the conditions for such behaviours. More importantly, the consequences of the behaviour are recorded. The main sources of information in a behaviour assessment include history, assessment interviews, direct observation and, where necessary, self-reports. Once the behaviour has been reliably observed, measured and recorded, it can be analysed according to its antecedents and consequences. The chain of events (antecedent–behaviour–consequence; A–B–C) forms the basis of behaviour analysis. Radical behaviourists insist that dysfunctional behaviours (i.e. responses) cannot be understood in isolation from the stimuli that trigger them and the consequences that follow from them. Thus, the complete stimuli–responses–consequences (S–R–C) event, or contingency, constitutes problem behaviour, not just the dysfunctional responses.

Behaviourism

The school of thought that arose from the learning theory and its applications outlined above has been called *behaviourism*. Radical behaviourists argued that classical and operant conditioning (together with modelling) form the building blocks of human and animal behaviour. J. B. Watson, the father of behaviourism, took an extreme behavioural view of human nature and development when he stated:

> *Give me a dozen healthy infants and my own specified world to bring them up and I will guarantee to take any one at random and train them to become any type of specialist I might select – doctor, lawyer, artist, merchant, chef and, yes, even a beggar man and thief – regardless of his talents, penchants, tendencies, abilities, vocations and race of his ancestors. There is no such thing as inheritance of capacity, talent, temperament, mental constitution and behavioural characteristics.*
>
> (Watson, 1925)

In behaviourism the core unit of study, as its name implies, is the overt observable behaviour. It is this feature of observing and measuring overt behaviour that is fundamental to behavioural approaches. The behaviourist rejected the view that mental phenomena such as motives, cognitions and emotions were worthy of study because they were unobservable. Skinner, one of the pioneers of behaviour therapy, regarded 'private events', such as thought processes and emotions, as irrelevant to the study of behaviour because they were regarded as unobservable, immeasurable and, hence, not scientific variables. In short, consciousness is antithetical to the strict behavioural model. Non-observable mental variables such as expectations, beliefs, memory and thought processes are discounted because they cannot be observed and, therefore, are held to be too unscientific to warrant serious consideration.

The behavioural model was not only applied to normal learning processes but was also thought to be applicable to abnormal behaviour to explain why and how it arose and was maintained. The symptoms of psychiatric disorders were understood by behaviourists as maladaptive learning. The model asserts that mental disorders arise as a result of maladaptive forms of learning. Behaviourism holds that if a behaviour can be learned, it can also be unlearned. Thus, changes to maladaptive behaviours are brought about by procedures designed to change antecedents or, more commonly, the consequences using the basic principles of classical and operant conditioning.

In its pure form, behaviour modification techniques have been more successful in children, mentally retarded populations and in residential and prison settings because the environment could be more reliably controlled in such situations. It has also been successfully employed in institutional settings, e.g. offending institutions, because environmental contingencies are more easily controlled in such environments. (Strictly speaking, behaviour therapy is the name given to behavioural interventions based on classical conditioning while behaviour modification techniques rely on operant conditioning paradigms. However, these two terms are often used interchangeably.)

Over the years, the radical behaviour model has undergone considerable revision and modification. More recently, behavioural approaches have been incorporated into cognitive behaviour interventions and pure behaviourism has fallen out of favour for a number of reasons:

- Radical behavioural approaches exclude, and in fact deny, the role of mental processes. Most contemporary behaviourists have moved away from this radical position and concluded that mental processes are, indeed, important, if not more important, in studying behaviour. The increasing popularity of cognitive theories of learning and cognitive therapies that focus on cognitions as intervening variables has given rise to cognitive behaviour theories and therapies.
- Another weakness of the behavioural model is the implicit assumption that behaviour depends exclusively on the environment. It ignores genetic contributions, individual predispositions and the active role of the individual in shaping the environment. By taking an extreme, deterministic position in the nature versus nurture debate, behaviourists present a one-sided view of human behaviour.
- The behaviourists' view is at best an over-simplification of what lies behind complex human behaviour. Although it may explain simple behaviour in animals, and in some situations in humans, it falls far short of accounting for complex human activities associated with learning, such as problem solving, abstraction, rule learning and concept formation.

Functional analysis

One particular form of behaviour assessment or analysis is *functional analysis* (also called functional behaviour analysis). Functional analysis emphasises the purpose, the behaviour serves the person. For example, a 'function' of agoraphobic behaviour may be avoidance of adult responsibilities such as work or family duties. Unlike radical behavioural approaches, functional analysis includes and often assigns a pre-eminent role to private events or non-observable cognitive variables. Private events, such as thoughts, feelings and physiological states, are not excluded from analysis and may, indeed, be

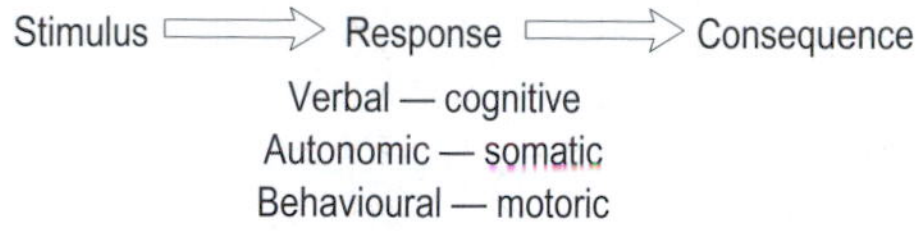

Stimulus ⇒ Response ⇒ Consequence
Verbal — cognitive
Autonomic — somatic
Behavioural — motoric

Fig. 1.7 Functional analysis. The three components of the responses (Lang, 1971)

the target of interventions. Functional analysis has been applied to maladaptive behaviours such as self-injury, stereotypic behaviour disorders and school refusal (in children). It has also been successfully applied to diagnostic categories such as anorexia nervosa, alcohol abuse, post-traumatic disorder and depression. These studies have shown that self-injurious behaviour, for example, is maintained by several reinforcing factors. One typology of the functions of self-injurious behaviour identified three possible reinforcement contingencies (Carr, 1977).

1. Positive reinforcement by social interaction and attention contingent on behaviour.
2. Negative reinforcement by removal of aversive social or academic demands, pain or discomfort.
3. Positive reinforcement by sensory stimulation or relief from strong emotions.

A subsequent study using a large sample of 152 people who showed self-injurious behaviour confirmed that indeed one of the three types of reinforcement listed above were critical in over 90% of the cases and interventions based on these findings were more successful in bringing about extinction of such behaviours (Iwata et al., 1994).

It should be clear by now that in functional analysis unobservable variables or private events enter the analysis in various ways, while in strict behaviour analysis private events, such as thoughts, feelings and physiological states, are excluded. More recently, a tripartite response analysis has been incorporated into the functional analysis design. Three related behavioural components have been proposed: verbal–cognitive, autonomic–physiological, and behavioural–motoric (Lang, 1971), as shown in Figure 1.7. This permits the study of each presenting complaint according to these criteria in a highly idiographic (person-specific) manner and suggest different treatment options.

OBSERVATIONAL LEARNING

Operant and classical learning fail to explain acquisition of complex behaviour sequences. For example, successive approximations cannot account for a blind person learning to speak after listening to someone speaking. In ordinary day-to-day situations both children and adults learn a great deal by simply observing others. Imitation or modelling occurs when individuals acquire or learn behaviours by observing other people's behaviours and their consequences.

A series of investigations, called the Bobo doll experiments, carried out by Albert Bandura and colleagues have become landmarks in the psychology of observational learning (Bandura, 1965). In the study preschool, children watched a five-minute film in which an adult model approached an adult-sized plastic doll, called the 'Bobo Doll', and attacked it by hitting, punching and kicking while aggressively shouting at it. Following this sequence, groups of children were shown a film with three different endings: one group saw another adult appear with food and drink and congratulate the model (model-reward group), another group witnessed the adult come in to reprimand and punish the model (model-punish group), and the third group was a control one where the film ended before the adult arrived (no-consequence group). Immediately after watching the film each child was allowed into a play room where a doll similar to the Bobo doll was placed together with other toys. The findings were remarkable:

- The most important finding was that *all* three groups showed substantially high levels of aggressive behaviour towards the doll. There was a distinct sex difference – boys produced more imitative aggression than girls.
- The model-reward group, which saw the misbehaviour rewarded, exhibited more aggressive acts than other groups.
- Children in the model-punish group showed relatively less aggression – this was particularly prominent in girls.

In a second stage of the experiment all three groups of children were offered rewards on reproducing the model's imitative response. All groups showed a considerable increase in punitive behaviour. Moreover, the introduction of reward to the observers (the children) completely wiped out the previously observed differences in performance in the three groups including the differences seen between boys and girls. The conclusions to be drawn from the experiment were obvious. It demonstrated that performance of aggressive behaviour is modelled by:

- Simple observation, modelling or vicarious learning.
- Observed consequences to the model (vicarious reinforcement or punishment).
- Available consequences to the observer (direct reinforcement).

The experiment further illustrates the distinction between *acquisition* of imitative behaviour and its *performance.* The fact that the punished group exhibited increased rates of imitative behaviour after receiving direct reinforcement goes to show that these children had initially learned the behaviour but its manifestation was evident only when they were rewarded for it.

According to Bandura, observational learning is not a simple repetition of observed behaviour, it is mediated by a number of cognitive factors:

- *Attention.* Focusing on certain aspects of the model's behaviour and not others.
- *Retention.* Committing the observed behaviour to memory.

- *Reproduction*. Repetition of the behaviour later.
- *Motivation*. The felt need to perform the above functions.

Much work has been carried out on the factors that influence observational learning. These can be generally grouped into: (1) characteristics of the model; (2) characteristics of the observer; and (3) response sequence or incentives available for performance of such behaviour. Observational or vicarious learning occurs best when:

- The model has high status and power or is attractive.
- The model is similar to the observer.
- The model is seen to be rewarded for the behaviour.
- The observer has a chance to practice the observed behaviour soon after watching the model perform it.
- The observer has low self-esteem or is dependent.
- The observer is reinforced for performing the imitative behaviour.
- The observer has already learned some components of the behaviour and has this in his or her repertoire.

Observational learning is ubiquitous in everyday life – children imitate adults, and most skills from learning to drive a car to the learning surgical techniques are acquired by close observation. The modelling effect has been shown to be a robust and important source of learning new behaviours in social situations. Research has repeatedly shown that aggressive behaviour in children is associated with harsh discipline, physical abuse and exposure to intra-familial violence. It has also been demonstrated that witnessing violent scenes of aggression on television is likely to lead to aggressive behaviour. Vicarious learning plays an important role in the acquisition of fears, anxiety and post-traumatic reactions. Anxiety reactions in children are often mediated by parental anxiety responses. Modelling is an important therapeutic tool in the treatment of phobias and a component of social skills training procedures.

A particularly worrying and potentially dangerous modelling effect is the effect of the presentation of suicidal behaviour in the media. There is overwhelming evidence to show that television reports of actual suicide and portrayal of suicide leads to 'copy cat' suicidal behaviour (Pirkis & Blood, 2001). The impact of the media on suicidal behaviour seems most likely when:

- The method of suicide is specified (especially when reported in detail).
- It is reported dramatically (for example with photographs of the deceased).
- The model/deceased and the observer are similar in terms of sex, age and nationality.
- The observer is young.

Often the reason for the suicide is oversimplified by the media attributing the act to single factors such as broken relationships, financial disasters or failure in examinations. The most common factor leading to suicide, mental illness, is often overlooked (Hawton et al., 1999).

OTHER TYPES OF COGNITIVE LEARNING

Over the past several years many other forms of cognitive learning have been studied. Cognitive learning is learning that involves mental processes such as thinking and development of decision rules. These are mentioned briefly below.

Observational learning. See above.

Insight learning. In most learning situations new learning occurs slowly. Consequently, learning is reflected in gradual improvements in performance. However, in some situations the solution to a problem comes in an instant, with a sudden grasp of a concept. This sudden awareness of a solution to a problem has been termed insight learning. This was demonstrated by Kohler, a Gestalt psychologist, as early as 1925. He observed that one of the chimpanzees that he was studying was able to reach a banana outside the cage using a stick and even join together two sticks to manoeuvre the banana towards him (Kohler, 1925).

Latent learning. Learning may take place in the absence of apparent reward and remain latent until a later date. In a series of experiments Tolman allowed rats to familiarise themselves with a maze (without any form of reinforcement). When food was made available later at one end of the maze, they could find their way to it as well as those who had received prior reinforcement and practice in the maze. Tolman hypothesised that the rats' previous experience in the maze was sufficient for them to form *cognitive maps* or mental layouts of the spatial relationships of the apparatus (Tolman, 1948).

Concept learning. Learning to form categorisations and organise one's thinking about objects and ideas requires abstraction, memory and other higher cognitive functions.

Rule learning. The relationship of concepts to one another is the basis of rules, some of which are explicit while others remain implicit and not stated.

Problem solving. Reasoning, solving problems and devising strategies are highly complex forms of thinking.

Learning to learn or meta-learning. This is almost the highest form of learning, where people understand their previous methods of learning so that they can be utilised in new situations.

SOCIAL LEARNING THEORY (SLT)

Albert Bandura (1986) extended and modified the scope of learning theory principles as applied to human beings in social situations. His theory, known as the *social learning theory* (SLT), is a social cognitive theory that attempts to provide a more complete picture of the process of learning. It is social in orientation because of its emphasis on the social and interpersonal context in which learning takes place. It is a cognitive model because it seeks to explain complex human learning and behaviour in terms of thought processes. Operant and classical forms of conditioning rely heavily on a limited range of principles established on the basis of experiments in animals, or, at best, on single case studies on humans. A particular weakness of theories of conditioning is that they singularly fail to account for the acquisitioning of novel or 'new' forms of behaviour. Bandura does not negate the role of classical and operant conditioning. He considers reinforcement to be facilitative rather than a necessary condition for learning.

The corner stone of SLT is the principle of *reciprocal determinism* between behaviour, personal factors and the environment. According to Bandura, these three factors operate as 'interlocking determinants of each other'. In other words, none of the three components can be understood in isolation from the others as a cause of human behaviour. This three-way interaction may be represented as follows:

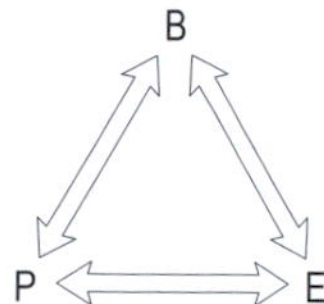

Where P is the person, E the environment and B the person's behaviour. The contribution of each of the factors is not just additive but interactive. For example, people not only react to external influences but actively select, transform and organise their environment – their behaviour influences, and is influenced by, the behaviour of others. Five-year-old Johnny may retaliate in response to perceived threats by another child and may experience chance success. This may be followed by his being the aggressor. Soon this would frighten off other children but attract other aggressive peers thus forming a gang of aggressive bullies. He may derive positive self-evaluation from the elevated status conferred on him. The resulting interactive cycle would lead to escalation of his aggressive behaviour. It is also important to remember that the relative contributions exerted by each of these interdependent factors differ with different settings and different behaviours.

In addition to the concept of reciprocal determinism, SLT emphasises three cognitive processes:

1. Observational or vicarious learning (see above).
2. Self-regulation.
3. Self-efficacy.

Self-regulation. According to Bandura, the ability to regulate one's behaviour involves self-observation, self-evaluation and self-reaction. Self-observation is the monitoring of oneself relative to others or in comparison with expected standards. Self-evaluation is a judgemental process, which attaches a particular value to one's performance. Positive self-evaluation is a potent intrinsic reinforcer. In depressed subjects, the perception of their performance and evaluation of behaviour is usually negative. Their self-reaction is often non-rewarding or self-punitive.

Self-efficacy. People hold beliefs about their own competence and self-mastery. They have judgements on what they are capable of. They expect certain outcomes and not others. Perceived self-efficacy is usually low in subjects with anxiety and phobic disorders leading to avoidance of feared situations.

Bandura's model of social learning is considered a highly significant development in learning theory. Applications of the SLT have been highly successful as a framework for understanding conduct disorders (in children) and aggressive behaviour and criminality in young people. Interventions based on SLT have been used in parent-training programmes and in residential forensic settings. Its application to aggressive behaviour is considered in Chapter 13.

REFERENCES

Abrahamson LY, Metalsky GI, Alloy LB (1978) Learned helplessness in humans: critique and reformulation. Journal of Abnormal Psychology, 87, 49–74.

Ayllon J, Azrin NH (1968) The Token Economy: a motivational system for therapy and rehabilitation. New York: Appleton-Century-Crofts.

Bandura A (1965) Influence of model's reinforcement contingencies on the acquisition of imitative responses. Journal of Personality and Social Psychology, 1, 589–595.

Bandura A (1986) Social Foundations of Thought and Action: a social cognitive theory. Englewood Cliffs, NJ: Prentice Hall.

Carr EG (1977) The Motivation of Self-injurious Behaviour: a review of some hypotheses. Psychological Bulletin, 84, 800–816.

Garcia J, Koelling RA (1966) Relation of cue to sequence in avoidance learning. Psychosomatic Science, 4, 123–124.

Hawton K, Simkin S, Deeks JJ, O'Conner S, Keen A, Alumen DG, Altmen DG, Philo G, Bulstrode C (1999) Effects of drug overdose in a television drama on presentation to hospital for self-poisoning: time series and questionnaire study. British Medical Journal, 318, 972–977.

Iwata BA, Pace GM, Dorsey MF, Zarcone JR, Vollmer TR, Smith RG, Rodgers TA, Lerman DC, Shore BA, Mazaleski JL, Goh H, Cowdery GE, Kalsher MJ, McCosh KC, Willis KD (1994) The function of self-injurious behaviour: an experimental–epidemiological analysis. Journal of Applied Behaviour Analysis, 27, 215–240.

Jones MC (1924) The elimination of children's fears. Journal of Experimental Psychology, 7, 382–390.

Kohler W (1925) The Mentality of Apes. New York: Harcourt Brace Jovanovich.

Lang PJ (1971) The application of psychophysiological methods to the study of psychotherapy and behaviour modification. In A Bergin & S Garfield (eds), Handbook of Psychotherapy and Behaviour Change. New York: Wiley.

Mowrer OH (1939) Stimulus response theory of anxiety. Psychological Review, 46, 553–565.

Ohman A (1993) Fear and anxiety as emotional phenomena: clinical phenomenology, evolutionary perspective and information processing. In M Lewis & J Hoviland (eds), Handbook of Emotions. New York: The Guilford Press.

Pirkis J, Blood RW (2001) Suicide and The Media: a critical review. Canberra: Commonwealth Department of Health and the Aged Care.

Rachman S (1977) The conditioned theory of fear acquisition: a critical examination. Behaviour Research and Therapy, 14, 57–60.

Rachman S, Hodgson RJ (1968) Experimentally induced sexual 'fetishism': replication and development. Psychological Record, 18, 25–27.

Rescorla RA (1968) Probability of shock in the presence and absence of CS in fear conditioning. Journal of Comparative and Physiological Psychology, 66, 1–5.

Rescorla RA (1988) Pavlovian conditioning: it's not what you think it is. American Psychologist, 43(3), 152–160.

Seligman MEP (1970) On the generality of the laws of learning. Psychological Review, 77, 406–418.
Seligman MEP (1975) Helplessness: on depression, development and health. San Francisco, CA: Freeman.
Skinner BF (1953) Science and Human Behaviour. New York: Macmillan.
Thorndike EL (1898) Animal intelligence: an experimental study of the associative processes in animals. Psychological Review (Monograph Supplement 2), 8.
Tolman EC (1948) Cognitive maps in rats and men. Psychological Review, 55, 189–208.
Watson JB (1925) Behaviourism (p. 82). New York: Norton.
Watson JB, Rayner R (1920) Conditioned emotional reactions. Journal of Experimental Psychology, 3, 1–14.
Wolpe J (1958) Psychotherapy by Reciprocal Inhibition. Stanford, CA: Stanford University Press.

FURTHER READING

Lieberman DA (2000) Learning: behaviour and cognition, 3rd ed. Belmont, CA: Wadsworth.

- A seminal text on learning, useful for reference purposes.

Martin G, Pear J (1999) Behaviour Modification: what is it and how to do it, 6th ed. Upper Saddle River, NJ: Prentice Hall.

- A useful book on behaviour therapy that describes its main principles and applications.

Rescorla RA (1988) Pavlovian conditioning: it's not what you think it is. American Psychologist, 43(3), 152–160.

- An in-depth discussion that provides an insight into the complex nature of classical conditioning

Mental abilities: intelligence and its relevance to psychiatry

2

'It has yet to be proven that intelligence has any survival value.'
Arthur C. Clarke

Psychology endeavours to address two broad aspects of human mental functioning: (1) those aspects that are *common* to all individuals and the general principles that are responsible for them (e.g. classical conditioning, memory and cognitive development); and (2) the ways in which individuals differ from one another. The latter, individual differences, are most prominent in three psychological domains: mental abilities; personality (and temperament); and motivation. We first consider one such area of individual differences – mental abilities.

Mental abilities, also called cognitive abilities, intellectual abilities and, more commonly, intelligence, have been notoriously difficult to define. For nearly a century a fierce and, at times, acrimonious debate has raged over the nature and concept of intelligence. In 1921 *The Journal of Educational Psychology* held a symposium at which they invited fourteen experts to define what they understood by intelligence. Each expert gave a different, often contradictory, conceptualisation of intelligence. Thus there appeared to be little consensus among researchers as to the philosophical nature of intelligence, let alone a universally accepted definition. Despite the fact that human intelligence is one of the most intensely researched subjects in psychology, there is great debate and much controversy as to how it is conceptualised, defined, analysed, studied and measured. The following definition is taken from the work of one of the experts in the field:

> *...the aggregate and global capacity to act purposefully, to think rationally and to deal effectively with the environment.*
>
> Wechsler, 1944

It is clear from the above definitions that intelligence usually includes three related abilities:

1. The *capacity to learn*, that is, to acquire, apply and manipulate knowledge.
2. The *ability for abstract thinking and reasoning* including analysis and generalising from learned information.
3. The *ability to adapt* and cope with new and novel situations and the capacity for problem solving.

It should be emphasised that intelligence is a *construct*, the contents, composition and boundaries of which varies according to the assumptions that various theorists adopt. Neither is it context-free – an individual's performance may vary from one situation to another and according to the domain that is under scrutiny. Conceptualisations of intelligence also vary across ethnic groups and cultures. One is considered intelligent if one excels in skills valued by one's own group. Western cultures place a high premium on scholastic abilities while some other cultures are known to regard abilities such as the skills involved in understanding others and the capacity to understand oneself as more important. Some Eastern cultures consider non-conventional cognitive competencies such as intellectual self-effacement and self-assertion (knowing when to speak up and when not to) an important aspect of intelligence (Sternberg et al., 1981).

In spite of the disagreements among different theorists, and perhaps as a result of it, a huge amount of research has been carried out and a wealth of knowledge has been accumulated over the last hundred years. Intelligence is one of the oldest subjects to be studied in the field of psychology. Sir Francis Galton (1883), a cousin of Charles Darwin, was one of the first to carry out scientific research into the field. He attempted to measure intellect by studying variables such as reaction time, auditory threshold, ability to estimate weight and similar measures. He believed that individuals with superior intellect (for Galton this meant individuals from the upper strata of society) exhibited enhanced perceptual and sensory skills. For example, one of his experiments involved judging the weight of gun cartridges with the subject blindfolded. His contention was that those from higher walks of life and their offsprings fare better at such judgements than those from lower classes. Galton also carried out studies of family trees of the famous scientific families at that time, and in his book, *Hereditary Genius: an inquiry into its laws and consequences*, published in 1869, he argued that genius ran in families. He was also one of the earliest workers in the field of twin studies. Together with his colleague Karl Pearson he developed a statistical technique, the Pearson product-moment coefficient for analysing the data that they obtained from the twin studies. Galton is considered to be the founding father of psychometrics, the study of measurement of mental or psychological factors.

In 1904, Charles Spearman, a British psychologist, examined children's abilities using complex tests. He pioneered the statistical procedure *factor analysis*. It is designed to locate a smaller number of dimensions or factors that underlie the relationship among a large number of variables. Factors are theoretical constructs or hypothetical variables derived from a set of data, and factor analysis portrays the degree of interrelationship among these variables (see Chapter 8). In the case of intelligence it involves studying the correlation among a series of ability tests in a large population. Spearman extracted a single factor, the general ability factor, which he called *g*, that he believed underlies all other abilities. Current research shows that conventional tests of intelligence are indeed correlated with one another.

In recent years, a number of scholars, influenced particularly by cultural considerations and stimulated by an interest in education, have argued that applying the psychometric model to the study of intelligence has adopted too narrow an approach and focused on those aspects of knowledge emphasised by Western educational systems. These new approaches consider intellect to be comprised of a variety of statistically and qualitatively independent cognitive abilities. As a result of the insights gained from recent work, our understanding of the construct of intelligence has undergone considerable change. Thus, a symposium held in 1986 (sixty-five years after the 1921 symposium) witnessed a significant shift in the conceptualisation of intelligence by experts on the subject (although disagreements as to the definition of intelligence were no better). In addition to the traditional three components – learning, reasoning and adaptation – the concept had been broadened to include a range of other skills and competencies.

Hence, there are two currently influential approaches to the study and understanding of intelligence:

1. *The Psychometric approach.* This is based on the assumption that most human abilities are underpinned and anchored on a basic and fundamental general cognitive ability or 'general intelligence' or *g*. This view is best known for the measurement intelligence – the intelligent quotient or IQ. In this approach, intelligence is thought to be almost a singular, although composite, attribute that can be studied, assessed and measured.

2. *Systemic approaches.* These attempt to explain intelligence in terms of specific mental processes that are used in the performance of individual tasks. These theories maintain that there are many different 'intelligences' or systems of abilities that are relatively independent of one another. These are new ways of thinking about mental abilities that have widened the concept of intelligence and have succeeded to a large extent in challenging the monolithic concept of psychometric intelligence, which had hitherto dominated the field. These approaches define intelligence rather differently. Two such definitions are as follows:

> *... the possession of knowledge, the ability to efficiently use knowledge to reason about the world and the ability to employ reasoning effectively in different environments.*
>
> Sternberg, 1985

> *... the ability or skill to solve problems or fashion products which are valued within a cultural location.*
>
> Gardner, 1983

In the following section the psychometric concept of intelligence is described in some detail followed by an outline of two systemic theories.

THE PSYCHOMETRIC CONCEPT OF INTELLIGENCE

The psychometric approach has monopolised the field for nearly a century. The most remarkable achievement of this method of investigation of human mental abilities has been the measurement of intelligence by tests yielding an index of intelligence, the intelligence quotient or IQ. Both the approach and its derivative, the IQ, has been upheld as the greatest achievement of psychology and also criticised relentlessly as unfair and unscientific. Thus far the psychometric method has proved most useful in clinical and other applied settings. An understanding of the basis of the psychometric approach is therefore crucially important in clinical practice – it is also important to be aware of its limitations.

The basic premise of the psychometric concept of intelligence is that all mental abilities are influenced by a *single* fundamental factor, *g*, or general ability. This singular pervasive ability is said to underlie most human abilities. The *g* factor is thought to be used to some extent in all intellectual tasks. The statistical concept of factor analysis forms the backbone of the psychometric approach (see Chapter 8 on psychological measurements). The essence of the psychometric method is that those who scored high on one set of tests, to a large extent, scored high on other tests. When an array of varied tests assessing, for example, spatial ability, verbal skills, abstract thinking and logical reasoning are administered to a population, the results of all of these tests are found to be positively related to one another. In short, most human abilities, Spearman and his followers contend, are positively correlated. It is argued, therefore, that each of these measures has in common a general factor, *g*, which accounts for this correlation.

The psychometric approach sees intelligence as an entity by itself that can be measured and studied. Although the nature of Spearman's *g* factor is far from clear, psychometric theory holds that *g* is necessarily involved in many different types of, if not all, abilities. Spearman held that while *g* was at the core of all abilities, a specific but minor component, *s*, described whatever ability was unique in carrying out a task (as in a specific factor for music or foreign language) and such specific factors were unrelated across tasks and were often a result of learning. Spearman's theory has, therefore, been sometimes called the 'two factor' theory (Figure 2.1A)

Proponents of the psychometric approach uphold the construct validity of *g* and have produced a vast amount of research as to its nature, source and associations. (Kline,1993). In the psychometric theory of intelligence, general intelligence or *g* is presumed to be a singular attribute that is common to all human beings and, hence, valid across various cultures. In addition, it is held to be biologically based and largely inheritable.

Cattell – fluid and crystallised intelligence

While Spearman viewed *g* as a unitary but complex entity, other workers in the field have sought to refine and advance the concept of *g*. Horn and Cattell (1966) have partitioned *g* into two components, 'fluid' and 'crystallised' intelligence (Figure 2.1B). These two factors have been extensively studied. *Fluid intelligence* (g_f) is thought to be the basic reasoning ability, the ability involved in extracting rules and relationships. It is the ability to solve problems that require speed of perception and information processing but little previous knowledge. It is the ability involved in new learning and novel problem solving that does not depend on formal schooling or acculturation. When arranging or grouping information according to a given rule or solving a novel problem for the first time we are using fluid ability. *Crystallised*

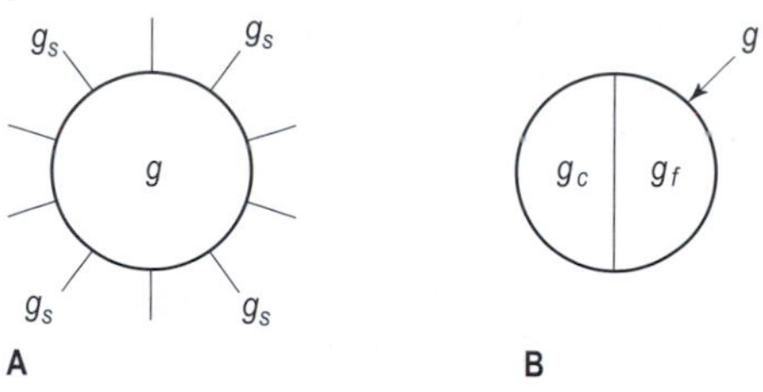

Fig. 2.1 (**A**) Diagrammatic representation of Spearman's 'two-factor' approach (g_s refers to specific intelligence); and (**B**) the concept of crystallised (g_c) and fluid (g_f) intelligence.

intelligence (g_c) is the product of investment of g_f in domains of learning such as vocabulary, general information and arithmetic skills. It involves the ability to remember and use information. It is more dependent than fluid intelligence on education and cultural background. Tests of verbal abilities are held largely to measure g_c.

The difference between fluid and crystallised intelligence is most apparent in the elderly, who show a decrease in fluid, but not crystallised, intelligence. Crystallised abilities, which include verbal abilities and knowledge hold up well or increase until old age, while fluid abilities decline after young adulthood. The ease with which children master computer technology and the number of middle-aged individuals who experience difficulties programming or using the video remote control testifies to the effect of ageing on g_f.

Thurstone – primary mental abilities (PMAs)

A contrasting approach to analysing mental abilities was undertaken by another influential researcher in the field, Louis Thurstone. He used a different method of factor analysis on a large sample of university students and applied a relatively large number of tests, sixty to be precise, covering a wide range of mental abilities but came to very different conclusions to those of Spearman. Instead of one overarching common factor he found seven distinct abilities, which he called *primary mental abilities* (PMAs). These were: spatial ability, verbal relations, word fluency, perceptual speed, numerical facility, memory and inductive reasoning (Table 2.1). His tests give a profile of a person's abilities rather than a global measure (Thurstone, 1938).

A central tenet of Thurstone's findings was that the PMAs were independent and separate showing no correlation with each other. Thurstone considered g to be essentially meaningless as it does not convey the strengths and weaknesses of the subject in the way that PMAs do.

Recently, however, there have been vigorous arguments as to whether or not PMAs can be further factor analysed to provide higher-order factors. Some psychometric theorists have reanalysed Thurstone's data and drawn conclusions very different from those of Thurstone and reported a certain amount of correlation between PMAs. Despite these findings, Thurstone's original work raises a disquieting question: how many basic mental abilities

Table 2.1 Primary mental abilities (Thurstone, 1938)

1. Spatial ability	Special relationships, visualising shapes
2. Verbal relations	Comprehension of meaning of words and verbal concepts
3. Perceptual speed	The ease with which visual details are detected
4. Numerical facility	Simple arithmetic problems
5. Word fluency	The speed in dealing with isolated words
6. Memory	Recall of paired words and word recognition
7. Inductive reasoning	Identification of rules or relationships in a set (e.g. series of numbers)

are there in man? Obviously there is no easy answer to the question; it depends on the type and number of tests that are considered important.

The issue of the number of second-order factors that could be extracted from scores on intelligence tests is more complicated. Horn and other workers (e.g. Hakstain & Cattell, 1978) have now expanded the $g_f - g_c$ theory to include six other abilities – short-term acquisition and retrieval (*Gsm*), broad speediness (*Gs*), broad visualisation (*Gv*), quantitative thinking (*Gq*), auditory intelligence (*Ga*) and long-term retrieval (*Gln*). A recent authoritative review of the subject has identified over 70 different abilities that can be discerned by currently available tests (Carroll, 1993).

Hierarchical models of intelligence

In an attempt to make sense of these seemingly confusing and contradictory findings, current psychometric approaches seeks to combine the g of Spearman, and the principles that underlie the primary mental abilities of Thurstone into a hierarchical organisation of cognitive abilities. In such an arrangement factors are placed at three levels: (1) a number of special-ability factors, similar to Thurstone's primary mental ability factors, derived from subtests such as tests of verbal or spatial abilities at the bottom of the pyramid; (2) a set of second-order factors extracted from these, which represent broad factors such as g_c and g_f in the middle; and (3) a single third-order factor, general cognitive ability, g, that occupies the apex of the hierarchy representing what all tests of cognitive abilities have in common.

Of the several hierarchical models that have been put forward, Carroll's *three-stratum model* is the most popular, but is by no means simple. Carroll (1993) reanalysed hundreds of studies carried out over half a century and arrived at six other second-level factors in addition to g_c and g_f (visual perception, auditory perception, general memory and learning, cognitive speed, processing speed and retrieval ability). In this model (Figure 2.2) the first-order factors include most of Thurstone's factors while the second-order factors encompass fluid and crystallised intelligence, as well as other six high-order factors. The model relies on the fact that at each level the factors are intercorrelated. The advantage of the model is that a person's cognitive abilities can be measured and described at each level of analysis.

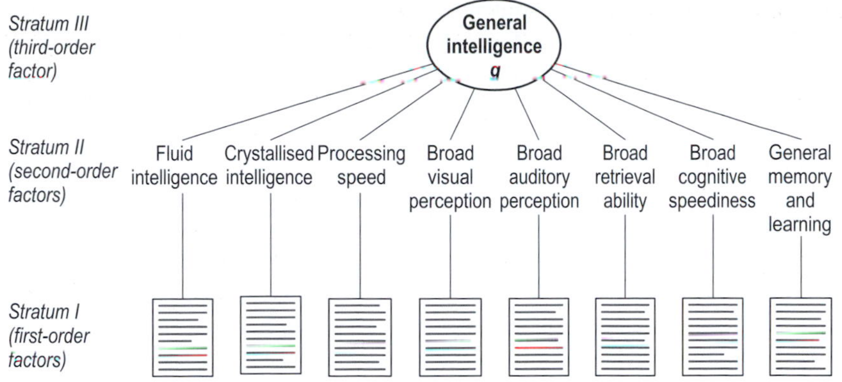

Fig. 2.2 An example of hierarchical representation of mental abilities (Carroll, 1993)

The main difficulty encountered with hierarchical models is that, although comprehensive and apparently sensible, the exercise becomes rather cumbersome and unwieldy, for example the battery of tests proposed by Carroll takes up to three hours to administer.

Measurement of intelligence – the psychometric approach

One of the main reasons for the success and popularity of the psychometric concept of intelligence is the ease with which this approach has been able to produce a single measurable unit of intelligence, the IQ. The two best-known tests of intelligence are the Stanford–Binet test and the Wechsler intelligence scales. The IQ and these tests of intelligence measure intelligence as defined by the psychometric approach. This caveat has to be kept in mind when using and interpreting the results of IQ tests. Tests based on other models are in their infancy and have not yet come into common use.

Stanford–Binet test

Testing of intellectual abilities has a long history. In 1905, the French psychologist Alfred Binet was commissioned by the French Government to devise tests to identify children who had learning difficulties. The aim was to provide special-educational help for such children. Binet and his co-worker, Theodore Simon, developed a set of age-graded tests grouped according to levels of difficulty in which most children of a given age could 'pass' the test items. They also introduced the concept of *mental age* (MA). Thus, a six-year-old child who responded correctly to all the test items normally completed by an average eight year old is said to have an MA of eight (and a chronological age of six). The Simon–Binet test (1905) became the first intelligence test to be published and used. In 1912, William Stern proposed that the scores on the Simon–Binet scale be divided by the chronological age of the subject to arrive at a 'mental quotient'. Louis Terman multiplied this ratio by 100 and called it the *intelligence quotient* (IQ). Thus was born the IQ, which continues to be used today. It was conceived as a ratio of the child's mental age (MA) relative to the chronological age (CA) calculated by the formula:

$$IQ = MA \div CA \times 100$$

This is called the *ratio IQ*. When, in 1916, Lewis M. Terman of Stanford University revised and refined the test, he incorporated the idea of the IQ and also made it applicable to adults as well. The Stanford–Binet test, as it came to be called, has undergone several revisions and has become one of the most popular tests of psychometric intelligence (Thorndike, Hagen & Sattler, 1986).

In the 1960 version of the test the ratio IQ score has been replaced by the *deviation IQ*, which, by definition, has a mean of 100 and a standard deviation of 16. The calculation of IQ is no longer based on the ratio of mental age to the chronological age. Instead the tests have been standardised on large populations. (Standardisation of a test refers to establishing how scores of a test are distributed among the population, see Chapter 8 on psychological measurements.) The scores usually show normal (Gaussian) distribution. The subject's raw scores are compared with norms derived from a large group of individuals of the same age. By definition, an IQ score of 100 is assigned to be the average score obtained by people in each age group. Thus a given IQ score is an index of a person's rank or deviation within the population of his or her age; it is a comparative measure of the performance of an individual in relation to the performance of others of the same age. (The fourth and current edition of the Stanford–Binet test, revised in 1986, (Thorndike, Hagen & Sattler, 1986) utilises the three-level hierarchical model of intelligence mentioned earlier.)

Wechsler intelligence scales

By far the best known and the most widely employed tests of intelligence are the Wechsler scales. David Wechsler has devised a family of tests designed for various age groups, all of which have undergone many revisions over the years:

- WAIS-III (1997) – Wechsler Adult Intelligence Scales – for ages 16 to 89.
- WISC-III-R (1991) – Wechsler Intelligence Scale for Children (Revised) – for ages 6 to 16 years, 11 months.
- WPPSI-R (1985) – Wechsler Pre-school and Primary Scale of Intelligence – for 3 to 7 years olds.

Wechsler intelligence scales consists of several subtests that are grouped to form two scales, the verbal scale and the performance scale. Each of the different versions yield three different scores: an overall or full scale IQ (FIQ), a verbal IQ (VIQ) and a performance IQ (PIQ). The items on each subset are arranged in order of difficulty, and administration is discontinued after a specified number of incorrect answers. In the verbal tests the subject is scored on the basis of the accuracy of their answers. These reflect knowledge of previously learned information. In performance tests the individual is provided with special material and is asked to arrange or manipulate them. For example, in the block-design tests the subject is asked to arrange coloured blocks to match geometric designs printed on cards. These tests aim to present the subject with unfamiliar and novel tasks to assess visuospatial capacity and speed of performance. The verbal tests are thought to be g_c loaded (except digit span) while performance tests are g_f saturated.

The most recent revision of the scale for adults is the Wechsler Adult Intelligence Scale – third edition (WAIS-III, Wechsler, 1997). It consists of seven verbal subtests and seven performance subtests (Table 2.2). It has retained 11 subsets from its predecessor, WAIS-R (1981) and added three new subtests. In the WAIS-III the main changes that have been made to the WAIS–R (1981) are:

1. Extension of the age range:
   - from 74 to 89 years.
2. Addition of three new subtests:
   - matrix reasoning (replaces object assembly in the performance scale);
   - symbol search (added to the performance scale);
   - letter–number sequencing (added to the verbal scale).
3. Addition of index scores:
   - a major structural change in WAIS-III is the addition of index scores. Factor analysis of WAIS-R had shown that there were three higher-order factors embedded in it. WAIS-III was devised with the explicit aim of producing subtests that would relate to the four hypothesised factors: verbal comprehension; working memory; perceptual organization; and processing speed. Results of factor analysis of WAIS-III data do indeed support the four-factor model. The addition of the four-factor indices is considered to be a major advancement, especially in the interpretation of individual profiles
4. Extension of the IQ range:
   - WAIS–III allows the test to measure IQ ranges from 45–155.

Administration and scoring of WAIS-III

WAIS is an individually administered test. It takes 60–90 minutes to complete the test. Some of the tests are timed, others are not. Unlike the previous version of the test, where the ‘reference group’ was between the ages of 20 and 40, WAIS-III now compares each individual score with that of an equivalent age group. Also, the current version has extended the age range from 16 to 89 (in the WAIS-R it was 16 to 74 years). The test has been standardised on a sample of 2250 US citizens. A Corresponding UK version, WAIS-III^{UK} (1999) that is normed on UK samples is available. The raw scores from each subtest are converted into standardized FIQ, VIQ and PIQ scores by the use of tables included in the test manual. The mean IQ for the FIQ, VIQ and PIQ is 100 with a standard deviation of 15.

Psychometric characteristics of WAIS-III

The average split-half reliability for IQ scores across the age groups is strong, ranging from 0.94 to 0.98. The test–retest reliability coefficients range from

Table 2.2 The Wechsler adult intelligence scale – third edition (WAIS-III; Wechsler, 1997)

Subtest	*Domain tested*
Verbal subtests	
Vocabulary	Word meaning
Similarities	Abstract reasoning
Arithmetic	Solving numerical problems
Digit span	Working auditory memory
Information	General knowledge
Comprehension	Reasoning ability, social judgement
Letter–number sequencing*	Attention, sequencing ability
Performance subtests	
Picture completion	Ability to grasp meaning, alertness to visual detail
Digit symbol-coding	Visual coding, processing speed
Block design	Analysis of abstract figures, spatial relations
Matrix reasoning*	Visual information processing, abstract reasoning
Picture arrangement	Abstract reasoning
Symbol search*	Visual processing speed, perceptual organisation
Object assembly	Spatial relationships, visual motor coordination
New WAIS-III four-factor structure	
1. Verbal comprehension	
2. Perceptual organization	
3. Working memory	
4. Processing speed	

*New subtests in WAIS-III.

0.95 to 0.97 for full-scale IQ. That is, the tests produce similar results in the same individual on repetition of the test. Individual subset reliabilities range from an average of 0.93 to 0.97. Thus, the reliability coefficients for WAIS-III are quite impressive. The convergent validity of the test, that is the correlation of the test with other tests purporting to measure intelligence, range from 0.80 to 0.90 meaning that the WAIS-III measures essentially the same constructs as the instruments measuring intelligence such as Stanford–Binet test. The fact that four factors (verbal comprehension, working memory, perceptual organization and processing speed) could be extracted by factor analysis is thought to be further evidence of the validity of WAIS-III.

The construct validity of the tests has been the centre of intense debate over the years and goes back to the definition of intelligence. The nature of *g* and what it means or stands for is not yet entirely clear. Those critical of psychometric definitions of intelligence have questioned the usefulness and applicability of intelligence tests.

It is also important to note that WAIS-III does not measure every possible construct that underlies intelligence. Also, since it is a measure of psychometric intelligence it carries with it the weaknesses of the psychometric concepts of intelligence and cognitive abilities. Nevertheless, Wechsler scales, the most commonly used intelligence test, have become the industry standard for measurement of cognitive abilities.

Interpreting WAIS-III scores

WAIS and similar intelligence tests are administered and interpreted by qualified psychologists with graduate or professional-level training in psychological assessment. The process of interpreting WAIS-III is a complex task that has to be carried out with caution because of the potential pitfalls. The main steps in the interpretation of the scores are:

1. Examining the FIQ.
2. Interpreting any VIQ–PIQ discrepancies.
3. Looking at the factor indices.
4. Looking at the pattern of scatter of subtest scores and interpreting subtest variability (profile analysis).

Interpretation of the full scale IQ

The FIQ is the single best indicator of global mental ability. It provides the person's relative standing in comparison with his or her age-related peers. The distribution of IQ scores in the normal population is discussed later. An FIQ score is statistically significant (at the 0.05 level) when it is 12 points below (or above) the mean (< 88). In practical terms, this means that the score has to be less than one standard deviation (15 points) below the mean to attain levels of statistical significance. But a statistically *significant* score does not mean that it is *abnormal*. Hence the clinical picture and other information need to be taken into account in interpreting the FIQ score.

Interpretation the FIQ–PIQ discrepancy

The next step in WAIS-III interpretation is to examine the extent of the difference between verbal IQ and performance IQ. The difference between the two scores has to be relatively large for it to be significant. On the WAIS-III, a significant difference (at the 0.05 level) between VIQ and PIQ is 9 points. Here again, although statistically significant, i.e. the scores are not due to chance error, studies in different age groups have shown that such discrepancies occur too frequently to be considered abnormal. Therefore discrepancies of more than 17 points (1.5 *SD*) are usually considered *abnormal*. Scores indicating PIQ > VIQ occur typically in learning disability (mental retardation) while a VIQ > PIQ profile is typical of Alzheimer's disease (AD). Most patients with AD show a VIQ > PIQ of more than 15 points. It should be noted that although the PIQ–VIQ difference is useful in assessing the severity of the patient's cognitive deficits, it is of little *diagnostic* significance in AD. Studies on patients with unilateral right-hemisphere damage have typically found VIQ to be 9 points higher than PIQ on average. However, given that there are wide variations in both scores, VIQ > PIQ should never be interpreted as diagnostic of right-hemispheric lesion, although it is consistent with it.

Interpretation of the subset scores

A detailed assessment of the scatter of scores in the subsets is best carried out by someone who is a specialist at the task. An uneven profile of subtest scores is typically seen in vascular dementia but may also occur in AD. The subtests can be grouped according to Horn and Cattell's fluid versus crystallized intelligence. g_f primarily includes digit span and matrix reasoning whereas g_c is measured by vocabulary and information subtests. An individual's performance on different subtests could also be compared to identify any conspicuous discrepancies and inconsistencies.

Raven's progressive matrices (RPM)

The matrices test is a purely performance-based test, which is said to be more useful in those with linguistic disadvantages. The RPM consists of a number of matrices that contain a logical pattern or design with a missing part. The subject's task is to select the appropriate missing part of the design from eight alternatives (Raven, 1938). The standard progressive matrices are comprised of sixty test items and the subject is first presented with simple problems in which he/she is asked to select one of a number of designs that will complete a given pattern. Once the subject has completed the first he/she proceeds to the next, and so on. The test becomes progressively more difficult, requiring abstract reasoning rather than simple pattern matching. The test loads on Spearman g factor and is said to be saturated with items measuring fluid ability (g_f). Unfortunately the test is not as culture free as it was once thought to be. Several studies have shown that the differences between white and coloured people in the USA on the RPM test scores are as large as those found on the traditional tests. In fact, it has been observed that ultimately no test can be culture free. Also, the educational level of the subjects has been shown to have a major effect on their performance in the test. The scale also has a complementary verbal scale, the Mill Hill vocabulary scale. Both these tests may be used with individuals as well as with groups.

One other test battery that needs to be mentioned is *the British ability scales* (Elliot, Murray, & Pearson, 1983). It is a collection of ability scales, which are used mainly in educational psychology to assess the abilities of children up to the age of 17 years. It has 23 scales with separate norms. Each subscale, ranging from word reading and copying to recall of designs, can be scored separately. The IQ can be measured from some of the subscales.

Stability of IQ

Intelligence test scores show a fair degree of stability over time. Several longitudinal studies have shown that children's scores remain largely stable throughout childhood and adolescence. Typically, the correlation coefficient of scores between the ages of 8 to 18 is about 0.7 to 0.8. A study of a large group of Canadian soldiers serving in the Second World War and then retested 40 years later showed the stability coefficient for verbal ability to be around 0.9 and that for non-verbal ability to be 0.6 (Schwarzman et al., 1987). Thus, minor variations apart, in general, IQ tends to be stable across the life span.

It is important to understand what stability of IQ test scores mean. While the child's overall performance increases with age, what remains stable is his or her score in comparison to individuals of the same age. Also, it is important to point out that the above figures are true for the *group* or *test population*. For the same individual, IQ tests administered years later show fluctuation by ±15 points or more. Several studies have shown that the high levels of stability of the scores do not apply to all members of the group; as much as one third of a group is likely to show a change by 15 points or more.

Predictive validity of IQ

IQ tests do, in fact, predict school performance quite well – the average correlation between IQ scores and school grades is about 0.5. Its predictive validity is higher for achievement in primary school (r = 0.60–0.70) but gets progressively less as one moves through secondary school (r = 0.50–0.60) to higher education (r = 0.40–0.50). (This may give a misleading impression, but it has to be remembered that an r of 0.50 accounts for only about 25% of the overall variance while the remaining 75% is determined by other factors.) School learning depends on numerous factors especially motivation, parental expectations and teaching practices, to name but a few. The socioeconomic status of the individual also influences the educational attainment but to a slightly lesser degree. Thus, children with a high IQ and from a better social background do better in education while the opposite is true of children with a lower IQ from a disadvantaged background. There is also a modest correlation between occupational status and IQ (r = 0.5) and work performance (r = 0.4). IQ shows a negative correlation with law abidingness (r = 0.2).

Group differences in IQ

Racial-ethnic differences. The subject of racial-ethnic differences in intellectual performance has been fraught with debate from the time intelligence testing began and continues unabated to the present. In the USA, numerous studies have consistently documented ethnic differences. In a statement endorsed by 52 academics known as experts in intelligence (Neisser et al., 1996), the mean IQ scores by group were reported as follows:

- Whites 100;
- African Americans 85;

- Hispanics between 85 and 100; and
- Asians and Jews somewhere above 100.

Research on Native Americans indicates the score to be around 90. This differential in IQ persists even when controlled for other factors like socioeconomic status. There is also evidence that differences in IQ scores between racial groups have been reduced in recent years. Second-generation immigrants' scores are higher than their parents' IQ. There has been a great deal of controversy around the race and IQ issue. It has now been convincingly demonstrated that the White–Black discrepancy in IQ test scores is not due to any particular characteristic of the tests or their administration. A task force of the American Psychological Association set up to review the debate on intelligence (Neisser et al., 1996) concluded that 'no adequate explanation of the differential between the IQ means of Blacks and Whites is presently available'.

A common misconception when referring to racial-ethnic group differences in measured intelligence needs pointing out. Group differences refer to average intellectual differences in performances of various groups defined through self-identification to racial-ethnic group membership. The range of individual differences *within* groups tends to be more than those *between* groups. The use of the term group differences in referring to patterns of IQ scores among racial-ethnic populations ignores the reality of overlap of individual scores between groups and perpetuates the myth that nearly everybody of one racial-ethnic group (e.g. White) performs higher than practically everybody of another group (e.g. African Americans).

Culture and IQ tests. There are two theoretical perspectives as to culture in psychology. One view holds that ability tests (and general principles of psychology) are intrinsically transportable from one culture to another. This approach, known as cross-cultural psychology, concerns itself with discovering both universals and cross-cultural variability in human mental characteristics, including abilities. Proponents believe that psychological variables in various cultures are universal and that psychometric tests provide a universal metric for comparative purposes (Poortinga, 1989). A competing view, called cultural psychology, sees psychological tests not as universal instruments but as cultural genres. When psychologists use tests developed in their own culture to test members of a different culture, testees often do not share the same presuppositions about values, knowledge and communication implicitly assumed in these tests (Greenfield, 1997). Cultural psychology maintains that before researchers assess intelligence in a new cultural context, they first need to find out the local definition of intelligence. The initial investigation into the indigenous definition of intelligence is considered to be a prerequisite to testing of intelligence when the cultural background of the testee is different from those for whom the test was devised. On the other hand, where the cultural definitions are the same, the test could be used with only minor modifications.

In a study carried out in Liberia, subjects were given an object sorting test in which they were provided with a list of names of objects and asked to categorise them into tools, food, clothing, implements, and so on. Participants were seen to make systematic errors. For example, rather than sorting objects into tools and foods, they persisted in grouping potato and knife together. When asked for the reason, they replied, 'This is what a wise man would do'. When it occurred to the researchers to ask, 'How would a fool do it?' They came up with neat linguistically based categories! The researcher's criterion for intelligent behaviour was the participants' criterion for foolish behaviour and vice versa (Cole et al., 1971). Thus, the test seems to have had entirely different meanings for the tester and the testees. Findings such as these emphasise both the need to understand the implicit assumptions that underlie our ideas of knowledge and the fact that these vary from culture to culture in subtle ways. In short, different societies and cultures have different theories of knowledge and this needs to be acknowledged when devising tests.

Cultural differences apart, we have witnessed massive technological advancements in the last few decades. The effect of a simple instrument such as the calculator on arithmetic abilities of children and adults is as good an example as any. As calculators have become ever-present, mental-arithmetic capabilities have become less important in schools and other settings. Presumably the ability to do calculations unaided by calculators or computers is not considered intelligent behaviour by society anymore. No doubt, the concept of intelligent behaviour is bound to continue changing as societies develop, change and undergo transformation.

Sex differences in IQ

Although, on average, the total IQ scores for men and women show no significant differences, substantial and consistent differences have been noted for specific abilities. Males typically perform better on visuo-spatial tasks (e.g. route finding), mathematical skills and motor tasks involving aiming, whereas females excel in verbal abilities, fine motor tasks, and perceptual thresholds (touch, taste, hearing and olfaction). But recent work has shown that verbal test scores for men have converged over the last two decades towards those of women. A similar trend for mathematical abilities to match those of men has been documented for women (Hyde, 1991).

Thus gender differences in IQ subtests may not be biologically based, as was once thought. Instead, it is now argued that the gender differences in the subtests may be related to the way boys and girls are socialised. However, one gender difference has persisted – the performance of males on visuo-spatial tests. It remains to be seen whether this too will show change with time as society undergoes further transformation.

Changes in IQ over time

Does IQ change? Can IQ be increased? One of the most striking findings in IQ studies has been the fact that mean IQ scores have been shown to have increased by 3 points per decade in the Western world over the last 50 years, resulting in an average increase of 15 points or one standard deviation over this period (Flynn, 1987). Known as the *Flynn effect*, this rise in IQ has been attributed to a number of factors, better nutrition, cultural changes, experience in problem solving, and so on. Interestingly, this steady increase in IQ is not reflected in intelligent behaviour, such as peaceful living and avoidance of conflicts and wars. In fact, it seems to have had minimal impact even on educational achievement over the years.

An alternative way of looking for possible changes in IQ is to examine the effect of intervention programmes to improve intelligence. Early intervention programmes designed to improve IQ scores have yielded good short-term results. Enrichment programmes carried out in the USA, such as Project Head Start in which children from disadvantaged backgrounds were exposed to stimulating experiences and received massive input for one or two years at primary school, have produced a rise in test scores during the course of the programme. But these gains are short lived and by the end of the primary school years there appears to be no difference in IQ when compared with controls (Zigler & Muenchow, 1992). (However, the benefits of Head Start are more far reaching than its effects on IQ – it has been shown to be effective in producing social, educational and personal advantages.) This and other evidence go to show that IQ scores are not immutable and fixed.

Genes and (psychometric) intelligence

Research into the genetics of IQ has produced a vast quantity of data and the conclusions have been unequivocal: the genetic contribution to psychometric intelligence, as indexed by the IQ, is substantial. The strongest evidence for this comes from twin studies. Although all twin studies have been subjected to criticisms of various kinds, over the past four decades research in several countries has yielded remarkably consistent results. These results hold up well, not only for full scale IQ but also for individual cognitive abilities such as verbal and spatial abilities. A representative set of figures from pooled data from many different studies is shown in Table 2.3.

Several conclusions may be made from the information in Table 2.3 (Bouchard & McGue, 1981):

1. The closer the genetic relationship between siblings, the greater their correlation between IQ scores (r for MZ > DZ > siblings).
2. Separated twins correlate quite substantially in IQ.
3. Monozygotic (MZ) twins reared apart resemble each other to a greater

Table 2.3 Findings regarding psychometric intelligence from twin studies (Bouchard & McGue, 1981)

	Correlation coefficient (r)
Monozygotic twins reared together (MZ)	0.86
Monozygotic twins reared apart (MZA)	0.72
Dizygotic twins reared together (DZ)	0.65
Dizygotic twins reared apart (DZA)	0.6
Siblings reared together	0.5
Siblings reared apart	0.2

degree than dizygotic (DZ) twins reared together. Collectively these three findings indicate that heredity makes a powerful contribution to IQ.
4. However, twins reared together show greater correlation in IQ scores than those reared apart, implying an environmental effect.

The pattern of correlations found is consistent with the pattern of correlations predicted on the basis of polygenic inheritance. That is, the higher the proportion of genes two family members have in common the higher the average correlation between their IQs. Thus, the phenotype (intelligence) is demonstrably directly related to the genotype. Estimates of heritability (h^2), the proportion of variance attributable to genetic difference in the sample being studied, typically works out to about 0.50 in children, meaning that approximately half, or 50%, of variability among individuals in the population under study is due to genetic differences. The literature on genetic studies is vast, and, in spite of the problems associated with twin studies, the findings show that around 50% of the variation in IQ is accounted for by genetic factors. However, it is necessary to exercise caution when interpreting these findings. *Heritability applies to groups or populations and not to individuals.* It would, therefore, be incorrect to interpret these findings to mean that in a given individual 50% of his or her intelligence is genetic and the rest is environmentally determined.

A surprising finding that has been reported in many different genetic studies is the developmental trend observed in heritability of IQ. The commonsense belief that as the child grows up and comes under wider influences from the school, peers and the community, environmental influences would be more important (with corresponding decrease in genetic contribution) has been shown not to be true. A robust finding from studies of twins at various ages has been that genetic influence on IQ *increases* with age. Heritability for IQ in infancy is around 20%, in childhood it is about 40% and in adolescence and adulthood it is 50%. A recent study of twins at the age of 80 years and older concluded that the heritability for IQ was around 60% (McClearn et al., 1997).

Environment and psychometric intelligence

The 'environment' includes a range of influences on intelligence, from family environment to schooling and peer pressure. Curiously, it has been genetic studies, twin and adoption studies that have provided the best evidence for the effect of environment on IQ scores. The role of environmental factors on cognitive abilities is more difficult to unravel because there are few accepted variable units to measure environmental influence. The non-genetic component ($1 - h^2$) is taken to be due to environmental factors. Evidence for environmental contributions to psychometric intelligence come from several sources:

1. Data from twin studies cited above
2. Pairs of unrelated children reared together show correlations in IQ in the order of 0.23 and the corresponding figure for adoptive parents and adopted children is around 0.20 indicating that environmental influences account for 20–25% of the variation in IQ (Plomin, 1988).

3. The substantial improvement in IQ scores repeatedly documented in children from deprived backgrounds when they are placed in stimulating environments is further proof of the contribution that environment makes to children's IQ.

The relative contributions of shared (e^2) and non-shared (c^2) environment has shown that shared environmental influences (aspects of the environment that family members experience in *common*) account for around 25%. Non-shared environmental influence (aspects of the environment that are unique to the individual) accounts for about 10% of the variation (Figure 2.3). Another striking feature is that shared environmental influences decline from childhood to adolescence and adulthood. In young adulthood shared environmental effects on IQ almost disappear and the correlation is almost zero, implying that the long-term effect of shared family environment is very little indeed.

Behavioural genetic explanations for individual differences in intelligence stress the importance of a third factor, the gene–environment interaction, in addition to the independent contributions made by genetics and environment. Human beings choose and shape the environment and are not passive recipients of environmental influences.

In summary, both heredity (nature) and environment (nurture) contribute to intelligence. Their relative contributions appear to be about the same, around 50% each. They interact in various ways and to partition the effect of genetic and environmental influences on psychometric intelligence appears to be more complicated than was once thought.

Effect of ageing on IQ

Contrary to popular belief, the decline in IQ with age is not large. This was clearly demonstrated by the Seattle longitudinal study of adult intelligence. It was an ambitious project that began in 1956 and recruited a random sample of 25 men and 25 women at five-year age intervals from 20 to 70. The 500 original participants were tested every seven years. New participants were recruited into the study every 7 years in the course of the study. The sample tested in 1994 included over 5000 subjects. Longitudinal data from the study showed that individuals' intelligence was relatively stable across this age

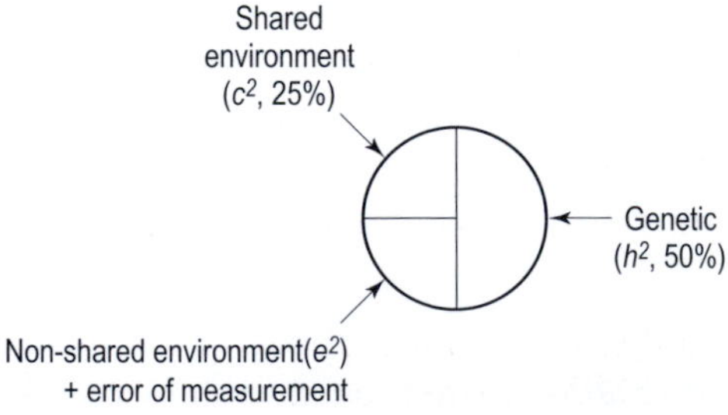

Fig. 2.3 Contribution of genetic (h^2), shared environmental (c^2) and unshared environmental (e^2) influences on children's psychometric intelligence in a population (the concept of heritability is applicable to populations and not to individuals)

range disproving the previous findings that intelligence follows a inverted U-shaped trajectory. The main finding was that in most individuals IQ generally increases till about the age of 40, remains stable until the age of 60, and then shows slight decline by age 70 (Schaie, 1994). It is now believed that intelligence shows relative stability across adulthood. The differences observed in previous studies in different cohorts appear to be a function of societal changes, especially education. There is also enormous variability among individuals.

Ageing has a differential effect on verbal and performance test scores with performance IQ falling more rapidly than verbal IQ (Figure 2.4). On the WAIS-III the IQ changes are as follows:

- Performance IQ peaks around 20–24 and begins to decline thereafter and after 65 years the average verbal-performance discrepancy is about 20 points in absolute terms, although this relative discrepancy will not be evident in their actual profiles (because their IQ scores are based on norms for their age group).
- Verbal IQ, when controlled for education, increases steadily from 20 to about 50, peaking at ages of 45 to 54 and then declines slightly in the 70s and 80s when it reaches the same level as in the 20s.

Distribution of IQ scores in the general population

The assumption behind the deviation IQ is that intelligence falls around a normal distribution. From Figure 2.5 it can be seen that 68% (two-thirds) of the population have IQs within one standard deviation of the mean (85–115), while 95% of the population have IQs within two standard deviations of the mean (70–130).

The IQ could also be expressed as percentiles where 100 corresponds to the 50th centile, an IQ of 110 to 75th centile, and an IQ of 90 falls at the 25th centile. For example, someone who has attained a score corresponding to the 80th centile has performed at a level such that only 19 persons out of 100 would perform better than him/her.

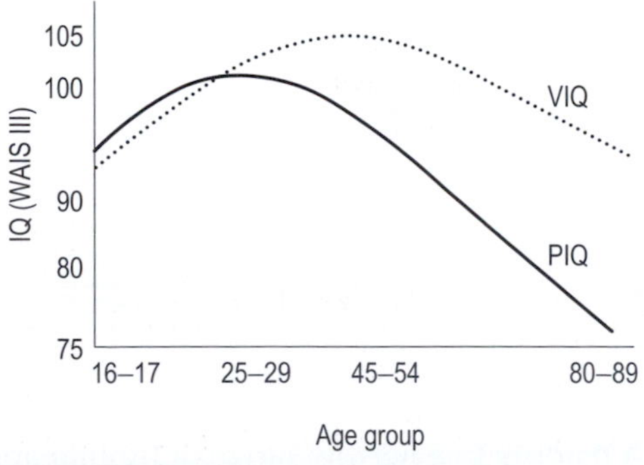

Fig. 2.4 Verbal and performance IQ from 16 to 89 years

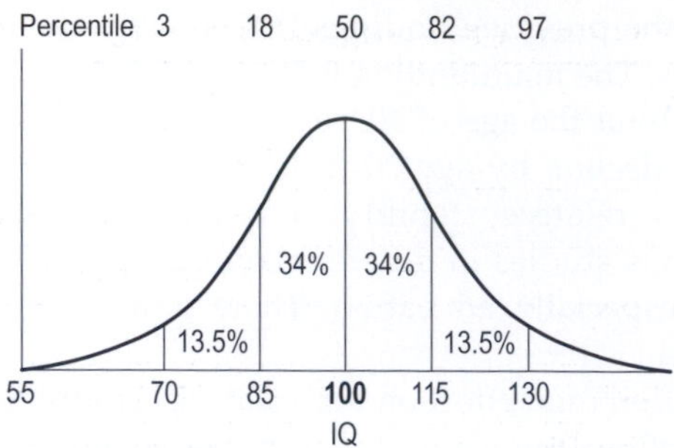

Fig. 2.5 The distribution of WAIS IQ scores in the normal population

Box 2.1 The 'knowns' and 'unknowns' about human (psychometric) intelligence (based on Neisser et al., 1996; Deary, 2001)

- Individual differences in cognitive abilities show a hierarchical structure. A general factor Spearman's *g* accounts for about 40–50% of the variance in a battery of varied tests of intelligence
- Psychometric intelligence is more than *g* because lower-order factors account for the rest of the variance
- Psychometric intelligence shows strong stability across adult life span
- Both genes and environment make substantial contributions to psychometric intelligence. The effect of shared environment in *adulthood* is very low in comparison to that made by non-shared or unique environment
- Psychometric intelligence differences are important predictors of educational outcomes, occupational status and workplace success
- The differences between intelligent test scores in Blacks and Whites does not result from any obvious bias in test construction and administration nor does it simply reflect differences in socioeconomic status. There is no support for a genetic interpretation. Explanations based on culture may be appropriate
- Although there are no important sex differences in overall intelligent test scores, substantial differences do appear for specific abilities. Males typically score high in visuo-spatial and mathematical skills, whereas females excel on a number of verbal measures
- There is more to intelligence than those aspects captured by psychometric intelligence. Other forms of intelligence such as creativity, wisdom, practical abilities and social sensitivity are not measured by conventional intelligent tests. Very little is known about them

Research into psychometric intelligence over more than a century has generated a vast quantity of data (and controversy). The main findings of research are summarised in Box 2.1. Ian Deary (2001) has provided a balanced account of our understanding of intelligence.

SYSTEMIC THEORIES OF INTELLIGENCE

The psychometric approach to intelligence has recently come under heavy criticism for several reasons. First, several current theorists argue that the concept of *g* (and IQ) apply to a narrow range of human abilities and do not tap into other systems of abilities. They argue that there are many different

Table 2.4 The psychometric and systemic approaches to intelligence

Psychometric approaches	*Systemic approaches*
Singular factor *g*	Multiple intelligences
Measured by IQ tests	Dynamic tests; no single test
Based on factor analysis	Base on varied approaches
'Culture bound'	More culture fair
Predicts scholastic achievements	Predicts occupational success, learning
Context – 'laboratory like' conditions	Contextualised to a variety of situations
A general theory	Modular theories

'intelligences' that are not sufficiently accessed by conventional psychometric tests like the WAIS. In recent scholarship on the subject there has been a distinct swing towards multifactorial models of intelligence (and away from hierarchical models). Second, the bias of IQ tests towards the dominant culture and culturally dependant knowledge has received considerable attention. It has been argued that intelligence tests are heavily biased in favour, and reflect the values, of white, middle-class society. IQ tests have been (mis)used to categorise children as having learning disabilities and thus deny them equal opportunities in education. Third, many workers in the field have produced evidence to show that a weakness of the psychometric method of measuring intelligence is that it is conducted under 'laboratory-like' conditions and not in the natural environment. A key objection raised by the new theorists is that psychometric tests of intelligence have to be contextualised. Their argument is that, for a measurement of intelligence to be valid, assessments need to be carried out in near-real-life situations rather than under laboratory conditions.

An elegant example of the use of intelligence in natural settings is provided by studies of child candy vendors on the streets of Brazil (Saxe, 1988). Children as young as 6 and 7 years, who had had no formal education, were found to be able to use various mathematical computations to earn a living. They were found to be performing complicated mathematical operations when purchasing and selling. At the buying phase they bought candy that would sell, and in determining the selling price they were seen to convert the wholesale price paid for a multi-unit box to a retail price for individual units while making sure that they were making a profit. At the time of selling they had to bargain with the customer, handle money and convert currencies. In addition they had to make allowances for inflation and compete with peers. The mathematics involved in candy selling is not abstract and it came as no surprise that on formal tests of intelligence they did well on problems similar to those encountered in selling but performed poorly on other conventional tests of intelligence.

This and other findings lend support to the new theories of intelligence, which view it as a system of interacting abilities rather than as a specific set of abilities. In addition, these theories are concerned more with the cognitive *processes* that underlie intelligent behaviour. They seek to identify, describe and assess the efficiency of the specific processes that individuals use when performing tasks. Three such theories are discussed below. Table 2.4 provides a summary of the differences between the psychometric and systemic approaches. Here we provide two examples from the many research studies that emphasise these viewpoints.

Gardner's theory of multiple intelligences

According to Howard Gardner (1983) intelligence is not a unitary concept, rather it includes a number of intellectual skills and abilities ('intelligences') that are relatively independent of one another, and what is measured by traditional IQ tests are those abilities that are valued by our particular culture and society. He described seven forms of intelligences: linguistic, logical–mathematical, spatial, musical, bodily–kinaesthetic, interpersonal and intrapersonal. He suggested that the first two were those valued at school, the next three valuable in the arts and the last two a sort of early emotional intelligence concept. Currently there are no tests for abilities based on Gardner's theory but assessments have been developed in some areas like movement (bodily–kinaesthetic intelligence). Assessments are based on the principle that subjects should be permitted diverse modes of response and multiple ways of demonstrating understanding and that for assessments to be fair they have to be carried out in near-natural settings.

Sternberg's triarchic theory of human intelligence

Robert Sternberg, a prolific researcher and writer in the field of intelligence (he has written more than fifty books on the subject), has persuasively challenged the wisdom of the psychometric approach. He has convincingly argued that psychological tests measure only part of the entire picture of what intelligence is. His theory, named the triarchic theory of intelligence (Sternberg, 1985), holds that there are three different aspects of intelligence that together account for human intellectual abilities (Figure 2.6).

- *Analytical abilities*. These refer to the strategies used in trying to solve familiar problems by comparing, analysing and evaluating elements or the relationships between them.

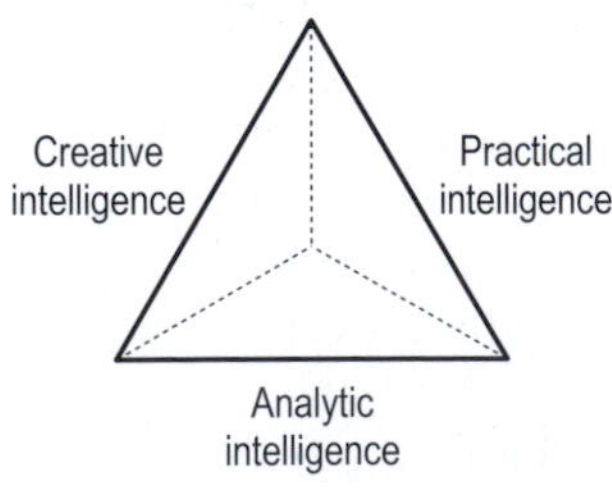

Fig. 2.6 The three types of intelligences according to the triarchic theory of intelligence (Sternberg, 1985). IQ tests measure analytic intelligence only

- *Practical abilities*. Abilities that involve application of existing knowledge to everyday practical problems.
- *Creative abilities*. Abilities required for new and imaginative ways of thinking about the problem or its elements.

Most psychometric tests measure only the analytic intellectual abilities. Practical intellectual abilities, which reflect the capacity to solve common-sense problems that a person encounters in day-to-day life is thought to be more important for success at work than analytic ability. Sternberg maintains that the three abilities are relatively independent but interact with one another. In addition, general intelligence is understood in terms of the *processes* used to arrive at the solutions to various kinds of problems. Assessing these domains requires different forms of tests, including multiple-choice items and essay questions in verbal, quantitative and pictorial domains.

The triarchic theory, mentioned in outline here, is a comprehensive and detailed model of intelligence backed by a large body of research (Sternberg, 1988). It is a bold attempt to explain three aspects (systems) of our intelligence (Figure 2.7):

1. Information processing aspects and the underlying *mechanisms* (*componential sub-theory*) including metacomponents (planning, monitoring and evaluating problem solving) and knowledge acquisition
2. Contextual aspects dealing with relationship between the individual and the environment (*contextual sub-theory*). Sternberg outlines three ways in which people apply their intelligence to life tasks:
   - by adapting to existing environment;
   - by shaping the environment;
   - by selecting a new environment.
3. Aspects that deal with our experience (*exponential sub-theory*). Included in this is the application of previous experience leading to automisation, the ability to perform tasks automatically, such as skilled reading and dealing with novel problems.

Sternberg's theory has generated a vast amount of research but the construction of tests of intelligence based on the theory have met with only limited

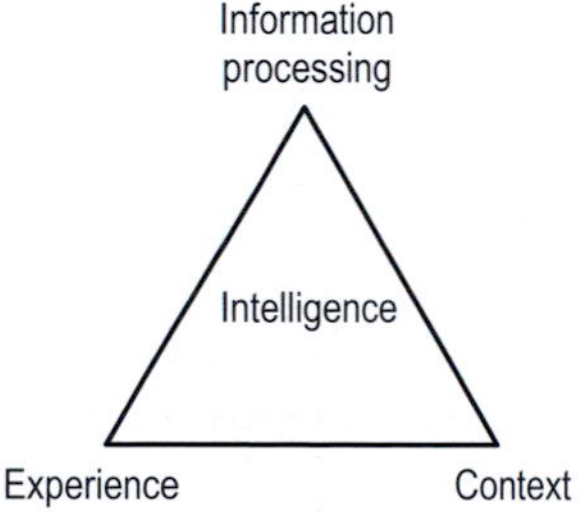

Fig. 2.7 A simplified representation of the triarchic theory of intelligence (Sternberg, 1988)

success. Questionnaires designed to measure practical intelligence have been developed in various domains, particularly in business management. The examinee is presented with work-related situations and asked to choose options for dealing with them. Sternberg has also produced evidence to show that tactic knowledge or practical intelligence is: (1) different from psychometric intelligence; and (2) that it is a better predictor of job performance than IQ tests (Sternberg & Wagner, 1993).

Bioecological view of intelligence

A recent entrant to the field of intelligence theories is the bioecological theory of Bronfenbrenner and Ceci (1994). Their theory is based on three sound findings from various studies including some of their own:

1. They subscribe to the view of intelligence as a modular or multiple resource system rather than a singular or, even, a hierarchical resource pool.
2. They assert that from the beginning of life there exists interaction between biological potential and environmental factors such that two individuals who are born with equal 'intelligences' may, by adolescence, be seen to have different intellectual profiles. Interaction between biologically determined cognitive potential and the ecological context results in changes that set a cascading effect in motion. The effects of environmental influences depend on the time when they occur in the course of lifespan development and they are specific to each type of cognitive ability.
3. They take a developmental perspective and, drawing on evidence, propose that specific cognitive abilities vary in their sensitivity to environmental influences. Interaction between the biological potential and environment is seen not as additive but multiplicative such that even small changes may lead on to a chain of events resulting in massive developmental transformation in abilities over time.

Other 'intelligences'

Recently there have been attempts to incorporate a new category of intelligence, called *emotional intelligence*, within the broad framework of human cognitive abilities. It has been defined as 'the ability to monitor one's own and others' emotions, to discriminate among them and to use the information to guide one's thinking and actions' (Salovey & Mayer, 1990). In essence, emotional intelligence involves:

- Self-awareness; knowing one's emotions.
- Managing emotions rather than emotions driving one's behaviour.
- Emotional self-control and self-motivation.
- Recognising emotions in others; empathy.
- Handling relationships and interpersonal effectiveness.

The concept of emotional intelligence has been popularised by Goldman (1996). Although the concept and its descriptions have an intuitive appeal, as a scientific concept it has been difficult to study. A number of tests have been constructed to measure emotional intelligence and its various components, but as yet most of the tests have been unable to capture the overall concept.

DISORDERS OF INTELLECT

Mental retardation (learning disability)

Mental retardation (MR) refers to *arrest* or incomplete development of the mind that occurs during a person's early development (birth to 18 years). By convention, an IQ score of less than two standard deviations below average (corresponding to IQ below 69) is used as a cut off point. The subaverage general intellectual performance is widespread and global (affecting all or most aspects of intellectual functioning). Although both ICD-10 and DSM-IV employ the term mental retardation for this diagnostic category, it is commonly referred to as learning disability (LD), especially in the UK. Irrespective of the precise terminology, there are three core criteria for learning disability:

- Significant impairment intellectual functioning (i.e. IQ below 69 on WAIS).
- Significant impairment of adaptive functioning.
- Age of onset before adulthood.

All three criteria must be met for a person to be considered to have learning disability. The concept of impaired functioning refers to the ability of the person to adapt to the daily demands of life. It is, therefore, related to a person's age and sociocultural expectations associated with his or her environment at any given time. It is essential that a measure of functional ability be used in addition to the intelligence test for two reasons:

1. Individuals within the low IQ range show considerable variation in their functional ability and this carries the danger of labelling well-functioning people as 'retarded'; and
2. Most IQ tests show 'floor effects', i.e. they are not sensitive below 3 or 4 standard deviations below the mean.

In addition to clinical assessments of level of self-care and daily living abilities, levels of adaptive functioning may be carried out through the use of rating scales to assess a wide array of domains such as the level of self-care (personal hygiene, ability to dress), daily living skills (using money, finding one's way around), communication and socialisation. *Vineland adaptive behaviour scale* is one of the most popular scales for assessment of adaptive functioning (Sparrow, Balla & Cicchetti, 1984). Assessment of the individual needs of the person with learning disability and identification of the necessary support to meet those needs, rather than reliance on psychometric testing, forms the essence of management of people who fall into this category. Psychometric

Table 2.5 Classification of Mental Retardation according to IQ and their occurrence in the group

Degree of mental retardation	*IQ*	*Prevalence in the MR group (%)*
Mild mental retardation	50/55–70	85
Moderate mental retardation	30/40–50/55	10
Severe mental retardation	20/25–35/40	3–4
Profound mental retardation	< 20–25	1–2

testing is neither sufficient, nor always necessary, to produce a meaningful assessment of a person with learning disability.

People with learning disabilities do not constitute a homogeneous group. However, there is general agreement that it consists of two groups:

1. A non-organic group, sometimes called familial or subcultural group, that is associated with mild MR (IQ 50 to 69) with relatively better adaptive functioning, poor environment and low genetic inheritance; and
2. An organic group with severe MR (IQ < 50) typically associated with organic causes, Down's syndrome being the commonest.

The degree of mental retardation is graded from mild to profound depending on the IQ as shown in Table 2.5. The more severe the degree of intellectual impairment, the greater is the likelihood of an underlying specific biological cause.

Specific learning disability (SLD)

In contrast to mental or intellectual retardation, SLD refers to impairment in one (or more) dimension(s) of performance for a given age and IQ. Specific reading retardation (SRR; dyslexia is a subgroup that comes under this umbrella term) is the commonest of this group. An arbitrary cut-off point of 2 *SD* below predicted level is used to identify these children. This is a heterogeneous group of disorders, thought to arise from abnormalities of cognitive processing that affect skills acquisition from early stages of development. In ICD–10 these disorders are called specific disorders of scholastic skills (SDSS). Global IQ is usually within the normal range but the achievement in the specific domain (reading, spelling or arithmetic skills) falls below that expected for a given IQ and age.

Dementia

The term dementia refers to a global *decline* in intellectual abilities. Alzheimer's disease (AD), the commonest cause of dementia, leads to an irreversible and rapid loss of intellectual and other cognitive functions. Most cases of dementia may be identified clinically. Tests such as the mini-mental state examination (Folstein, Folstein & McHugh, 1975) are often helpful. However, application of a test such as WAIS may show that in Alzheimer's type dementia:

1. The full scale IQ (FIQ) may be lower than that expected on the basis of educational/occupational attainment.
2. Nonverbal abilities are likely to be more impaired than verbal abilities. Verbal/performance IQ discrepancy on WAIS of greater than 15 points is found in about half (not all) patients with AD. What this means is that the WAIS should be used in combination with specific tests of memory, e.g. Wechsler Memory Scale (WMS, see Chapter 7), if it is to be useful in the diagnosis of AD.
3. Uneven profile of subtest scores (this is more common in vascular dementias).
4. Current IQ is lower than the premorbid IQ estimated from National Adult Word Reading Test (NART, Nelson & Willison, 1991) or other similar test that assesses premorbid IQ.

The NART is a 50-item single-word reading test, all of which are irregular (such as naïve, debt, bouquet and psalm) and cannot be pronounced using the usual rules of spelling. The supposition is that the test makes minimal demands on current cognitive capacity and depends on prior or premorbid ability, because the testee must have prior knowledge of the words' pronunciation. Premorbid IQ is estimated on basis of errors made. NART error scores can be converted to an IQ on the WAIS-III by using a special formula. Its validity as an index of prior intellectual functioning has been well established (Crawford et al., 2001).

Psychopathology in persons with learning disability

In addition to the consequences resulting from impaired cognitive and social functioning, the psychiatric implications of learning disabilities are two-fold. First, it has been repeatedly shown that the prevalence of psychiatric morbidity is markedly increased in children and adults with learning disabilities. For example, in the Isle of Wight study, Rutter and colleagues (1976) found that among children between the age of 9 and 11 years, the occurrence of psychiatric disorders was around 20% (and 7% in the general population). A Swedish study found that among adults with LD, 33% with mild LD and 70% with severe LD had a psychiatric disorder (Gostason, 1985). The mental disorders included a wide range from anxiety to schizophrenia.

Second, in those with borderline learning disability *and* a major mental illness the prognosis tends to be poorer than those with normal intelligence. Borderline learning disability is the term used to refer to persons with an IQ in the range 70–85 (i.e. 1–2 standard deviations below the mean). Although this group is not recognised by ICD-10 as a distinct category, it is included in the DSM-IV under a V code (clinically significant factors). This includes 18% of the population and, although the majority show no deficits and live independently in the community, when mental illnesses occur in those with borderline intellectual functioning they tend to be hospitalised for longer periods resulting in inappropriate occupation of beds, and are harder to rehabilitate (Hassiotis et al., 1999). The poor prognosis in this group has received considerable attention in the recent past.

REFERENCES

Bouchard TJ, McGue M (1981) Familial studies on intelligence. Science, 212, 1055–1058.

Bronfenbrenner U, Ceci SJ (1994) Nature–nurture reconceptualised in developmental perspective: a bioecological model. Psychological Review, 101, 568–582.

Carroll JB (1993) Human Cognitive Abilities: a survey of factor analytic studies. Cambridge: Cambridge University Press.

Crawford JR, Deary IJ, Starr J, Whally LJ (2001) The NART as an index of prior intellectual functioning: a retrospective validity study covering a 66-year interval. Psychological Medicine, 31, 451–458.

Cole M, Gay J, Glick J, Sharp DW (1971) The Cultural Context of Learning and Thinking. New York Basic Books.

Deary IJ (2001) Looking Down on Human Intelligence: from psychometrics to the brain. Oxford: Oxford University Press.

Elliot CD, Murray DJ, Pearson LS (1983) The British Ability Scales (rev. ed.). Windsor, UK: Nelson–National Foundation for Educational Research (NFER).

Folstein M, Folstein S, McHugh P (1975) Mini-Mental State: a practical method of grading the cognitive state of patients for the clinician. Journal of Psychiatric Research, 12, 189–198.

Flynn JR (1987) Massive IQ gains in 14 nations: what IQ tests really measure. Psychological Bulletin, 101, 171–191.

Galton F (1883) Enquiries into Human Faculty and its Development. London, UK: Macmillan.

Gardner H (1983) Frames of Mind: the theory of multiple intelligences. New York: Basic Books.

Goldman D (1996) Emotional Intelligence. London: Bloomsbury.

Gostason R (1985) Psychiatric illness among mentally retarded: a Swedish population study. Acta Psychiatrica Scandinavia Supplementum, 318, 1–117.

Greenfield P (1997) You can't take it with you: why ability assessments don't cross cultures. American Psychologist, 52(10), 1115–1124.

Hakstain RN, Cattell RB (1978) Higher stratum ability structure on a basis of 20 primary abilities. Journal of Education Psychology, 70, 657–569.

Hassiotis A, Ukoumunne O, Tyrer P, Piachaud J, Gilvarry C, Harvey K, Fraser J (1999) Prevalence and characteristics of patients with severe mental illness and borderline intellectual functioning. Report from the UK 700 random controlled trial of case management. British Journal of Psychiatry, 175, 135–149.

Horn JL, Cattell RB (1966) Refinement and test of the theory of fluid and crystallised intelligence. Journal of Education Psychology, 57, 253–270.

Hyde JS (1991) Half the Human Experience: the psychology of women. Lexington, MA: Heath & Co.

Kline P (1993) Intelligence: the psychometric view. London: Routledge.

McClearn G E, Johnson B, Berg S, Pedersen NL et al. (1997) Substantial genetic influence in cognitive abilities in twins 80 or more years old. Science, 276, 1560–1562.

Neisser U, Boodoo G, Bouchard TJ, Boykin AW, Brody N, Ceci SJ, Halpern DF, Loehlin JC, Perloff R, Sternberg RJ, Urbina S (1996) Intelligence: knowns and unknowns. American Psychologist, 51(2), 77–101.

Nelson HE, Willison J (1991) National Adult Word Reading Test Manual, 2nd ed. Windsor, UK: NFER–Nelson.

Plomin R (1988) The nature and nurture of cognitive abilities. In RH Sternberg (ed.), Advances in Psychology of Human Intelligence. Hillsdale, NJ: Erlbaum; 1–23.

Poortinga YH (1989) The equivalence of cross-cultural data: an overview of basic issues. International Journal of Psychology, 24, 737–756.

Raven JC (1938) Progressive Matrices. London: Lewis.

Rutter M (1976) Isle of Wight studies, 1964–1974. Psychological Medicine, 6, 313–332.

Salovey P, Mayer JD (1990) Emotional intelligence. Intelligence, Cognition and Personality, 9, 185–211.

Saxe GB(1988) The mathematics of child street vendors. Child Development, 59, 1415–1425.

Schaie KW (1994) The course of adult intellectual development. American Psychologist, 49, 304–313.
Schwarzman AE, Gold D, Andres D, Arbuckle TY, Chaidelson J (1987) Stability of intelligence: a 40-year follow-up study. Canadian Journal of Psychology, 41, 244–256.
Sparrow SS, Balla DA, Cicchetti DV (1984) Vineland Adaptive Behaviour Scales. American Guidance Service, MN: Circle Pines.
Sternberg RJ (1985) Beyond IQ: a triarchic theory of human intelligence. Cambridge: Cambridge University Press.
Sternberg RJ (1988) The Triarchic Mind: a new theory of intelligence. New York, Viking.
Sternberg RL, Wagner RK (1993) The *g*-ocentric view of intelligence and job performance is wrong. Current Directions in Psychological Science, 2, 1–4.
Sternberg RL, Conway BE, Ketron JL, Bernstein M (1981) People's conception of intelligence. Journal of Personality and social Psychology, 41, 37–53.
Thorndike RL, Hagen EP, Sattler JM (1986) The Stanford–Binet Intelligence Scale, 4th ed. Chicago, IL: Riverside Publishing Company.
Thurstone LL (1938) Primary Mental Abilities. Chicago, IL: Chicago University Press.
Wechsler D (1944) The measurement of adult intelligence, 4th ed. Baltimore, MD: Williams & Wilkins.
Wechsler D (1997) The Wechsler Adult Intelligence Scale, 3rd edn. San Antonio, CA: The Psychological Corporation.
Zigler EF, Muenchow S(1992) Head Start: the inside story of America's most successful educational experiment. New York: Basic Books.

FURTHER READING

Deary IJ (2001) Looking Down on Human Intelligence: from psychometrics to the brain. Oxford: Oxford University Press.

- An outstanding book that takes stock of the subject, a 'spring cleaning' of the research area.

Sternberg RJ (ed.) (2000) Handbook of Intelligence. Cambridge: Cambridge University Press.

- One of the fifty-odd books by one of the greatest living researchers in the field.

Neisser U, Boodoo G, Bouchard TJ, Boykin AW, Brody N, Ceci SJ, Halpern DF, Loehlin JC, Perloff R, Sternberg RJ, Urbina S (1996) Intelligence: knowns and unknowns. American Psychologist, 51(2), 77–101.

- The report of a task force established by the American Psychological Association. The task force was able to arrive at a unanimous decision on the various controversial issues around IQ. The report summarises their findings. Worth its weight in gold.

Personality and its importance to psychiatric practice

3

'No man is an island, entire of itself, every man is a piece of continent, a part of the main.'
John Donne, *Devotion Upon Emergent Occasions,* 1624

People resemble and differ from one another in various ways both physically and psychologically. For example, all individuals have the same body parts (face, head and limbs) but each person also has a unique and easily recognisable appearance. Likewise every person has a characteristic manner of thinking, feeling, behaving and relating to others. Some people are typically introverted, and reserved, others are extroverted and outgoing. Some are invariably conscientious and organized, whereas others are consistently carefree. All of us can describe other people that we know in a few phrases or sentences. Despite the fact that everyone has an intuitive understanding of what is meant by personality, it is difficult to capture it in a single definition. The task is further complicated by the fact that it means different things to different personality psychologists depending upon the framework that they use to understand its nature. It is not surprising, therefore, that more than fifty definitions of personality have been proposed since the subject began to be studied scientifically. In fact, Gordon Allport, a pioneer in the study of personality, reviewed fifty definitions of normal personality in his book, *Personality: a psychological interpretation* (Allport, 1938).

For the sake of simplicity we will refer to two commonly used definitions of personality (derived from various sources):

> *Personality is an individual's distinctive and enduring patterns of thoughts, feelings and behaviour in his/her relationship with the environment.*
>
> *Personality refers to a reasonably stable pattern of behaviour including thoughts and actions that distinguish people from one another.*

These definitions encompass and emphasise three aspects of personality as it is currently understood:

1. That personality is unique and distinctive to the individual (as much as physical appearance). Although people may show the same characteristics such as emotionality, aggression or conscientiousness, these manifest in different degrees and combinations that are distinctive to the individual.
2. That personality is relatively stable across time (in adults) and situations. Important aspects of adults' personality are thought to remain unchanged during their life span. Even though maturation and life experiences influence the way one feels and behaves, for the major part of one's life personality remains highly stable and enduring.

3. That personality characteristics manifest in our relationship with the environment, especially in interaction with others. Different situations may generate different patterns of behaviour in the individual. For example, a person may be submissive towards his superiors at work and be dominant (and even aggressive) towards his spouse. In this case constancy has to be sought for certain types of behaviour in certain types of situations. In fact, variability in behaviour patterns in different situations could be viewed as a personality characteristic.

Our understanding of normal personality has become more sophisticated over the last few decades in response to, and as a result of, fierce controversies generated by the views put forward by early workers in the field. Before examining the various theories of personality it is useful to distinguish between two fundamentally different approaches through which all personality theories could be understood.

Nomothetic and idiographic approaches

Nomothetic methods of study. These (in Greek, *nomos* = law) are concerned with aspects of personality that are common to all people. They focus on how people are alike on different personality variables. Typically they involve the study of personality variables in a population or group by comparing the individual's profile of variables with the population 'norms'. Most contemporary personality research has been of the nomothetic variety. These methods of study assume the personality differences to be *quantitative* variables that are common to all the individuals, and that they are normally distributed in the population showing the typical bell-shaped spread.

Idiographic methods. These centre around the study of the person and his/her uniqueness and individuality (in Greek, *idios* = person or own). They focus on the way people are different and view the differences as *qualitative*. They do not require comparing the person with others, the unit of study is the individual and there is no need (or methods) for comparison. They are concerned with the real individual rather than the average or typical person. These approaches consider that most, if not all, aspects of personality are fundamentally idiosyncratic to the individual and that generalised theoretical approaches are deceptive.

Psychoanalytic theories (Freudian, and post-Freudian.), humanistic approaches (Rogers, Maslow) and personal construct theory (Kelly) are idiographic theories that emphasise the subjective experience of subjects. Contemporary trait theories of personality (Cattell, Eysenck, Costa & McRae), in fact most measurements in psychology, adopt the nomothetic approach. Table 3.1 summarises the main features of the two approaches.

In clinical practice a combination of idiographic and nomothetic approaches are used. Faced with a patient presenting with features of, say, depression, the clinician assesses them against a list of symptoms and signs known to occur in a group of patients with depression (nomothetic approach). Next the clinician proceeds to make an evaluation of how and why

Table 3.1 Nomothetic and idiographic approaches

Nomothetic approach	*Idiographic approach*
Variable centred	Person centred
Compared with others (normative)	Compared with self (ipsative)
Studies group norms	Studies individual norms
'People have lots in common'	'Everyone is different and unique'
Sees individual differences as quantitative	Sees individual differences as qualitative
Unit of study is the group or population	Unit of study is the single case
Common tests: WAIS, EPQ, NEO-PI-R	Repertory grid, Q-sort, projective tests

this particular patient experiences these symptoms at this particular time of his/her life, taking into consideration normative and non-normative life events, current stresses, childhood experiences, and so on (the idiographic approach). Indeed the application of nomothetic findings from research to the idiographic peculiarities in the patient is the essence of good clinical practice.

Theories of personality

The field of personology (the study of personality) abounds with theories. Of all the theories of personality, it is the trait theories that have dominated the field over the last few decades and produced a large number of empirical research findings that have helped to refine the theoretical concepts that underpin them. Table 3.2 provides a list of the better-known theories.

This chapter seeks to provide an outline of the main personality theories. Trait theories receive greater mention because of the important position they occupy in current literature. Psychoanalytic theories are discussed in Chapter 13.

Table 3.2 The main theories of personality

Theory type	*Proposer*	*Examples*
1. Type theories:	W. H. Sheldon, C. Jung	
2. Psychoanalytic theories:	S. Freud, Post-Freudians	
3. Phenomenological theories:	C. Rogers, G. Kelly	Personal construct theory
4. Interactionist theories:	A. Bandura W. Mischel	Social learning theory Person situation theory
5. Narrow band theories:	J. B. Rotter M. Friedmann & R. H. Roseman	Locus of control theory Type A and Type B behaviour patterns
6. Trait theories:	R. B. Cattell H. J. Eysenck P. T. Costa & R. McCrae	Sixteen personality factors (16PF) Three factor theory (PEN) Five factor model (FFM)

Personality types

Throughout history there have been many attempts to classify human beings in terms of differences in their character or temperament. *Personality types* refer to categories of personality descriptions so that individuals can be grouped as falling into one or other type. The earliest observations of behaviour patterns conceived of four temperaments that were thought to be qualitatively different. Thus Hippocrates and Galen described four personality 'types' based on presumed excess of the type of body fluid: sanguine (cheerful and optimistic); choleric (aggressive and quick tempered); phlegmatic (slow and lazy); and melancholic (sad and pessimistic). Kretschmer (1936), a German psychiatrist, following a similar scheme, described three *body types* each associated with a mental illness: pyknic (affective illnesses); asthenic (schizophrenia); and athletic (no mental illness). Sheldon (Sheldon & Stevens, 1942) investigated the relationship between temperament and body types and found that certain body types were associated with distinct temperaments:

- *Ectomorphs* were tall with long limbs, showed *cerebrotonic* characteristics (socially inhibited and lonely).
- Mesomorphs were stocky and muscular with a *somatotonic* temperament (active, assertive and athletic).
- *Endomorphs* were fat, rounded and 'pear shaped' and exhibited a *viscerotonic* temperament (amiable, happy and sociable).

Needless to say the body and personality types are not supported by research and were gross oversimplifications, given the state of knowledge at the time that they were described.

The concept of personality types received a boost through the descriptions of 'extraversion' and 'introversion' by Carl Jung (1875–1961). These words, already in use in English literature, were employed by Jung to denote the person's attitude towards the world. Extraverts are said to show an interest in the outside world and be excited by it; they are supposed to be outgoing, sociable, impulsive and carefree. Introverts, in contrast, are interested in internal ideas and thoughts. They are, therefore, introspective, reserved and responsible. Sometime later Jung proposed two other pairs of psychological types: thinking versus feeling, underpinned by how a person perceives the world; and intuition versus sensation, based on how a person appraises the world. A commonly used personality inventory popular with business and personnel choice, The *Myers–Briggs type indicator* (Myers, 1975), is based on Jung's six personality types.

PHENOMENOLOGICAL APPROACHES

Phenomenology is the study of subjective experience. It is concerned with events and happenings as one experiences them. It does not deny the objective reality of events or the existence of unconscious mental processes, rather it is concerned with the study of *subjective* experiences known only to ourselves, and how they are perceived and experienced. The best-known figures in the field are Abraham Maslow, George Kelly and Carl Rogers. Maslow's contribution is outlined in Chapter 5, on motivation. The theories of Kelly and Rogers are briefly discussed below.

George Kelly's theory of personal constructs

Kelly's theory of personality holds that individuals perceive, interpret and conceptualise the world in widely different ways. Kelly's hypothesis is that each person's behaviour and personality is the direct result of the ways in which he or she perceives and understands the world and other people. There are no objective realities or 'absolute truths', only interpretations that people place on them. According to Kelly, people are 'naïve scientists', attempting to make sense of the world. Like scientists, they make personal observations and form hypotheses. These personal hypotheses help them make sense of the world and their experience. The specific hypotheses people have of their world, which vary from individual to individual, are called *personal constructs*. He called these *personal constructs* emphasising that they are unique to the individual. Based on the personal constructs the individual interprets events, makes predictions and anticipates events.

Kelly's theory, as expounded in his seminal work, *The Psychology of Personal Constructs* (1955), puts forward one fundamental postulate and eleven corollaries. His fundamental postulate is that: 'A person's processes (thoughts, feelings, experiences, and so on) are psychologically channelized by the ways in which he anticipates events'. The corollaries describe properties of constructs and their organisation.

Constructs are stable but not fixed and undergo change as a result of experience. Constructs are dichotomous in nature and are bipolar, for example, happy–sad, friendly–unfriendly, honest–dishonest, and so on. Each person is thought to evolve a construction system, some are hierarchically organised while others are not. Thus, constructs are, in Kelly's words, 'useful concepts, convenient fictions and transparent templates' that guide one's perception and behaviours. Since reality is always experienced from one perspective, which is unique to the person, there are numerous other means of interpretation, different realities or alternative constructions.

According to Kelly, psychopathology results from a faulty or dysfunctional construct system. He defined a psychological disorder as 'any personal construction which is used repeatedly in spite of consistent invalidation'. Thus anxiety arises when the person's construct system does not coincide with reality. Similarly, guilt is said to result when one's actions are not in keeping with one's core constructs. Therapy based on personal construct theory aims to help the client to revise, modify or change their construct system. Psychotherapy therefore involves enabling the client to see things from a different perspective, to loosen their constructs or adopt alternative constructs. The techniques used to bring about these changes involve experimentation, homework, role-play and fixed-role therapy. For example, Kelly would redefine a person's idiot–genius construct as unskilled–skilled and ask the client to act the fixed-role sketch for a period of time.

Kelly devised a technique called the role construct repertory test, later called the *repertory grid technique*, or Rep Grid for short, to explore the nature and contents of an individual's personal construct. It essentially consists of the following steps (Figure 3.1). Try it for yourself.

1. Write a list of names of persons who are important in your life. It could include abstract descriptions such as controlling person or a brief description of the person (e.g. disliked person). Usually the list consists of ten *elements*.
2. Next consider three people (elements) from the list. They are designated by circles in the first row of the grid under their names. Decide how two of them are alike in an important way and different from the third. Place an X in the circles corresponding to the names of two people who are alike leaving the remaining circle blank.
3. Write a word or a brief phrase describing the way in which the two people are *alike* in the similarity or emergent pole column (e.g. loving, caring, supportive).
4. Similarly, write a word or phrase in the contrast or implicit pole column describing the way in which the third person is *different* from the two who are alike (e.g. conditional love, rejecting).
5. Repeat the procedure for the succeeding nine rows considering various triads in turn.

Congratulations! You have just completed the Rep Grid. The labels on the similarity–contrast pole in each row indicates the bipolar constructs that you use in social relationships. The completed grid of twenty constructs gives a map of *your* constructs.

The Rep Grid provides the therapist with an insight into the *subject's* construct system and his or her subjective reality and provides important clues as to how the individual evaluates people and events. A number of computer programmes have been developed that 'measure' the distance between constructs or between 'elements'. The Rep Grid is a unique idiographic tool that gives a picture of how people create their world-views. The method has been

Elements	Self	Mother	Sister	Teacher	Friend	Brother	Partner	Happy person	Disliked person	Competent person	Constructs	
											Similarity pole	Contrast pole
1	⊗	⊗					○				Competent	Incompetent
2		⊗			○		⊗				Easy going	Tense
3	○				⊗		⊗				Anxious	Relaxed
4		⊗	⊗	○							Fun loving	Serious
5		⊗			○				⊗		Thoughtful	Dismissive
6			⊗	○	⊗						Caring, loving	Closed, rejecting
7		○	⊗					⊗			Calm, restful	Impulsive
8	⊗		○				⊗				Self-centred	Generous
9	○		⊗		⊗						Bright	Dull
10	⊗			○			⊗				Affectionate	Cold

Fig. 3.1 The repertory grid

put to good use in unlikely fields such as market research (comparing and contrasting various products) and in management (in analysis of leadership styles). An imaginative use of the test has been in the analysis of thought disorder in patients with schizophrenia. Departing from the principle of allowing the subject to choose the elements and constructs, Bannister and Fransella (1967) employed standardised elements and constructs to understand the thinking processes of thought-disordered patients. The elements and constructs were chosen by the authors and applied to a normal population and the patients' performance on the constructs were compared with those 'norms'. This is an outstanding example of a nomothetic test based on an idiographic theory.

Kelly was well ahead of his time. His ideas of personal constructs and constructionism have been reinvented by cognitive psychology as schemas and scripts. An influential body of knowledge known as social constructionism (which holds that all knowledge is derived from mental constructions of members of a social system) owes its origins to the pioneering work of George Kelly.

Carl Rogers' person-centred approach

Carl Rogers developed his theory from his experience with psychotherapy clients. His approach was radically different from those who went before him and attempting to summarise it in a few pages is to do injustice to his contribution to the field of psychology and psychotherapy. His groundbreaking work, *Client-centred Therapy* (Rogers, 1951), is necessary reading for anyone interested in psychotherapy. He was primarily interested in the private world of the individual that he termed the *phenomenal field*, to denote everything the person experiences at a given time. The phenomenal field is known only to the individual and defies measurement. Unlike psychoanalysis, Rogersian theory and therapy is primarily concerned with the present and seeks to understand how the person perceives the world in the present. A defining characteristic of his approach is the overwhelming belief in personal growth. According to Rogers, man has one basic tendency – to actualise. *Self-actualisation* refers to the drive people have to attain self-development, maturation and growth. Self develops from one's perceptual and phenomenological field. An important contribution to development of self is how the subject is evaluated by others, particularly by parents and later by peers. *Positive self-regard* develops from positive evaluations of self by others. A child experiencing love from his parents perceives himself as lovable and worthy of love. The child comes to understand that positive regard from others often comes with conditions attached to it, thus he learns about *conditions of worth*. The 'self' formed on the basis of these perceptions is organised into a self-concept.

Sometime experiences may get distorted in the way that they are experienced. Parents' or other peoples' experience may be perceived as if based on one's own: 'I perceive my parents experiencing this behaviour as bad' is distorted and symbolised as 'I perceive this behaviour as bad'. Any experience that is inconsistent with the structure of self may be perceived as a threat. The role of therapy is to examine these inconsistencies so that the structure is revised to assimilate and include new experiences. This leads to the greater acceptance of self.

Therapy based on Rogers' theory is known as *client-centered therapy*. It is a non-directive form of therapy, in that the therapist makes no interpretations or suggestions and provides no advice or reassurance. The main aim of the therapist is to help the client discover the distorted self-concepts that inhibit self-development. Rogers places great emphasis on the therapist–client relationship. This relationship is based on three cardinal principles:

1. *Genuineness*. The therapist must be genuine. This means that they must have ongoing access to their own internal processes – their own feelings, moods and attitudes.
2. *Accurate empathy*. The therapist must continually try to understand the client's experience *from the client's point of view*. It is the capacity to think and feel oneself into the inner life of another person that is important. It is our life-long ability to experience what another person experiences, albeit to an attenuated degree.
3. *Unconditional positive regard*. Rogers compared this attribute to that of a parent's love towards its child. By a myriad of actions the parent gives the message that, even though from time to time the child is likely to evoke feelings of anger, disapproval or disgust, the child is basically loved and loveable. This does not mean that the therapist has to be paternalistic or sentimental but that the therapist gives the client a great deal of room to be a separate and independent person.

These are considered to be necessary preconditions for growth and self-actualisation in the therapeutic process. The client-centred approach is popular in counselling, psychotherapy and in group therapy (sometimes known as encounter groups).

The Q-sort. Carl Rogers and his co-workers used an idiographic measurement technique called the *Q-sort method* to study the self-concept. The distinguishing feature of the Q-sort is that it measures personality characteristics within an individual ideographically and not the differences between people as nomothetic methods do.

The Q-sort is a set of statements that describes different aspects of personality (Block, 1978). The test consists of a series of statements about self printed on separate index cards. The subject arranges (sorts) the card into a series of piles on the basis of the degree to which the statements describe him or her (e.g. 'I am generally confident', 'I think of myself first'). The subject is asked to sort the cards into seven or nine categories along a continuum from 'not at all like me'. (with a value of zero) to 'very characteristic of me' (with a value of 9). Intermediate categories contain statements that apply to various degrees. An important feature of the Q-sort is that it requires the tester to assign a specified number of statements to each category. For example, the subject is asked to place exactly four items in category 9 (the most descriptive items), and twelve items in category 8 (the next most descriptive) and four items in category 1 (the least descriptive). In psychometric terms, the cards are arranged into a fixed distribution, similar to the normal curve. The psychometric advantage of the forced distribution is that the subject's decision to place the card in one pile rather than another depends not on comparison with *other people* but on how they judge the characteristic to apply to self, relative to *other items*. It is this feature, the focus on the individual, that makes the Q-sort truly idiographic. The commonest research use of Q-sort has been to assess the person's self-concept in the Rogerian sense.

The usefulness of the Q-sort technique depends on the selection of the set of characteristics for study and research. A standardised set of 100 items describing human personality was developed by Block (1978). Known as the California Q-set, it employs idealised depictions (prototypes) of clinical descriptions such as 'optimally adjusted individual' and 'paranoid person'. An imaginative use of this method of study is the *Shedler–Western assessment procedure-200* (SWAP-200) for the assessment and classification of personality disorders (Western & Shedler, 1999)

TRAIT-BASED APPROACHES TO THE STUDY OF PERSONALITY

All languages use various words to describe people. Descriptions of people as quiet, lazy, friendly, aggressive, and so on, are universal. Allport and Odbert (1936) compiled a list of almost 18 000 English words that described personal qualities. From this huge list it was possible to group words that have similar meaning and arrive at a smaller number of broad dimensions that describe personality. For example, descriptions such as hard working, industrious, meticulous and painstaking may be brought under the umbrella term 'conscientious'. By systematically working through all or most of the adjectives one could arrive at a small number of personality dimensions that are both necessary and sufficient to describe the main essentials of any individual's personality. The assumption here, known as the lexical hypothesis, is that important differences in personality among individuals are encoded as single terms in most languages. A refined method is to devise questionnaires based on the lexical or other personality theory and ask individuals to rate themselves (self-reports) and then submit the scores to factor analysis. Factor analysis is the technique most commonly used to identify multiple traits from scores derived from questionnaires, and it is described in more detail in Chapter 8.

Using these methods, personality psychologists have been able to develop a general scientific theory of traits. The trait approach has become the most dominant method of studying personality, and in the rest of this chapter we will focus predominantly on trait approaches to personality. There is now a growing consensus as to the nature and characteristics of personality traits as well as the number of traits required to describe and understand human personality. But first, what are traits?

A commonly accepted definition of personality traits is that they are relatively stable personal predispositions that give rise to consistent patterns of functioning and behaving in a range of situations. Several aspects of this definition are of particular importance.

First, traits are *dispositions*. They refer to characteristics that are latent and may not always be manifest. To say that a person is aggressive (a trait) is not to say that he/she will invariably be aggressive in all circumstances. For example, aggression may be evident in the form of domestic violence in a man who is meek and mild at work. It should be noted that trait descriptions do not specify the circumstances that result in the manifestation of the trait. Thus, the expression of the trait is contingent upon some set of eliciting conditions. All major traits interact with the situational variables to produce particular behaviours. Thus a trait represents a predisposition to respond and both the person and the situation make relative contributions towards behaviour.

Second, traits are *descriptions* of predispositions to act in particular ways. Often traits have been erroneously used to *explain* behaviour. For example, an aggressive person may be said to be violent *because* he is aggressive. The circularity of the statements is obvious. Although not very apparent, the term may be used to imply causality in everyday usage and clinical situations. Traits are descriptive terms and are not explanatory. Traits provide one of the ways of *describing* human personality characteristics. For instance, trait anxiety is associated with state anxiety only under certain conditions. They are not causal agents themselves, their effect on behaviour is not straightforward and depends on a number of variables, especially situational factors.

Third, the reference to 'patterns of behaving' in the definition is not incidental. Descriptions of traits involve some generalisation or reference to aggregates of behaviours in different situations. This association of trait with general rather than specific behaviours is evident in everyday concepts of the term, where trait descriptions are usually qualified by words such as 'usually', 'generally speaking' or 'largely', indicating that the descriptions involve a collection of behaviours. Thus traits are, at best, descriptive constructs that encapsulate the aggregate behaviour patterns of individuals. The clinical significance of this is that traits are poor predictors of single *acts* of behaviour. Prediction of risk based on traits alone is risky business! What is more, the predictive value of traits is notoriously poor in other areas of functioning too. For example, even the best trait-based personality tests do not predict job performance (Blinkhorn & Johnson, 1990).

The above discussion of what a trait is, and what it is not, is meant to point out the limitations of the concept of traits before discussing the various trait theories. This is particularly important because current trait theorists assert that a consensus is emerging around the basic structure of personality (see later). Moreover, personality disorders, as defined in the DSM-IV and ICD-10, are claimed to be based on traits! Nevertheless, as one authority on personality has pointed out, 'there are fundamental problems with the trait concept, and that the trait model is not the only personality model to recognise consistency and coherence in functioning' (Pervin, 1994). Next, we consider the various trait theories of personality.

Cattell's sixteen primary personality factors (16 PF)

Raymond Cattell (1950) studied data from self-reports, reports of significant others, and observations of behaviour and subjected these to factor analysis. He identified sixteen robust primary personality factors or dimensions (Table 3.3).

Table 3.3 The sixteen personality factors assessed by 16 PF

Factor	*Trait description*	
	High	*Low*
A	Outgoing	Reserved
B	Higher intelligence	Low intelligence
C	Stable	Emotional
E	Assertive	Humble
F	Happy-go-lucky	Sober
G	Conscientious	Expedient
H	Venturesome	Shy
I	Tender-minded	Tough-minded
L	Suspicious	Trusting
M	Imaginative	Practical
N	Shrewd	Forthright
O	Apprehensive	Placid
Q1	Experimenting	Conservative
Q2	Self-sufficient	Group-tied
Q3	Controlled	Casual
Q4	Tense	Relaxed

For Cattell these sixteen factors, which he called these source traits, form the basic elements of an individual's personality. He believed that everyone possesses the same 16 traits but to a greater or lesser extent. But Cattell's theory is more extensive than the 16 traits. He describes other groups of traits that have different properties. Although a trait theorist, he acknowledged the complex interaction between traits, situations and abilities. The *sixteen personality questionnaire* (16 PF) that he and his colleagues developed is a self-report personality questionnaire that has been widely used in research and to some extent in practical settings. Despite the fact that Cattell has consistently argued for the need to describe personality in terms of his 16 primary factors, later workers have extracted five second-order factors from the 16-PF scales: extraversion; neuroticism; tough poise; independence; and control (Krug & Jones, 1986).

Eysenck's three-factor (P-E-N) theory

Eysenck put forward an elaborate theory of personality, backed up with a large amount of research. Although his theory, known as the three-factor or the P-E-N theory, has lost some ground recently to the new arrival, the five-factor model, it is worthy of consideration in some detail because it led to a substantial amount of research. In Eysenck's theory, personality traits are hierarchically organised with specific but narrow traits at lower levels in the hierarchy and global but broad superordinate factors or domains at the top (Eysenck & Eysenck, 1985).

Eysenck's three high-order factors are: extraversion–introversion; neuroticism–stability; and psychoticism–impulse control. These three second factors, confusingly called types, are derived from Eysenck's personality questionnaire, a self-reported questionnaire consisting of several yes/no items (e.g. 'Do you like going out a lot?' or 'Do you long for excitement?). The questionnaire has been subjected to a number of revisions resulting in the current version, which is called the Eysenck personality questionnaire–revised (EPQ-R) (Eysenck & Eysenck, 1991). First-order factors are derived from specific responses to the items in the questionnaire. The first-order factors have been found to be correlated and three second-order factors, which Eysenck called types, have been extracted: extraversion (E); neuroticism (N); and psychoticism (P). Thus the type is the superordinate conception that occupies the apex of the hierarchy and the first-order factors occupy the lower level.

The types or second-order factors described by Eysenck (Figure 3.2) are:

- *Extraversion–Introversion*. The typical extravert is sociable, outgoing, enjoys social activities, takes risks and loves excitement and change. Introverts tend to be quiet, serious, reserved and enjoy solitary pursuits like reading.
- *Neuroticism–Stability*. Those with high neuroticism scores are usually anxious and prone to worry and psychosomatic symptoms. They are emotional and their judgement is affected by emotions. At the other end of the pole, those with low N scores are calm, more relaxed and emotionally stable. They recover quickly from emotional upheavals. More recently this dimension has been called emotionality.
- *Psychoticism–Impulse control*. People high on P show attributes such as callousness, aggression, coldness, hostility and lack of empathy. This dimension has also been called tough-mindedness – superego control.

Eysenck emphasised that the three dimensions are: (1) normal personality factors found in all populations that are 'normally' distributed in the population, except for P where there is a marked skew towards low scores; (2) high scores on the types may predispose individuals to psychiatric disorders; and (3) the E and N scores are independent of each other and can be represented orthogonally. Depending on the scores an individual can be 'placed' relative to both dimensions. Those with extreme scores fall in the periphery while the normal population scores aggregate around the centre. Eysenck claimed that the three dimensions of E, I and P 'have predictive and explanatory power across a heterogeneous collection of real-life situations'. He claimed that it was possible to locate psychiatric diagnostic categories within the dimensional framework. Those with anxiety disorders such as obsessive-compulsive disorder, general anxiety disorder, phobias and depression have high I and N scores, while those with psychopathic disorder and hysterical disorder show high E and N scores (Figure 3.3).

Eysenck's theory and research goes further than describing the structure of normal personality. It has given rise to a large body of psycho-physiological and experimental studies as well as genetic research. In particular, his work asserts that the P-E-N dimensions are (1) biologically based; and (2) largely heritable (Eysenck & Eysenck, 1985).

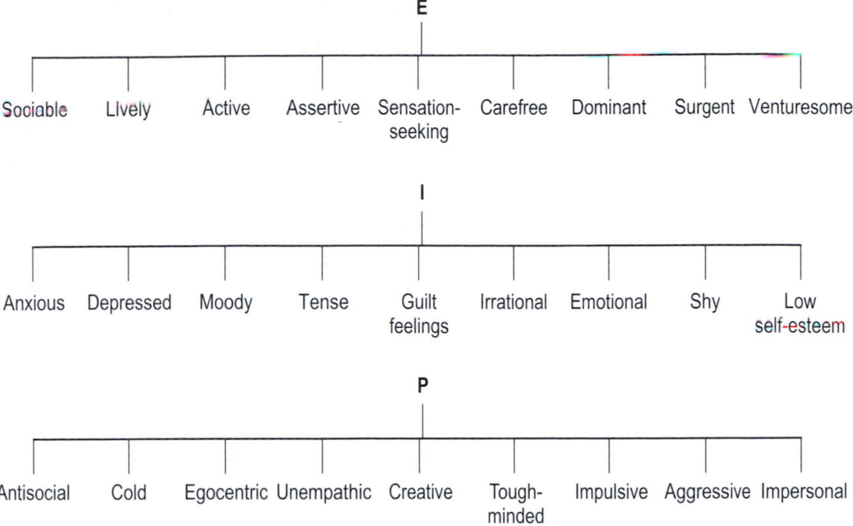

Fig. 3.2 The hierarchical structure of extraversion (E), introversion (I) and psychoticism (P)

Biological basis of Eysenck's three types

Eysenck invoked the concept of arousal to explain the neurological basis of E and N dimensions. Arousal refers to a continuum of states of activity of the organism ranging from sleep through wakefulness to high excitement or emotion. Many factors increase arousal, including hunger, intense stimuli and stimulant drugs such as caffeine and amphetamines, whereas sleep deprivation, sensory deprivation and depressant drugs, including alcohol, are thought to lower the arousal levels. According to Eysenck, the biological substrate of cortical arousal is located in two neural systems:

1. The cortico-reticular loop. Incoming ascending afferent pathways project onto the cortex but also send collaterals to the ascending reticular acti-

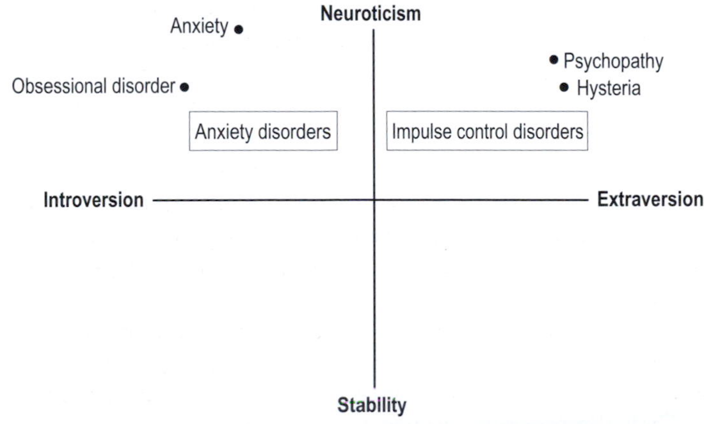

Fig. 3.3 Eysenck's extraversion, neuroticism and associated conditions

Table 3.4 Features of extroverts and introverts (Eysenck & Eysenck, 1985)

Extravert	*Introvert*
ARAS under-aroused, inhibited	ARAS over-aroused, excited
Excitement-seeking, easily bored, risk-taking, 'stimulus hungry'	Self-contained, retiring, prefer calming activities, show 'stimulus aversion'
Poor at vigilance tasks	Better at tasks requiring concentration
Susceptible to sensory deprivation	Less susceptible to sensory deprivation
Easily sedated (e.g. with Amytal)	Sedation difficult
CNS stimulants improve performance	Sensitive to stimulants
Higher pain threshold	Less tolerant to pain
Poor classical conditioning; S–R link not easily achieved	Condition better; more responsive to rewards and punishments

vation system (ARAS). Arousal is thought to be associated with the activity of the cortico-reticular loop. Eysenck asserted that extraverts have habitually *low* cortical arousal while introverts tend to be over-aroused. People are said to behave in ways that keep them at their own optimal level of arousal. Thus extraverts (who have a 'sluggish' ARAS) seek strong external stimulation to raise their arousal levels whereas introverts (who have a overactive ARAS) avoid such stimulation and seek calming activities. Psycho-physiological findings related to the extraversion–introversion dimension are summarised in Table 3.4 (Eysenck & Eysenck, 1985).

2. ***The visceral-cortical loop.*** This comprises the feedback loops between the limbic system and the cortex. Arousal in this system is associated with autonomic and emotional responses. The neuroticism–stability dimension is thought to reflect the activity level of this system. The system is thought to be highly aroused in those with high N scores making them more liable to anxiety and susceptibility to fear and distress.

These postulations have been put to test in numerous studies resulting in a large volume of research. Unfortunately, the results have been inconsistent and not always in keeping with the theory. The very concept of arousal has been questioned. Arousal is not a unitary construct and conventional measures of arousal – heart rate, EEG and skin conductance – show very little correlation with one another. The highest correlation between any two of the measures was a mere 0.16. There is little evidence to support the association of neuroticism and autonomic nervous system arousal.

P is the least studied of the three dimensions and there is little empirical support for the dimension of psychoticism. Eysenck half-heartedly attempted to link it to variations in levels of androgens. In spite of extensive research into Eysenck's theory, the evidence for correlates of personality types so neatly postulated by Eysenck remains patchy and unconvincing.

Heritability of Eysenck's three factors

Traditional behaviour genetic studies have consistently found substantial heritability estimates for Eysenck's E and N factors. Eysenck (1990) pooled data from six, large, twin studies conducted in different countries and concluded that the additive genetic effects for the three factors is around 50%. Heritability of P has been doubted on account of the questionable validity of the P scale of the EPQ. Independent analysis of similar data has confirmed the findings for the E and N factors. In short, all studies agree that over half the variance in extraversion arises from genetic factors.

The five-factor model (FFM, 'the big five')

During the last two decades rapid progress has been made towards a consensus on the structure of personality. Gradually, agreement has been growing about the number of high-order factors needed to account for the major personality features. Most workers in the field of personality now seem to agree that the *five-factor model* (FFM) provides a good enough framework for the comprehensive description, study and assessment of personality. The emergence of the five robust factors, called 'the big five', has been hailed as a major advancement in personality psychology, although it is not without detractors. Of the many five-factor models that have been put forward, the five-factor theory of Costa and McCrae has achieved prominence. Their FFM, discussed below, has been backed up by a massive amount of empirical research and a deluge of publications. Moreover, most other trait schemes seem congruent, but not equivalent with, the FFM. Costa and McCrae's FFM has the name of the 'grand theory of personality traits'.

The FFM contends that the five global-level orthogonal factors, corresponding to the second-order factors, are both necessary and reasonably sufficient for describing personality. The five factors, called domains, are: neuroticism (N); extraversion (E); openness to experience (O); agreeableness (A); and conscientiousness(C) – remembered easily by the mnemonic OCEAN. The NEOA and C dimensions correspond to the second-order factors of Eysenck and Cattell's primary traits.

1. ***Neuroticism (N).*** This dimension represents individual differences in the tendency to express distress. In broad terms, it is the tendency to see the world as threatening. Those with high N scores experience chronic negative affects such as guilt, self-consciousness and depression.

2. ***Extraversion (E).*** This is the general tendency to confront and engage the world. Those high on E tend to be venturesome and assertive while those low on E are reserved, quiet and retiring (introverts).

3. ***Agreeableness (A).*** This involves the more human aspect of the person with characteristics such as kindness, emotional support to others, nurturance and altruism at one pole and hostility, indifference and self-centredness at the other pole. Those high on A are likeable and friendly.

4. ***Conscientiousness (C).*** This refers to the will to achieve, diligence, thoroughness as well as being ethical and governed by conscience.

5. ***Openness to experience (O).*** This includes such characteristics as intellect, imaginativeness, the need for variety, experience and ideas. It is not equivalent to measured intelligence. Individuals low on O are said to favour conservative values and judge others in conventional terms while those who score high on O are rated as having wide interests, enjoy aesthetic pursuits

Table 3.5 Five-factor model of personality: domains and facets (Costa & McCrae, 1992)

Domain	*Facet*
Neuroticism	Anxiousness, Angry hostility, Trait depression, Self-consciousness, Impulsiveness, Vulnerability
Extraversion (vs. introversion)	Warmth, Gregariousness, Assertiveness, Excitement seeking, Positive emotions
Openness (vs. closedness)	Fantasy, Aesthetic feelings, Actions Ideas, Values
Agreeableness (vs. antagonism)	Trust, Compliance, Altruism, Modesty, Tender-mindedness
Conscientiousness	Competence, Order, Dutifulness, Achievement-striving, Self-discipline, Deliberation

and are unconventional in their thinking. This has been considered as the most controversial domain.

The FFM is a hierarchical theory, like that of Eysenck, with each second-order factor being made up of six lower-order traits or facets (Table 3.5). The five factors are measured by the neuroticism, extraversion, openness, personality inventory-revised (NEO-PI-R, see Chapter 8).

In spite of the extensive work that has been carried out on the five domains and their facets there is still some overlap in their definitions. For example, angry hostility included under neuroticism is closely related to the negative description of agreeableness. Similarly, the impulsiveness facet of neuroticism is at odds with the generally accepted Eysenckian concept of extraversion (Eysenck includes impulsivity under the psychoticism domain). A clearer specification of facets seems necessary. There is some doubt as to the definition of the fifth factor, openness to experience. Some consider it primarily as a factor of intellect, while others see it essentially as a need for variety in action, intellectual curiosity and liberal values.

Despite its shortcomings, the FFM has received extensive support from several lines of research. The model's claim to cover the entire universe of personality traits rests on four achievements:

1. There is broad agreement about an individual's levels on the five factors between self-reports and reports by peers or spouses, with correlations between all five dimensions in the region of 0.45.
2. The robustness of the five factors has been firmly established in factor analysis of self-ratings in numerous cross-sectional and longitudinal studies. Cross-cultural studies using translations of NEO-PI-R have shown the five factors to be present in all human groups that have been studied. For example, Costa and McCrae compared American five-factor structure with those found in six non-English speaking cultures – German, Portuguese, Hebrew, Chinese, Korean and Japanese samples – totalling 7134 individuals. All five factors were reproduced, even at the level of secondary

Table 3.6 Heritability of the big five factors (pooled data from various sources) – heritability of intelligence and height are given for comparison

Trait/characteristic	*Correlation coefficient for MZ*	*Correlation coefficient for DZ*	*Heritability (h^2)*
Extroversion (E)	0.50	0.20	0.60
Neuroticism (N)	0.41	0.24	0.34
Openness (O)	0.51	0.14	0.37
Conscientiousness (C)	0.41	0.23	0.18
Agreeableness (A)	0.47	0.11	0.72
Intelligence	0.85	0.60	0.50
Height	0.90	0.50	0.80

loadings. They concluded that the five-factor personality structure is universal (McCrae & Costa, 1997).

3. The big five factors have been discovered in constructs offered by other personality theories. Different systems of trait descriptions can be mapped on to the big five with considerable ease. The five factors appear to be inherent in a wide variety of standard systems of personality description, including Cattell's sixteen factors, Eysenck's three factors and Jung's personality types (as measured by Myers–Briggs type indicator). Although Eysenck has claimed that the FFM does not represent an improvement on his three factors, Costa and McCrae have produced evidence of convergent and discriminant validity of Eysenck's scales and their NEO-PI-R. According to their studies, the E and N domains on the two models are essentially the same and the negative pole of Eysenck's P factor corresponds to a combination of C and A of the FFM (Costa & McCrae, 1995).
4. The five factors show moderate to high degrees of heritability (Table 3.6).

The FFM offers an extremely general framework for the classification of traits. Because the five factors occupy a large space in the universe of personality, domains such as extroversion and neuroticism are not of much use in the prediction of specific behaviours in particular situations. Narrower trait (facet) measures occupying a lower level in the hierarchy, such as friendliness, may be more homogeneous and be better predictors of behaviour. An adequate description of personality functioning, for example the description of premorbid personality, requires more specific information than that can be derived from the five general factors. It has been argued that, because of its inherent limitations, the FFM should be viewed as *one* important model in personality studies and not as *the* model of personality (McAdams, 1992).

SITUATIONALISM AND INTERACTIONISM

The basic assumption of trait theories that traits are enduring predispositions that predict a substantial proportion of variance in behaviour came under heavy fire from Walter Mischel, an influential figure in personality psychology. His research findings and arguments, forcefully expressed in the landmark book *Personality and Assessment* (Mischel, 1968) had a devastating effect on trait theories of personality. Often called situationalism, this view challenged trait theories for ignoring the well-known fact that individuals' behaviour varies from situation to situation.

Mischel based his arguments on the *inconsistency* of peoples' behaviour: a person may be sociable in one setting and retiring in another, conscientious in one situation but not in another. This aspect of human behaviour had been demonstrated in several studies long before Mischel took issue with trait theories. For example, a well-known study carried out in the 1920s investigating the trait of honesty in children, clearly showed that, when given the opportunity to cheat, children did indeed indulge in cheating and deception. In this experiment, children were given intelligence tests, the sheets were collected and copied by the experimenter and handed back to the children to mark their own answers. The children gave themselves higher marks. The intercorrelation between the experimenter's scores and the children's' scores was as low as 0.2 (Hartshorne & May, 1928). This and the findings of many other studies are at odds with the central assumption of trait theories – that traits are dispositions stable across time and situations. Mischel showed that, in a study of aggression and withdrawal in children, the children showed more trait-relevant behaviours only when the demands of the situation were high. Similarly, extraverts have been shown to perform better on tasks of verbal ability in stimulating environments, while introverts do better under non-stimulating conditions.

The 'person versus situation' debate that raged fiercely in the 1970s highlighted a number of deficiencies in the trait theories. First, as Mischel demonstrated, the correlation between traits and corresponding behaviour seldom exceeds 0.3, indicating that it accounts for only 9% of behaviour variance. This finding has been replicated in numerous studies and is difficult to dispute. Indeed 'the 0.3 barrier' has proved to be a difficult hurdle for trait theorists to cross. Second, traits, on their own, are of little use in predicting behaviour. Large-scale studies on Eysenck's extroversion factor show very little correlation with, for example, those behaviours predicted by theory. Third, workers attempting to partition the test-score variance to person, situation and person–situation interaction, using analysis of variance, have attributed, on average, only 12% of variance to personality factors (Bowers, 1973).

Interactionism takes the view that human behaviour is the result of the person (P), the situation (S) and their interaction (P × S). This view emphasises the dynamic, continuous and reciprocal process of the interaction between the individual and the environment. According to this approach, human behaviour is the result of multilevel and multidimensional interaction between P and S. Neither personality factors nor situational factors alone determine behaviour, nor is it a combination of each of these that produces behaviour but the interaction between these two factors. Endler and Magnusson (1976) have summarised the basic elements of the interactionist approach as follows:

1. Person–situation/environment is a reciprocal process. Individuals both influence and are influenced by the environment. The environment is not a passive factor either.
2. Individuals are intentional, *active* agents in the interactional process. They

act upon the environment by choosing, changing, modifying and reshaping it.

3. On the person side of the interaction, cognitive variables, especially the meaning one assigns to the situation, are important determinants of behaviour.
4. On the situation side, the environment provides not only stimulation but also information to which individuals respond depending upon the psychological meaning they attach to the situation.

Since Mischel's assault on trait theory, both the protagonists and antagonists have moved from their polarised positions to middle ground. Mischel himself has recently changed his position from his original situationalist standpoint to one that accommodates the role of the person's cognitive attributes, Costa and McCrae (1994), the main authors of the FFM, have introduced a model of personality development that includes what they term 'basic tendencies' and 'characteristic adaptations'. 'Basic tendencies' refer to dispositions or traits that interact with the environment to produce 'characteristic adaptations'. The latter conjunction involves elements that are relatively fixed (i.e. characteristic) and others that are fluid (i.e. influenced by the environment). Therefore 'characteristic adaptations' are the material that mental health professionals deal with, and they deserve our attention.

The main message for the clinicians is that they need to be aware of the use of personality measures and descriptions at different levels of abstraction depending on the level of precision required for the given task. Broad traits such as the big five serve to predict broad classes of behaviour, but are not as good as lower-level traits at predicting *specific* behaviours. For example, a measure of big five factor conscientiousness will predict whether or not a person will arrive at a meeting on time with less precision than a measure of the highly specific trait of punctuality. Matching the level of abstraction of the personality measure to the behaviour predicted is especially important in clinical work when predicting the risk of offending.

Does personality change? The reader may recall that personality and personality traits were described as stable and enduring, implying that they showed little change during adult life. Although Costa and McCrae (1994) assert that personality is stable ('set like a plaster') and does not change after 30 years, others have produced evidence to show that personality is malleable in adulthood (Helson & Wink, 1992). Here again, the discrepancy is largely due to the level of personality organisation that has been studied. According to the authors of the big five, the median correlation for measures of the big five assessed across time points three to thirty years apart is 0.65. Ten-year stability coefficient for E ranges from 0.7 to 0.84, while for N it was shown to be 0.58 to 0.69. Those who have studied different personality units such as life tasks and psychobiographies report that personality is much more open to change than the trait theorists lead us to believe.

One of the strong arguments in favour of the trait concept of personality is that traits show a considerable degree of heritability. Pooled data from twin studies involving thousands of twins do indeed show that most personality traits, including the big five, exhibit a moderate degree of genetic influence

Box 3.1 Features of personality traits

- Traits are descriptions of dispositions to feel, act and behave in particular ways.
- Conceptually, traits refer to broad second-order factors.
- Eysenck held that personality could adequately be captured by three factors (E, N and P); current theories hold that the big-five factors are more suitable for describing and studying personality.
- Traits are relatively stable across adult life.
- Genetic studies have shown that Eysenck's three factors and the big-five factors are moderately hereditable.
- Traits, by themselves, are of little use in predicting behaviour. Situational factors are important determinants of much human behaviour.
- Identification of abnormal personality traits may be more useful in studying personality disorders (see later).

(Table 3.6). In the last 30 years, behaviour genetic studies on MZ and DZ twins reared together and apart have arrived at some robust conclusions: (1) personality traits are to a considerable extent heritable; (2) personality traits cannot be attributed to shared environmental influences; (3) non-shared environmental influences, like illnesses and having different peer groups, play a major part in determining personality; and (4) the above three findings apply to all five big-five factors.

In conclusion, personality involves more than a collection of traits and predispositions. It is the sum total of the patterning that each person develops as a way of dealing with the traits that he or she is endowed with, the social context that he or she encounters and the experiences that he or she has received (Rutter, 1987). The main features of traits are summarised in Box 3.1.

CLINICAL APPLICATIONS

Personality has significant implications for clinical work. For example, a marked change in personality is important especially if it has occurred within a short period of time. Onset of psychiatric illnesses, organic brain changes (including head injury and dementia) and drug misuse are important causes of recent personality change. Premorbid personality and the level of functioning before the onset of psychiatric disorder have an important bearing on the prognosis and course of the disorder. In the following section we address three areas of clinical importance.

Eliciting premorbid personality

Assessment of premorbid personality requires, in addition to self-description, collateral information from people who know the person well (e.g. spouse, friend, co-worker). Historical information such as educational attainments, employment history and personal history (e.g. close relationships) is useful in gaining an understanding of the subject's personality and level of social functioning. As noted by Eysenck, certain psychiatric disorders are associated with certain personality types. In eliciting premorbid personality from the subject, open-ended questions followed by probes are often useful. Following the probes, it may be necessary to give a short list of common adjectives to describe personality, especially in those patients who are not very forthcoming. For example, in a patient showing antisocial behaviour one needs to ask about his temper in general followed by questions about difficulties in impulse control as well as other difficulties or problems that his angry outbursts have led to (police involvement, loss of friends, or tensions in marriage). A scheme based on the FFM is outlined in Box 3.2.

Case example

In a postgraduate examination a candidate had seen a patient who showed the typical features of paranoid schizophrenia but was found to be very anxious during the interview, something the candidate had observed and made a point of reporting. Subsequently, when he was asked to think of reasons as to how the anxiety features in this patient could be explained, the candidate seemed baffled (because extreme anxiety is unusual in chronic schizophrenia). He attempted to explain it on the basis of possible akathesia or a reaction to his hallucinations and delusions. But the real reason was that the patient had always been an anxious individual from a young age especially when meeting people new to him. The candidate had forgotten to ask about the premorbid personality, probably because of the candidate's own anxiety!

Personality factors in the prediction of risk

How useful are personality traits in predicting future risk to self and others? Unfortunately, personality factors and personality assessment measures are of little use in the prediction of risk in patients with suicidal or violent behaviour. But the P × S model of interactionism provides a useful framework for assessing risk, particularly in the analysis and prediction of violence. Although all methods of risk assessment are fraught with problems, a frame-

Box 3.2 A scheme for eliciting premorbid personality

- How would you describe yourself as a person?
- How would others (friend, spouse) describe you?
- How would you describe your general mood, pretty even, up and down or mostly low? Do you get worried easily? When under a lot of stress do you go to pieces? Do you get anxious and tense more easily than others? Would you describe yourself as a nervous person? (N)
- How would you describe your temper? Do you often get into arguments with others? Do you think you have difficulties controlling your temper? Have you regretted having lost your temper? Have you got into trouble because of your temper? (A)
- Would you describe yourself as outgoing, active, and wanting to be where the action is? Or are you reserved and prefer to do things alone? Do you like to have a lot of people around you? (E)
- Do you tend to be well organised and meticulous? Do you strive for excellence in most things you do? (C)
- What sorts of things interest you (pastimes, hobbies)? Do you like trying new things or do you tend to stick to things you are used to? (O)

work that takes into account personal, situational, historical and illness-related factors has been found useful (Monahan, 1981). Interpersonal violence cannot be predicted with any degree of certainty by personality tests, checklists or diagnostic labels. A systematic application of all available knowledge should include the following (mnemonic – DISH):

- *Dispositional factors.* This includes personality traits and level of intelligence.
- *Illness related factors.* Delusions, especially of a persecutory nature, command hallucinations.
- *Situational or contextual factors.* Current-life situation, stresses, current emotional state, substance misuse.
- *Historical factors.* Past history, especially previous violence.

Personality and psychiatric disorders

It is generally acknowledged that the personality of the individual plays a crucial role in the origin, course and prognosis of the psychiatric disorder. There are four ways in which personality may be associated with psychiatric disorder (Akiskal, Hirchfield & Yerevanian, 1983):

1. The personality of the subject may predispose the individual to the disorder (*the vulnerability or pathogenic model*) and set in motion processes that may cause development of psychopathology. Neuroticism is the trait that has been shown most strongly and consistently to be linked to depression, anxiety and stress-related symptoms. High N also predicts minor symptoms and high scores on Goldberg's *general health questionnaire*. A number of studies have clearly demonstrated an association between psychosomatic disorders such as non-ulcer dyspepsia, chronic fatigue syndrome, irritable bowel syndrome and chronic pain syndromes and high N – often they also have low E (high I). The stress–vulnerability model of disorders holds that when under sufficient stress a subject with a predisposition or diathesis to the illness displays symptoms of the illness. High E, however, has been shown to be a protective factor against depression and anxiety.
2. The personality of the subject may influence the form and course of a disorder (*the pathoplastic model*), even though personality trait is not a cause or component of the disorder. The prognosis of many psychiatric conditions is indeed influenced by the person's personality. For instance, a patient with schizophrenia whose previous personality has been sound carries a better prognosis than one who has always been withdrawn and odd.
3. The personality of the individual may be due to the effect of repeated episodes of the illness (*the complication or scarring model*). Psychopathology may influence the course of personality development. Schizophrenia or head injury can lead to personality deterioration and poor social functioning. One reason for the poor prognosis of adolescent-onset schizophrenia is that it often has a devastating effect on personality development resulting in lasting damage to the person's personality structure.
4. The personality may lie on a continuum with the disorder (*the spectrum or*

dimensional model). Thus, psychopathology may represent the extreme end of a continuously distributed trait. Many workers, mostly psychologists, believe that some, if not all, mental disorders are exaggerations of personality traits. Another way of stating their case is to say that they see the vulnerable personality as attenuated mental disorders. There is a powerful argument for conceptualising some forms of anxiety, depression and phobia as extreme variations of normal personality traits. The argument for dimensional classification of mental disorders is most striking in the case of personality disorders (see below).

How useful are formal personality measurements in clinical practice? The answer is that their value is quite limited. Measures of normal personality described above (e.g. NEO-PI, EPQ) have made little impact on day-to-day clinical work. There are many reasons for this. Most tests are too long and take considerable time to complete, and they are open to deliberately misleading answers. The self-reports are highly dependant on the subjective awareness of the patient. For instance, the question, 'Do you consider yourself friendly?' requires a certain amount of insight as to how others view him or her, and this may be deficient in some patients. Many clinicians would agree that personality tests do not provide any more information than clinical examination and observation. Their predictive value is notoriously low. However, personality tests have established an important place for themselves in research and, because of their high interrater reliability and the high validity of their constructs, have contributed enormously to our knowledge base in personality. A more fruitful approach has been the identification and measurement of abnormal personality traits

Abnormal personality traits

Various groups of workers have systematically attempted to identify abnormal personality traits in patients diagnosed as having personality disorders. Livesley, a prolific researcher in the field, has successfully identified some of the dimensions underlying each of the individual personality disorders. He and his colleagues have developed the *dimensional assessment of personality pathology–basic questionnaire* (DAPP–BQ; Livesley, Jackson & Schroeder, 1992) to assess abnormal personality traits. It is a 290-item self-report measure consisting of 18 separate scales measuring lower-order traits. There is considerable convergence between the Livesley factors and other measures of abnormal personality traits. In recent work, there appears to be an emerging consensus around the core abnormal personality traits. Livesley and co-workers have also been able to extract four higher-order factors from the 18 factors. They have labelled these factors as emotional dysregulation, dissocial behaviour, inhibitiveness and compulsivity.

Other researchers in the field of abnormal personality have attempted to study abnormal traits in a single personality disorder category. Hare and colleagues have studied antisocial personality disorder in forensic populations and produced a valid measure of the underlying concept of psychopathy. Hare's *revised psychopathy checklist* (PCL-R; Hare, 1991), containing 20

Table 3.7 Items in PCL-R (Hare, 1991)

Factor 1	*Factor 2*
Glibness/superficial charm	Need for stimulation/proneness to boredom
Grandiose self-worth	Parasitic lifestyle
Pathological lying	Poor behaviour control
Conning/manipulative	Early behaviour problems
Lack of remorse or guilt	Lack of realistic long-term goals
Shallow affect	Impulsivity
Callous/lack of empathy	Irresponsibility
Failure to accept responsibility for actions	Juvenile delinquency Revocation of conditional release

items, is shown in Table 3.7. As its name suggests, it consists of a checklist of items that is scored by the clinician on the basis of a combination of best available evidence from extensive review of notes, collateral information and a semi-structured review. The PCL-R measures a unitary construct, psychopathy, and extreme scores reliably discriminate between recidivists (repeated offenders) and non-recidivists. Factor analysis of the items has produced two oblique factors, Factor 1 measuring a callous and remorseless lifestyle and way of relating to others, and Factor 2 a socially deviant lifestyle. Factor 1 identifies the central personality characteristics of psychopathy and Factor 2 represents the antisocial behaviours contained in antisocial personality disorder in DSM-IV (Table 3.7). Norms are available for prisoners and forensic populations. Use of the instrument requires special training.

Personality disorder

Personality disorders (PD) are described in ICD-10 as '*deeply ingrained and enduring behaviour patterns* manifesting themselves as inflexible responses to a broad range of personal and social situations; they represent extreme or *significant deviations* from the way the average individual in a given culture perceives, thinks, feels and particularly relates to others; such behaviour patterns tend to be stable and to encompass *multiple domains* of behaviour and psychological functioning; they are frequently, but not always, associated with various degrees of subjective distress and problems in social functioning and performance'. The DSM-IV definition of PD is almost identical. Both systems of classification stipulate that the patterns of deviation are persistent and stable and that the onset can be traced back to adolescence or early adult life. It is worth noting that the DSM classificatory system places PDs on a separate axis, Axis II, together with mental retardation and has a different axis, Axis I, for clinical syndromes. There is considerable debate as to how the two axes should be conceptualised.

The ICD recognises nine personality disorders and the DSM–IV has ten categories. Moreover, in the latter they are arranged in three clusters as shown in Table 3.8.

Table 3.8 Personality disorders classification in ICD-10 and DSM-IV

ICD-10	*DSM-IV*
	Cluster A: Odd–eccentric
Paranoid	Paranoid
Schizoid	Schizoid
	Schizotypal
	Cluster B: Dramatic–emotional
Dyssocial	Antisocial
Impulsive	Borderline
Histrionic	Histrionic
	Narcissistic
	Cluster C: Anxious–fearful
Anxious	Avoidant
Dependent	Dependent
Anankastic	Obsessive-compulsive

Of all the psychiatric disorders included in the major classificatory systems, the ICD and DSM, the nosological status of PDs has been the most contentious. Psychiatrists have long been uncomfortable with the category of PD. Some of the major problems are:

1. Categories and criteria are not empirically based and are often inconsistent with empirical findings from cluster and factor analysis. Multivariate analysis of the diagnostic criteria yields factors that do not correspond to either the ICD or DSM diagnostic categories.
2. Personality-disorder categories are often overlapping and heterogeneous. Many patients who receive a diagnosis of one personality disorder often receive as many as four other personality-disorder diagnoses. For instance, nearly 95% of patients meeting the criteria for borderline PD meet the criteria for a second PD and about 50% meet the criteria for a third. In short, comorbidity is the rule rather than the exception and categories are not mutually exclusive.
3. The instruments that are used to assess PD do not meet the criteria that are normally expected in personality research, they show poor test–retest reliability at intervals greater than six weeks (Zimmerman, 1994).
4. Clinicians find direct questioning derived from PD criteria unhelpful and to draw inferences rely largely on the history provided by the patient and informants about relationships and functioning (Western, 1997).

A fundamental question is whether PDs are best classified dimensionally or categorically. Dimensions of personality, such as the big five are normally distributed in the population and it has been argued that PDs represent those at the extremes of the distribution curve. Categorical models, on the other hand, assumes discontinuity between the distribution in the normal population and in groups with PDs. That is, PD is thought to be *qualitatively* distinct from normal personality. Therefore we find ourselves in the paradoxical situation where dimensional approaches are the universally accepted currency in describing and measuring normal personality, whereas categorical approaches remain the dominant and officially accepted way of describing PDs.

But there is now an emerging consensus that a dimensional approach may be more appropriate for describing abnormal personality or PD. As research findings from recent work has grown, it has become increasingly evident that PDs are not *qualitatively* distinct from normal personality functioning but are simply maladaptive, extreme variants of personality traits. For example, inhibitedness, a Livesley high-order trait of abnormal personality, can be viewed as an exaggeration of passivity and aloofness of introversion, a FFM factor. Thus the trait structure appears to be stable across clinical and non-clinical populations and is, therefore, consistent with dimensional representations of PDs.

Empirical research based on the FFM appears to hold great promise for investigation of normal–abnormal personality correlates because of its robustness and the universality of the model. An important study by Livesley (Livesley, Jang & Vernon, 1998) has demonstrated remarkable congruence of domains of normal and abnormal personality functioning. This study provides evidence that: (1) traits of PDs are continuously variable; and (2) the dimensional model of normal personality, the FFM, is closely congruent with a model derived from PD or abnormal personality symptoms. The four higher-order traits of PD strongly resemble dimensions of normal personality as described in the FFM. The FFM factor neuroticism is essentially equivalent to the emotional deregulation factor of Livesley; FFM introversion factor is highly congruent with inhibitedness factor; FFM antagonism (polar opposite of agreeableness) corresponds to dissocial component; and FFM conscientiousness closely corresponds with compulsivity. The only FFM factor for which no equivalent was found in PD characteristics was openness/closeness to experience. Commenting on these findings, Widiger, an authority on PD aptly remarked, 'Four out of five ain't bad' (Widiger, 1998). Thus, Livesley's work strongly suggests that the domain of personality pathology can be explained reasonably well within the five-factor model.

It has been proposed that antisocial, dependent, schizoid and compulsive personality disorders are variants of the big-five factors extraversion, neuroticism, openness to experience and conscientiousness respectively. But the

Table 3.9 Predicted relationship between big-five dimensions and DSM personality disorder clusters

	Cluster		
Dimensions	*A (paranoid)*	*B (antisocial)*	*C (anxious/avoidant)*
Extraversion	–	+	–
Neuroticism	+	+	+
Agreeableness	–	–	+
Conscientiousness		–	+
Openness		+	–

relationships between the normal personality factors and PDs may not be simple. For example, from the perspective of the FFM borderline PD involves primarily excessive neuroticism (N) and antagonism (A). Neuroticism captures borderline pathology such as angry hostility, depression and emotional lability while antagonism encapsulates the oppositional, argumentative and manipulative tendencies (Widiger & Costa, 1994). These are summarised in Table 3.9. The FFM factor agreeableness was the only dimension of big five to be shown to correlate significantly with the PCL-R in a sample of prisoners. In these terms, psychopathy would be closely related to the polar extreme of the dimension A, antagonism.

The inescapable conclusion is that PDs are not qualitatively distinct from normal personality functioning – they are maladaptive, extreme variations of common personality traits. The implications of these findings are clear – categorical methods of classification of PDs are no longer tenable. The major classificatory systems, DSM and ICD, could be expected to incorporate these findings in their forthcoming revisions. Tyrer has proposed a simple dimensional system of classification of personality disorders (see Table 14.1).

NARROW-BAND THEORIES OF PERSONALITY

Some theories of personality restrict themselves to specific aspects of personality functioning and focus on one or two dimensions. Two such theories are mentioned here.

Type A and B behaviour pattern

Friedmann and Rosemann (1974) studied personality factors associated with coronary heart disease (CHD) and described a constellation of stable personality factors, which they called Type A behaviour pattern. After correcting for other variables such as smoking, high cholesterol and hypertension, they found Type A behaviour pattern to be an important risk factor for CHD.

Type A behaviour is characterised by the triad of *hostility, time urgency* and *competitiveness*. Type B behaviour pattern refers to the lack of Type A behaviours. Semi-structured interviews have been used to assess Type A/B behaviour. The Western collaborative group study showed that Type A personalities were twice as likely as Type B personalities to develop CHD over a ten-year period. This finding lead to the conclusion that Type A behaviour pattern was an independent risk factor comparable with traditional risk factors for CHD such as family history of CHD, smoking and hypertension (Review Panel on Coronary-Prone Behaviours and Coronary Heart Disease, 1981). Type A subjects have been found to show disproportionately elevated blood pressure when made to work under stressful conditions. Psychological interventions aimed at reducing Type A behaviour pattern have been shown to reduce the risk of CHD. Over the last two decades the Type A theory has been refined and of the three components of Type A pattern hostility has been shown to be the most important. The 'hostility complex', as it is now called, refers to a more specific and stable tendency to react to a broad range of frustration and provocation inducing events with anger, annoyance and disgust (Williams, 1987). Hostility is not a unitary concept either. There appears to be at least three aspects to hostility: hostile attitude; experienced hostility; and expressed hostility (Whiteman, Fowkes & Deary, 1997).

In the tradition of Type A research, various researchers have attempted to identify a single personality type associated with breast cancer. The concept of Type C or cancer personality has been developed to describe a style of personality characterised by denial and suppression of negative emotions. Type C individuals are described as conflict-avoiding, nice and friendly, but often harbouring internal resentment which cannot be safely expressed (McKenna et al., 1999). The precise mechanism by which the denial–repression factor affects the development of breast cancer awaits further research.

Locus of control theory

An influential theory, advanced by Rotter (1966), postulates a construct, named locus of control, as an important mediator of how people feel and behave especially in stressful situations. According to the locus of control theory, some individuals believe that they have personal control (internal locus) over events in their life whereas others attribute outcomes of events to outside factors such as luck or other people (outside locus). Locus of control is believed to be a stable attribute of an individual. Rotter's I–E scale is a self-administered measure designed to evaluate an individual's locus of control. People with a predominantly external locus of control have been shown in some studies to be prone to stress-related emotional symptoms, poor job satisfaction and low self-esteem, but the results have been rather mixed.

REFERENCES

Akiskal HS, Hirchfield PM, Yerevanian BI (1983) The relationship of personality to affective disorders: a critical review. Archives of General Psychiatry, 40, 801–810.

Allport GW (1938) Personality: a psychological interpretation. New York: Holt.

Allport GW, Odbert HS (1936) Trait Names: a psycholexical study. Psychological Monographs, 47, (1, No. 211).

Bannister D, Fransella F (1967) A grid test of schizophrenic thought disorder. Barnstaple, UK: Psychological Test Publications.

Blinkhorn S, Johnson C (1990) The insignificance of personality testing. Nature, 348, 671–672.

Block J (1978) The Q-sort Method of Personality Assessment and Psychiatric Research. Palo Alto, CA: Consulting Psychology Press.

Bowers RS (1973) Situationalism in Psychology: an analysis and a critique. Psychological Review, 80, 307–336.

Cattell RB (1950) Personality: a systematic. theoretical and factual study. New York: McGraw-Hill.

Costa PT, McCrae R (1992) Revised NEO Personality Inventory (NEO-PI-R) (NEO-FFI) Professional Manual. Odessa, FL: Psychological Assessment Resources.

Costa PT, McCrae R (1994) Set like a plaster? Evidence for stability of adult personality. In TF Heatherton & JL Weinberger (eds), Can Personality Change? Washington, DC: American Psychological Association; 21–40.

Costa PT, McCrae R (1995) Primary traits of Eysenck's P-E-N system: three and five factor solutions. Journal of Personality and Social Psychology, 69(2), 308–327.

Endler NS, Magnusson D (1976) Towards an interactional psychology of personality. Psychological Bulletin, 83, 956–974.

Eysenck HJ (1990) Genetic and environmental contributions to individual differences: the three major dimensions of personality. Journal of Personality, 58, 245–261.
Eysenck HJ, Eysenck MW (1985) Personality and Individual Differences: a natural science approach, New York: Plenum.
Eysenck HJ, Eysenck MW (1991) The Eysenck Personality Questionnaire – Revised. Sevenoaks, UK: Hodder & Stoughton.
Friedmann M, Rosemann RH (1974) Type A Behaviour and your Heart. New York: Knopf.
Hare RD (1991) Manual for the Hare Psychopathy Checklist – Revised. Toronto: Multi-Health Systems.
Hartshorne H, May MA (1928) Studies in the Nature and Character, Vol. 1. Studies in deceit. London: Macmillan.
Helson R, Wink P (1992) Personality change in women from early 40s to early 50s. Psychology and Aging, 7, 46–55.
Kelly GA (1955) The Psychology of Personal Constructs: a theory of personality (2 Vols.). New York: Norton.
Kretschmer E (1936) Physique and Character (2nd edn.). New York: Trubner.
Krug SE, Jones EF (1986) A large-scale cross validation of second order personality structure defined by the 16PF. Psychological Reports, 59, 683–693.
Livesley WJ, Jackson DN, Schroeder ML (1992) Factorial structure of traits delineating personality disorders in clinical and general population samples. Journal of Abnormal Psychology, 101, 432–440.
Livesley WJ, Jang KL, Vernon PA (1998) Phenotypic and genetic structure of traits delineating personality disorder. Archives of General Psychiatry, 55, 941–948.
McAdams DP (1992) The five factor model in personality: a critical appraisal. Journal of Personality, 60(2), 329–362.
McKenna M, Zevon M, Corn B, Rounds J (1999) Psychosocial factors and the development of breast cancer: a meta-analysis. Health Psychology, 18(5), 520–532.
McCrae RR, Costa PT (1997) Personality trait structure as a human universal. American Psychologist, 52(5), 509–516.
Mischel W (1968) Personality and Assessment. New York: Wiley.
Monahan J (1981) The Clinical Prediction of Violent Behaviour. Washington, DC: US Government Printing Office.
Myers IB (1975) Manual: the Myers–Briggs type indicator. Palo Alto, CA: Consulting Psychology Press.
Pervin LA (1994) A critical analysis of current trait theory. Psychological Inquiry, 5(2), 103–113.
Review Panel on Coronary-Prone Behaviours and Coronary Heart Disease (1981) Coronary-prone behaviours and coronary heart disease: a critical review. Circulation, 63, 1199–1215.
Rogers CR (1951) Client-centred Therapy. Boston, MA: Houghton Mifflin.
Rotter JB (1966) Generalised expectancies for internal versus external control of reinforcement. Psychological Monographs, 80, 1–28.
Rutter M (1987) Temperament, personality and personality disorder. British Journal of Psychiatry, 150, 443–458.
Sheldon WH, Stevens SS (1942) The Varieties of Temperament: a psychology of constitutional differences. New York: Harper & Bros.
Western D (1997) Divergence between clinical and research methods of assessing personality disorders: implications for research and evaluation of Axis II. American Journal of Psychiatry, 154, 895–903.
Western D, Shedler J (1999) Revising and assessing Axis II. Part 1. Developing a clinically and empirically valid assessment method, American Journal of Psychiatry, 156, 258–272.
Whiteman MC, Fowkes FGR, Deary IJ (1997) Hostility and the heart: it's the hostility in type A personality that matters, but which element of hostility? British Medical Journal, 315, 379–380.
Widiger TA (1998) Four out of five ain't bad. Archives of General Psychiatry, 55, 865–866.

Widiger TA, Costa PT Jr (1994) Personality and personality disorders. Journal of Abnormal Psychology, 103, 78–91.
Williams R (1987) Refining the type A hypothesis: emergence of hostility complex. American Journal of Cardiology, 60(27), 27–32.
Zimmerman M (1994) Diagnosing personality disorders: a review of issues and research methods. Archives of General Psychiatry, 51, 225–245.

FURTHER READING

Bannister D, Fransella F (1980) Inquiring Man: the psychology of personal constructs (2nd edn.). Harmondsworth, UK: Penguin.
- A highly readable book on personal construct theory.

Matthews G, Deary IJ (1998) Personality Traits. Cambridge, UK: Cambridge University Press.
- A scholarly work on the subject.

Livesley WJ (ed.) (1995) The DSM-IV Personality Disorders. New York: Guilford.
- An edited authoritative text dealing with all the controversies and confusions over this most elusive group of disorders.

Emotions and emotional disorders

4

'The most beautiful things in life cannot be seen or even touched. They must be felt with the heart.'
Helen Keller

Emotion is one of those mystifying terms that elude definition. All of us know what it is to experience an emotion such as sadness, joy or anger. Yet, when we are asked to say what an emotion is, we can hardly describe it. Similar problems of definition have bedevilled the scientific study of emotions. Currently there is no accepted definition of emotion and there continues to be intense argument as to what components constitute an emotion. Definitional problems apart, it is a curious fact that although emotions are an integral part of human existence and experience and emotional disturbances form the very essence of clinical psychology and psychiatry, we know little about the basis and regulation of our day-to-day emotions. Indeed, in comparison to our knowledge and understanding of physical phenomena such as blood pressure or body temperature, our understanding of emotions is rather primitive. Even by standards in psychology, our understanding of emotion is somewhat rudimentary.

What distinguishes emotions from non-emotions? What differentiates one emotion from another, for example loneliness and sadness, or sympathy and empathy? How many emotions are there in humans and how are they organised? How are emotions regulated? Very little is known about emotions to answer these questions with any degree of certainty. Where there is a dearth of facts theories are plentiful. In the case of emotions the field is replete with theories, so much so that a recent book enumerates 150 theories of emotion (Strongman, 1996). The situation is even more grave when it comes to our understanding of the relationship between normal and abnormal emotions. Is depression an extreme form of sadness or are they qualitatively different? Such vexed questions remain largely unanswered. Nevertheless, this field has been an area of intense study and we are beginning to develop a rudimentary explanation of what constitutes emotions as well as developing approaches to understanding the emotional process. Before attempting to describe the various approaches to the understanding of emotion it would be useful to clarify the terms that will appear in this chapter: feelings; affect; mood; and emotions.

FEELINGS, AFFECT, MOOD AND EMOTIONS

The terms feelings, affect, mood and emotions have been used loosely, and sometimes interchangeably, in both psychology and psychiatry. There is a growing consensus that they should be defined more rigorously and scientifically in order to communicate effectively and advance our knowledge in the field of emotions.

Feelings. In lay terms this refers to sensing, experiencing or being conscious of a process. It has also been used more specifically to refer to sensory perceptions and is therefore akin to touch, pain and pleasure. In the study of emotions, it has been used to describe one component of emotion, the intrapsychic subjective experience that provides the *qualia* to emotions. In this usage *feelings* denote the 'inner psychic experience', the elemental, non-observable and subjective aspect of emotions. It is in this sense that the word is used in this chapter. The scientific study of subjective feelings and experiences is known as phenomenonology.

Affect. This is one of the most misused words in psychology and psychiatry. It has been used synonymously with mood as in affective disorders (meaning disorders of mood). It has been also used to denote the observable aspect of emotions seen during the mental state examination. Thus, in DSM-IV affect is defined as the visible and audible manifestations of the patient's emotional response to external and internal events, such as thoughts, ideas, evoked memories and recollections. It has also been used by some emotion theorists, confusingly in our view, to describe the non-cognitive aspect of emotion, making up the non-observable 'feeling' component of emotion. Phenomenologists seem to ascribe a similar meaning when they describe affect as 'waves of emotion', the moment-to-moment feeling state, often shifting rapidly in response to a variety of objects or situations (Fish, 1967). This description is more akin to those of feelings than to other emotional phenomena.

But the commonest usage of the term has been in a more general way. *Affect refers to all things emotional.* All emotion-related phenomena may be subsumed under the broad umbrella of affect. It encompasses sentiment, preferences, emotions, moods and affective traits under its broad rubric. This is in keeping with the use of the word affect in mainstream psychology, where it has been viewed as a component of the tripartite division of mental functions together with cognition and conation (see Chapter 6). It is in this general sense the term is employed in the rest of this chapter and throughout this book.

Emotion. As indicated above, emotion has proved to be notoriously difficult to define and authors who have attempted to define it, have done so according to their favourite theory underpinning emotion. Research on lay people's commonsense definition of emotion has helped clarify the properties that constitute an emotion. Most people's understanding of emotion is that it is: (1) an internal state rather than external; and (2) a feeling state as opposed to bodily cognitive or behavioural state (Fehr & Russell, 1984).

These findings notwithstanding, the contemporary conceptualisation of emotions is as a multicomponent phenomenon comprised of at least five components: subjective; cognitive; physiological; behavioural; and expressive. A non-controversial definition of emotion would therefore be that *it refers to subjective feelings that have physiological, cognitive and behavioural components*. There is fierce debate as to which of these aspects deserve to be considered primary. Despite these controversies, there is implicit agreement on some of the underlying features of emotions. Emotions are specific mental states that are:

- sudden in onset and relatively short lived;
- experienced as intense; and
- triggered by some stimulus or event.

An example would be anger triggered by an insulting remark that results in an intense but momentary feeling of anger. Although the resentment may last longer, the experience anger is acute, episodic, transient and usually intense.

Mood. Mood refers to a relatively sustained and pervasive emotional state that is longer lasting – for hours, days or weeks. Moods are more enduring and stable than emotions. While emotions are brief and phasic moods are chronic and sustained. Unlike emotions, moods are not usually related to (or directed at) a specific object, an identifiable event or stimulus – mostly there is no immediate cause or environmental antecedent. This contrasts with emotions, which are usually brought about by a stimulus salient to the subject. A useful way of distinguishing between the two is to attempt to elicit the emotion-producing antecedents by asking questions such as 'Why is the subject sad/happy at this moment?' If a preceding event, memory or object comes to mind, 'He/she is sad/happy because ...', it is most likely to be an emotion. On the contrary, if one cannot think of any immediate cause for the mental state, it is more likely to be a mood.

The relationship between emotion and mood is best captured by the weather–climate metaphor: emotions are more like the rapidly changing weather whereas moods are akin to the more persistent pattern of climate. Mood states are usually of low intensity, longer lasting and often occur for no particular reason, as in the case of depression or generalised anxiety. The distinction between mood and emotion is not always as clear cut or patently obvious as the above account suggests. There are obvious exceptions, such as jealousy, which although classed as an emotion is relatively long lasting. Similarly, depressive mood episodes may be precipitated by specific events such as losses. Nevertheless, it has to be emphasised that emotion and mood, as much as we know them, are distinct and different from each other but the relationship between them is far from clear. Because of the long duration and persistent quality, moods influence other psychological qualities such as memory, thinking and attributions more than emotions do. Emotions and moods are analogues to the Gestalt concept of figure–ground relationship (see Chapter 6), emotions are figural while moods occupy the background. Table 4.1 summarises the main differences between emotion and mood.

COMPONENTS OF EMOTIONS

Researchers in the field of emotion agree on the multicomponential nature of emotions – their arguments have been about which of the components is central or primary. There is also general agreement that emotions consist of at least five interdependent, interconnected phenomena: feelings; physiological/bodily changes; cognitive processes; action tendencies; and emotional expression.

Fear, for example, comprises an event that is perceived as threatening (cognitions), accompanied by an increased heart rate, sweating and dilatation

Table 4.1 Emotion and mood

Emotion	*Mood*
1. Acute	1. Long lasting/sustained
2. High intensity	2. Low intensity
3. Antecedent present	3. Antecedent usually absent
4. Brief	4. Chronic and enduring
5. Phasic	5. Diffuse
6. Metaphor: weather, figure	6. Metaphor: climate, background

of pupils (bodily physiological changes) and characteristic facial changes (emotional expression) as well as a unique psychic feeling of fear (subjective experience or feeling) and a tendency to flight or fight (action tendencies or action readiness). In addition, fear is evoked by certain characteristic stimuli, such as threats to the subject's welfare.

Feelings – the emotional experience

The inner, subjective experience is the non-observable component of emotions. It refers to the specific feeling tone that accompanies each emotion. Each emotion is said to have a distinct quality, for example anger and fear are experienced as qualitatively different. Although not all emotion theorists agree on the distinction of each emotion, a respectable body of opinion, called 'feeling theories' hold that feelings form the most central component of emotions and that other processes – cognitions, bodily changes, action tendencies and emotional expressions – result from and follow the subjective feeling of the emotion. According to this view feelings are the very substrate or indivisible core of emotions. A major feature of emotional feelings is that they are experienced as either positive or negative, pleasurable or unpleasurable. This aspect of feelings has been called *valence* of the emotion. Because of the subjective nature of the experience, this component of emotions is usually the most difficult to study; the usual method of study is by diary records of the feelings that experimental subjects experience.

Autonomic reactions and bodily changes

Emotions produce autonomic responses in the body in the form of changes in heart rate, blood pressure, skin temperature, changes in pupils and so on. All 'excited emotions' such as anger and fear lead to sympathetic arousal pattern characterised by increased heart rate, increased sweating and respiration, constriction of skin blood vessels leading to pallor, dilatation of pupils, decreased gastrointestinal activity, and dry mouth. One way in which sympathetic activation is measured in the laboratory is by the galvanic skin response (GSR), which is a record of the variation in skin conductance brought about by sweating. In the past, some studies suggested that each of the main emotions produced specific autonomic response patterns and conversely emotions were thought to be capable of being identified by distinct autonomic 'signatures'. Although some differences do exist in the way heart rate, respiration and GSR change in response to different emotional experiences, these do not reflect characteristic patters for each emotion and there are no physiological changes or profile of changes that can be regarded as unique for each emotion. In short, none of the discrete emotions such as anger, fear, sadness, happiness and disgust can be identified by autonomic activity alone as indexed by changes in heart rate, blood pressure, respiration and GSR (Cacioppo et al., 2000).

Facial and bodily changes – emotional expression

Emotions are accompanied by observable body behaviour – facial, vocal, gestural and postural changes. Unlike physiological changes that are generalised, emotional expression bears a consistent relationship towards specific emotion. Charles Darwin's classic work *The Expression of Emotions in Man and Animals*, published in 1872, gives a descriptive analysis and evolutionary perspective on emotional expression. Infants and children as young as one month of age have been shown to both express and comprehend emotions such as anger and sadness. Emotional expressions, especially facial cues, are to a large extent unlearned and universal. Most emotions are associated with characteristic facial expressions. For example the 'sad face' shows raised forehead, pulled down corners of the mouth, brows drawn upwards and together, and drooping eyelids. Vocal cues are based on three perceptual dimensions: loudness; pitch; and time. In sadness, for example, speech is typically soft, low pitched and slow with prolonged silences. Bodily emotional expressions are as common as facial expressions and include behaviours such as being physically energetic, jumping up and down in joy, or assuming a slumped, stooping posture in sadness.

Facial expressions have been studied in great detail using sophisticated coding systems, video recordings and electromyography of facial muscles. Although facial expressions can be suppressed, modified or faked, video studies show that in the first few seconds (five seconds at the most) facial expressions reflect what one genuinely feels. After this, willed action may mask these emotional expressions (Ekman, 1992).

Action tendencies

Emotions are accompanied by impulses to act in ways appropriate to the particular emotion. Such action tendencies or action readiness may be acted upon, in which case it leads to observable behaviour (such as attack, or avoidance in the case of fear) or may not even be recognised (as in the case of increased muscle tension occurring in anger). Indeed some theories have defined emotions on the basis of action tendencies. Different emotions have different forms of action readiness: anger (aggression); sadness (withdrawal); fear (protective action); surprise (looking for cause); disgust (rejection and withdrawal); and love (proximity seeking).

Cognitive appraisal

Cognitive interpretation and evaluation of the emotion provoking event is an important – for some theorists the *most* important – component of emotion. Emotions are only rarely elicited directly by emotion producing stimuli. Many emotions are the result of the appraisal of the situation and its relevance to the subject. The same event or situation may be experienced differently and provoke different emotions depending on the individual's appraisal of the context in which the event occurs. A prick sustained in the dark may cause little distress if it is thought to be a thorn prick, but would cause extreme fear and panic if it was considered to be a bite from a poisonous snake. In the former instance, the interpretation of the event is a rather innocuous one while in the latter instance it is appraised as potentially fatal. Cognitive processes are thought to mediate between the actual environmental stimuli and the emotional experiences. Cognitive theories of emotion hold that cognitive evaluation, interpretation and attributions constitute important, if not the most important, component of emotion. Typically research in this area has consisted of asking subjects to keep records of emotions experienced (emotion diaries) and then identify particular appraisal patterns (favourable/unfavourable, controllable/uncontrollable, self/other responsibility, etc.).

Emotional elicitors

Emotions are experienced in relation to other things – events, situations, people, actions, memories, and fantasies. One is sad *about*, afraid *of*, or angry *at* something or someone. Events, or conditions that give rise to emotional responses, therefore deserve as much attention as the various components of emotions. Antecedents that lead to emotional responses are to be found in day-to-day human social interactions. Some such elicitors may be innate (fear of snakes, heights, etc.) while others arise from conditions of association or learning.

Although researchers have attempted to study the 'intrinsic emotion-producing stimuli', the situations that evoke emotions are complex and complicated. One way of overcoming these difficulties has been to identify

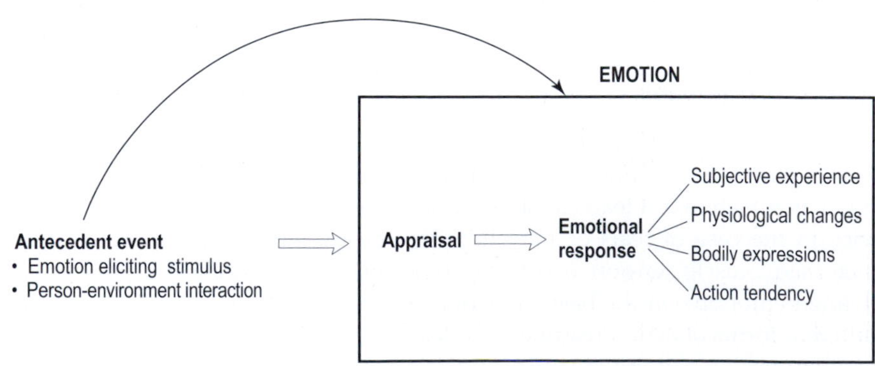

Fig. 4.1 The emotional process

distinctive 'themes' that are consistently found to be correlated with each emotion. Some of these 'core relational themes' are considered later.

The processes involved in the production of emotion may be summarised as follows: the emotion eliciting antecedent event or stimulus leads to cognitive appraisal of the situation followed by the emotional response, which consists of subjective experiences, physiological changes, bodily experience of feelings and action tendencies (Figure 4.1). It is now generally accepted that the stage of appraisal may be bypassed in certain situations where emotional responses are automatic and occur instantly and are beyond one's awareness. The main theories of emotion are considered next.

THEORIES OF EMOTION

Physiological theory of James and Lange

One of the earliest theories of emotion, proposed by William James (1890), postulates that body responses to stimuli and their perception is the basis of emotions. A Danish physician, Karl Lange put forward similar views about the same time. Since then it has been known as the James–Lange theory and has generated other theories as well as much research. The theory argues for the converse of the lay idea of emotion that sees bodily changes as a consequence of emotions. In James' words, 'The bodily changes follow directly from the *perception* of the existing fact and that our feelings of the same changes as they occur *is* the emotion' (James, 1884). The assertion here is that events or stimuli cause physiological changes in the body and the perception of this reaction *is* the emotion. This is summarized in Figure 4.2. According to James, 'we are afraid because we tremble ..., we feel sad because we cry'. The main thrust of the theory is that afferents from the receptors produce changes in the viscera and skeletal muscles and the feedback that comes from them is the emotion itself. James and Lange assumed the existence of discrete emotions and that each emotion involved a unique physiological response.

Although there is little evidence to support James–Lange's theory, two pieces of evidence lend some credence to it. Recent work showing the significance of facial expression in the experience of emotion (the facial feedback theory) is an offshoot of James–Lange's theory (Laird, 1974). It has been found that under experimental conditions, subjects mimicking facial expressions for corresponding emotions produce the autonomic changes seen in emotional states and also experience some subjective feelings akin to the emotions that were mimicked. Another piece of evidence of the theory comes from other studies that have demonstrated that patients with high spinal injuries show

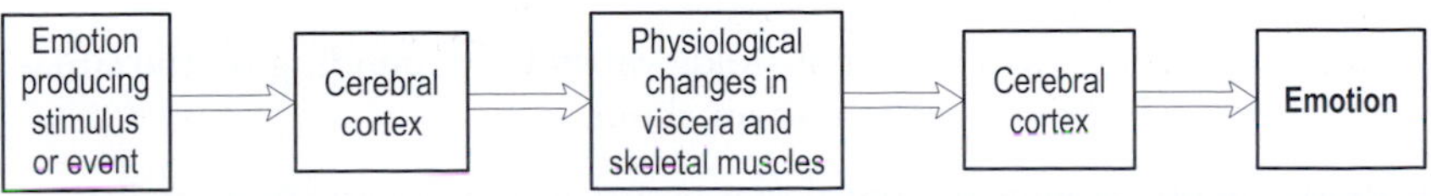

Fig. 4.2 James–Lange (physiological) theory of emotions. 'Perception of the bodily changes is emotion'

diminished emotional responsiveness (Hohman, 1966). Although the James–Lange theory has been of much heuristic value and stimulated much research in emotions and its correlates, there is very little support for the original suppositions and contemporary approaches do not afford physiological changes much importance.

Cannon–Bard theory of central activation

Walter Cannon and Philip Bard rejected the view that physiological arousal alone leads to perception of the emotion. According to them, emotion-producing stimuli concurrently and simultaneously lead to the activation of the autonomic nervous system (producing changes in smooth muscles, glands and heart rate) and the cerebral cortex (where emotion reaches consciousness). They believed that both pathways involve the thalamus, which mediates between the environmental stimuli and the cortex on one hand and the autonomic system on the other. Discharge from the thalamus was supposed to lead to excitation of the cortex and autonomic nervous system as shown in Figure 4.3 (Cannon, 1929). These two pathways and processes were thought to be independent of each other. From a neurophysiological point of view this theory is grossly inaccurate, for we now know that the limbic system is the brain structure most intimately involved in the generation of emotions. Moreover, there is little evidence for the occurrence of autonomic changes and the subjective experience of the emotion at the same time.

Cognitive theories of emotion

Cognitive theories of emotion hold that cognitive variables such as expectations, evaluations, memories and appraisals of the intrinsically emotion-producing stimuli or events are the very essence of emotions. Such cognitive evaluations are seen as both necessary and sufficient conditions for emotional experience. Cognitive theories of emotion currently occupy a commanding position in the conceptualisation of emotional processes. Of the many cognitive theories of emotion two are outlined here: Schachter and Singer's cognitive labelling theory and Lazarus' cognitive appraisal theory.

Schachter's cognitive labelling theory

A major contribution to our understanding of emotion comes from a series of classic experiments devised and conducted by Schachter and Singer in 1962. Their theory, also know as the two factor theory of emotions, proposes that:

1. Emotional states are characterised by general arousal of the sympathetic nervous system; and
2. We interpret and label these physiological states depending on the situational cues we believe brought them about.

In short, the physiological arousal that occurs following an emotional trigger is given a name according to our own interpretation of that emotional stimulus and situation. Thus, the same state of arousal could be labelled in

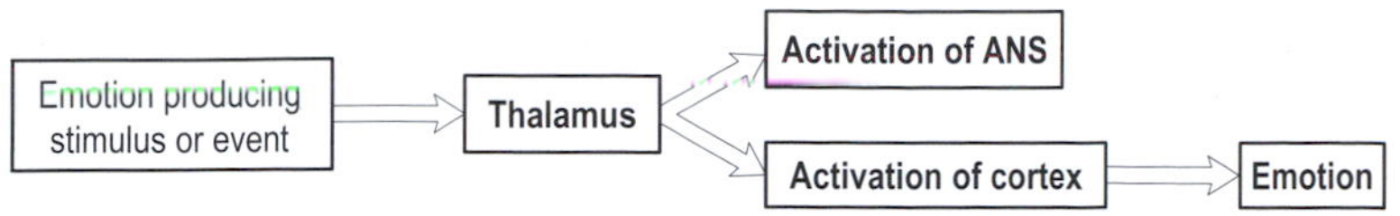

Fig. 4.3 Cannon–Bard theory of central activation

many ways depending on the situation and individual's interpretation of the circumstances. Simply stated, the theory postulates that an emotional state consists of a state of arousal combined with a cognition that permits labelling of the emotion.

Schachter and Singer (1962) devised an experiment in which subjects were told that they would receive an injection of a vitamin to test its effects on vision. In reality the subjects were injected with adrenaline with the explicit aim of increasing arousal. There were four groups in all:

1. An *informed* group who were told about the physiological effects adrenaline would have on them.
2. A *misinformed* group who were given misleading information and were told that it would result in itching, numbness and headache.
3. An *uninformed* group who did not receive any information about the effects of the injection.
4. A *control* group that received injections of saline.

Each subject was individually placed with a confederate ('stooge') who acted in one of two ways: in one condition he acted happy, excited and euphoric and in the other he was irritating, hostile and behaved angrily. The purpose of the experiment was to find out how subjects responded emotionally to the confederates' behaviour under normal conditions and in the adrenaline induced condition of high arousal. The results of the study showed that, in the euphoric situation, the informed and misinformed groups reported experiencing more happiness than the uninformed subjects. Similar results were obtained in those exposed to the angry conditions. The findings were taken to mean that under conditions of arousal individuals turn to environmental cues to explain what they were feeling (Figure 4.4).

Although the analysis of Schachter and Singer's results have been interpreted differently and replications of the study have produced variable results, by emphasising the central role of cognitive factors as mediating variables interposed between the emotion-producing event and the experience of

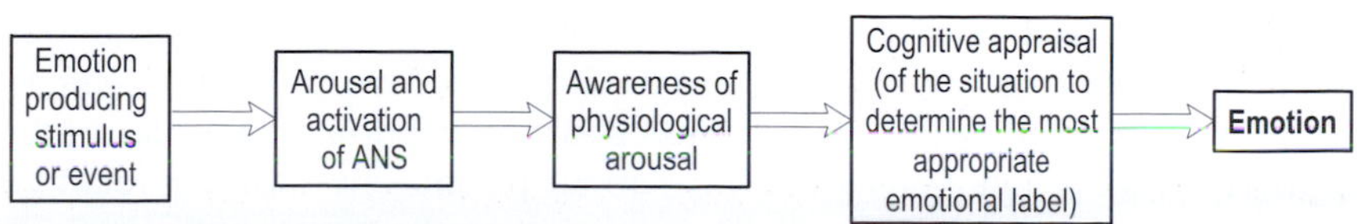

Fig. 4.4 Schachter and Singer's cognitive labelling theory of emotion

emotion, their experiments were a turning point in our understanding of emotions. In general, all the available evidence supports only a partial form of Schachter's theory. We have to turn to other cognitive theories for a more complete explanation.

Lazarus' cognitive appraisal theory

Over the last twenty years, Lazarus' has developed an overarching theory of emotion that stresses the importance of cognitive factors, especially appraisal, as a way of understanding the emotional processes. By incorporating coping mechanisms, over the years he has expanded his ideas into a grand theory of emotions (Lazarus, 1991).

The fundamental premise of Lazarus' theory is that *cognitive appraisal* forms the core to all emotional processes. Appraisal consists of continuous evaluation of the significance of what is happening for personal well being. It involves interpretation of the perceived event or situation ('what is happening?') followed by evaluation ('what are the implications for me?'). It encompasses environmental realities on one hand and personal beliefs, expectation and goals on the other. For Lazarus each emotional reaction is a function of a particular kind of appraisal. Emotion is viewed as being generated by such evaluations of specific person–environment relationships, hence appraisal is seen as a necessary and sufficient condition. The appraisal is said to imbue an event with meaning and personal relevance to the subject. Different emotions correspond to different appraised contingencies rather than the objective properties of the situation. Moreover, individuals differ in the way that they appraise the same event or situation. As a result, appraisal theories of emotion are capable of accounting for individual variations in emotional experiences. Lazarus considers that appraisal occurs in two sequential steps:

1. Primary appraisal. This refers to an evaluation of the relevance of an event or encounter ('does it matter to me?'), whether there is potential for emotion depends on how important or salient the event is to the subject. If appraised as harmful the resulting emotion will be a negative one while if appraised as beneficial the emotion will carry a positive valence. Other dimensions useful for distinction between different emotions is the kind of relevance to the individual, such as responsibility, self-esteem, controllability, and so on.

2. Secondary appraisal. This concerns the coping actions that are available to the individual. Issues such as accountability or responsibility (self or other), control, coping potential and future expectations ('will I be able to manage?') influence the way that people experience different emotions.

Lazarus' theory (also called cognitive-motivational-relational theory of emotions) is an elaborate network of concepts and includes other major elements in addition to cognitive appraisal. One such concept is *core relational themes*. Lazarus emphasises causal antecedents as important variables in the appraisal process. Emotions are always about person–environment relationships that involve harm or profit. The emotion-producing stimuli are never simple but result from the person–environment interaction in social situations. Each emotion is said to involve a distinctive core relational theme. Typical core relational themes for various emotions are as follows:

- Anger – offence against self.
- Sadness – experiencing loss.
- Happiness – realisation of goal.
- Fear – facing threat or damage.

These themes are, according to Lazarus, universal in human experiences. Hence appraisal theories substitute situation for stimulus. Describing antecedents as situations allows for different emotional meaning to be attached to the same event.

Over the last 30 years, his theory has grown into a complex model of emotions, stress and coping underpinned by substantial research and has the advantage of being applicable to real-life situations. It encompasses personality (example beliefs and values) and environmental (situations, stimuli) variables as antecedents that are appraised by individuals resulting in emotional states, which are accompanied by coping processes. This chain of events is outlined in Figure 4.5.

Lazarus–Zajonc debate

Lazarus' theory, though extensive in its sweep and well researched, has not gone unchallenged. The assertion that emotions need cognitive appraisal as a precondition was most forcefully challenged by several workers, notably Zajonc (1980). This controversy, known as the Lazarus–Zajonc debate, was about whether emotions and cognitions were independent (though interdependent) processes, as Zajonc would have us believe, or whether emotional responses depend on cognitive processes, as asserted by Lazarus and colleagues. Zajonc has produced some persuasive arguments backed up by a substantial amount of research to show that:

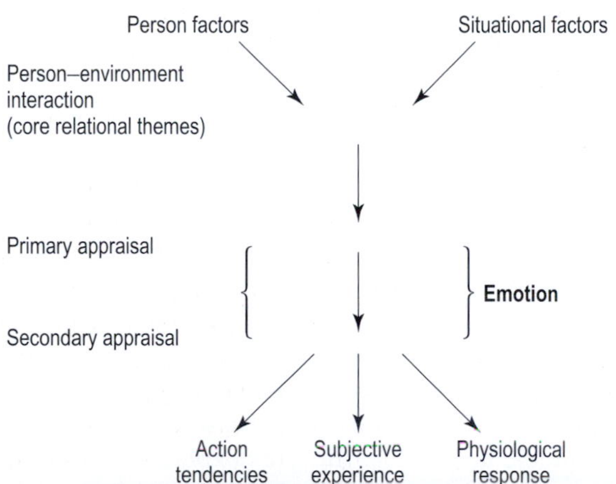

Fig. 4.5 Lazarus' cognitive appraisal theory of emotion

1. Emotional reactions can be established in the absence of conscious awareness.
2. Emotional states can be induced by non-cognitive and non-perceptual procedures such as drugs, hormones and electrical stimulation of the brain.
3. Separate neuroanatomical structures can be identified for emotion and cognition.
4. Some emotions are triggered instantly before cognitive mediation is possible and infants show emotions such as anger and disgust.

There is now incontrovertible evidence to support the existence of preconscious automatic cognitive processes in the production of some emotional reactions. This is a radical departure from the traditional understanding of cognition as those processes that deal mainly with conscious processes, such as thinking, reasoning and knowing (see Chapter 6). Our current understanding of emotional processes is summarised in Figure 4.1.

NUMBER OF EMOTIONS AND THEIR NATURE

How many emotions are there and how do emotions differ from one another? Are there discrete, basic, universal motions or are they best characterised as points within a two-dimensional space? One way of verifying this notion of basic emotions is to study emotions in diverse cultures. This is precisely what Paul Ekman and colleagues did.

Primary emotions

In a well-known study carried out by Ekman and colleagues, photographs of actors who posed to express certain emotions were showed to individuals from literate (American, Swedish, Japanese and Kenyan) and preliterate (New Guinea tribes not exposed to outsiders) cultures and they were asked to identify the emotions portrayed. Seven emotions were readily identified by all groups: *happiness*, *surprise*, *anger*, *fear*, *sadness*, *contempt* and *disgust*. In another part of the study, the workers asked a group of New Guinea tribesman to portray emotions that were appropriate to certain situations, for example when a child had died. When these photographs were shown to American college students they were able to identify the emotions with a high degree of accuracy (Ekman, 1982). Based on these and other findings, Ekman argued that these emotions are largely independent of culture and are 'elemental and pure'. They are present from early infancy and are thought to reflect neural dispositions for primary emotions. Thus cross-cultural research has convincingly demonstrated that a small set of emotions, called *primary emotions*, has universal distinctive signals that are recognised as such by members of most societies, from industrialised to preliterate ones, across the world (Box 4.1). According to Ekman, these seven emotions are expressed on the face in the same way in every culture. These universal facial expressions, it is argued, are innate and not learnt. This explains why congenitally blind people show the same facial expressions for each of these emotions as sighted people do (Ekman, 2003).

Box 4.1 Universal primary emotions shown in facial expressions in various cultures (Ekman, 1982)

- Happiness
- Surprise
- Anger
- Sadness
- Fear
- Disgust
- Contempt

While facial expressions are basically the same across various nationalities, they are not entirely culture free. In interpersonal situation, non-verbal emotional expression is, to an extent, rule governed. There are also culture-specific rules that encourage, or discourage, the expression of emotions or specific emotions. Such *display rules* are prescriptive and proscriptive norms for emotional manifestations that are learnt early in life (Ekman & Friesen, 1975). Cultural norms about how emotions ought to be expressed in different social contexts influence the way in which individuals in a particular society show their emotions. For example, in collective societies, members are more restrained in showing anger in the presence of elders.

Those who argue for a dimensional representation of emotions have produced evidence for a two-dimensional classification of emotions. This issue remains one of the hottest debates in the field of emotion. Future neuroimaging techniques may hold the key to confirming or refuting the primary emotion theory. Support for the discreetness of emotions comes from recent positron emission tomography (PET) studies, which demonstrated convincingly that different brain structures are involved in happiness and sadness (George et al., 1995). This study, carried out on healthy female volunteers, showed that induction of transient sadness is associated with increase in cerebral activity in the limbic and paralimbic structures, whereas the most significant changes observed in transient happiness is a widespread *reduction* in secondary association cortex in the temporoparietal and right prefrontal areas.

EMOTIONAL STATES, TRAITS AND THEIR ORGANISATION

States and traits

Emotional states are transient 'internal conditions' and have to be distinguished from traits. While traits are stable predispositions, states are unstable and change from situation to situation. A person high on trait anxiety may have a general predisposition to experience frequent transient states of anxiety, whereas most people are subject to states of anxiety at certain times, for example at interviews or in examination situations. As a trait, anxiety is a chronic enduring condition that characterises how a person feels in most

Table 4.2 States and traits

State (e.g. state anxiety)	*Trait (e.g. trait anxiety)*
Transient internal mental state	A general predisposition
Momentary, unstable	Stable and enduring
Sensitive to situational changes	Relatively stable across situations and across time

aspects of his/her life regardless of the situation. As a state, anxiety is a temporary, short-lived feeling that all people experience under certain conditions. Thus traits are stable over time but traits show fluctuations. States, but not traits, are sensitive to situational factors (Table 4.2).

The state–trait anxiety inventory (STAI; Spielberger, 1883) is a well-known questionnaire that includes 20 trait and 20 state items for anxiety. The state items ask the subject to describe how they feel at a certain moment (for example, when completing the questionnaire). Items include such statements as: 'I feel tense', 'I feel jittery'. The trait items refer to how the subject feels generally. Items are rated on a four-point scale. The trait scale measures anxiety proneness of the subject. A person scoring high on trait scale can be expected to respond to psychological stress with higher levels of state anxiety than a person with a low trait anxiety score. Research has shown this to be the case. For example, in one study when the STAI was applied before, during and after the test, subjects high on trait anxiety were shown to have high state anxiety when sitting for an examination (Kendall et al., 1976).

EMOTION AND COGNITION

Emotions colour, distort and influence perceptions, thoughts, memories and interpretations of events in a number of ways. Some of the known influences of emotions on cognitions are:

Emotion and selective encoding. Several experiments have demonstrated that high levels of anxiety and depression are associated with biased encoding favouring negative information. Anxiety is strongly associated with attention to threatening stimuli while depression appears to show no such link.

Emotion and selective interpretation. Anxious and depressed subjects show a definite bias towards estimation of future negative events as well as subjective evaluations concerning current life circumstances. They have also been shown to rate their performance in social situations negatively. It is thought that these patterns of judgement reflect interpretative negative thoughts that favour negative interpretation of ambiguous information.

Emotion and selective memory. Depression, but not anxiety, is associated with recall of negative information regarding self. There has been some debate as to whether the selective memory bias is the result of emotional states or enduring personality traits. Three pieces of evidence show that it is the emotional state, i.e. mood, that largely mediates the bias in memory favouring negative information. First, it has been demonstrated that induction of negative mood produces selective recall of emotionally negative material from the past

(Teasdale & Barnard, 1993). Second, studies examining patients recovering from depression have found the negative bias reduced or abolished. Third, it has been shown that diurnal variation in levels of moods shown in clinical depression are associated with corresponding changes in recall of emotionally negative information (Clark & Teasdale, 1982).

Cognition–Emotion: what is the relationship?

In psychology, the relationship between emotion and cognition has been a topic of hot debate for some time. Cognitive and information-processing models have consistently argued that emotion is the logical sequel of appraisal of the environment, whereas 'the feeling theorists' assign a primary role to emotion. Following the Zajonc–Lazarus debates of the 1980s, there has recently been an increasing rapprochement between the two camps. It has been shown that some emotional responses arise after minimal or no cognitive processing. These and other observations have brought about a redefinition of cognition that includes pre-attentive processing. Now it is believed that some of the critical processes involved in cognitions are automatic, non-conscious and effortless. Most cognitive psychologists now believe that cognitions involve both intentional and automatic processes.

It has been suggested that two semi-independent pathways may be involved when an individual encounters a situation. One of these pathways corresponds to the cognitive appraisal/information processing model and the other, which occurs *simultaneously*, is an emotion-processing mechanism that determines the emotional 'feeling' state of the emotion. There is also emerging consensus that cognitive processing is not equally relevant to all emotions – different emotions vary in the level of processing involved. Simple fears probably require less cognitive processing than sadness, which requires higher-level processing

On available evidence it would seem reasonable to conclude that emotions and cognitions are interdependent and that there exists a reciprocal relationship between the two. Thus, certain types of interpretations or evaluations act as antecedents to emotional states but those emotional states themselves increase the likelihood of these very cognitions (Teasdale, 1983). The debate is far from over and is leading towards attempts to formulate new paradigms. As pointed out by Rachman (1997), one of the foremost workers in the field of cognitive behaviour therapy research, in the near future we can look forward to a theory of cognitive–emotional processing that embraces the interplay between affect and cognition.

EMOTION AND COMMUNICATION

Emotions are more than private psychological experiences. An important aspect of emotional experience is the expression of emotion for various forms in interpersonal communication. Indeed some have argued that the primary function of emotion is to communicate feelings and needs to other people in social interactions with family, friends, strangers or enemies. People tend to communicate emotions in a variety of verbal and non-verbal ways.

Monitoring another person's behaviours for emotional cues is central to everyday personal interactions.

Brief and subtle facial expressions. Indeed, emotions do produce automatic and instantaneous non-verbal displays that reflect the person's true emotional state, especially in the first few seconds of interpersonal exchange (called emotional 'leakage') before intentional and voluntary censorship change the expression. Ekman (2003) has described two types of subtle facial changes:

1. *Micro expressions*, brief expressions lasting about 0.2 seconds, where the person is trying consciously or unconsciously to conceal an emotion; and
2. *Subtle expressions* that last longer but are faint and therefore easily missed.

Recognising these facial changes in clinical encounters provides clues to how patients are feeling at that point in time. Since emotions never tell you their cause, it is the clinician who has to take steps to acknowledge the emotion that is expressed and also make gentle inquiries about what the cause may be.

On receiving an emotional communication from another person, the recipients inevitably respond with various types of emotional communication of their own. These interactive patterns govern the exchange of social messages. Understanding such emotion-based communications is a key factor in the relationships between doctors and patients, psychotherapists and clients and parents and their children.

Emotions are thought to have evolved in human beings because they were adaptive and had survival advantage. They have served as a universal communications system to promote group cohesion of humans. Anger displays have subserved the function of warning off potential enemies while fear reactions produce immediate warning signals to other members of the group as well as to the self. There is growing evidence to suggest that hard-wired neurological networks exist between emotions and their expression, especially non-verbal expression.

Emotional matching. Emotional communications are often subtle. It is a well-known fact that other people's emotions influence our own emotions and behaviours. For example, it has been shown that when mothers pretend to be depressed and assume a depressive face this produces a similar expression in their infants. Such *emotional matching* appears to be a ubiquitous phenomenon, especially in close and intimate interactions between individuals, for example between married couples, good friends and in therapeutic encounters between clients and clinicians. This extraordinary influence, albeit non-conscious, that the emotions of one person exert on the emotional state and behaviour of another underlies all empathetic feelings. Psychoanalysts have been aware of this phenomenon for a long time and have variously called it projection or projective identification.

NORMAL EMOTIONS, MOODS AND EMOTIONAL DISORDERS

The relationship of normal emotions (and moods) to psychopathology and emotional disorders is not clear. In some disorders the abnormal mood states form the major part of the condition. Someone suffering from depression, for example, experiences a pervasive mood of intense sadness for an extended period of time from weeks to months. In other disorders, such as post-traumatic stress disorder, conduct disorder and anxiety, emotions are an important component of the condition. In spite of the obvious relationship between normal and abnormal emotions, our understanding of emotional disorders, on the basis of what we know about normal emotions, is rather deficient and wanting.

Normal fear

Fear is one of the commonest emotions experienced by man and animals. It is also one of the primitive reactions in all higher organisms as evidenced by the demonstration of infants' fear of heights (see Chapter 12) and the 'hawk effect' seen in newly hatched ducks and geese at the sight of predators (see Chapter 11). There is no doubt that man and animal have an innate biological propensity to react to some situations and stimuli fearfully. This innate tendency to fear some stimulus configurations more than others has been called *preparedness* (Seligman, 1971). Examples of the kind of stimuli that provoke fear independent of experience include encounters with snakes, spiders, rats, mice and other 'creepy crawlies'. Sudden loud noises, fast approaching objects and moving at great speed (e.g. falling) also produce fear instantaneously. Such innate fears appear to be generated automatically and almost instantaneously. There is no doubt that the situations that elicit fear are potentially dangerous and hence the fear response has obvious survival advantage. It is interesting to note, however, that dangerous weapons, such as guns, do not produce similar fear reactions.

While a small number of fears may be inborn, to a large extent most of the fears experienced in day-to-day life are learnt. All studies on the epidemiology of fears have consistently shown that women show fearfulness of more situations than men. A more recent study of the incidence of fears in normal populations is the ECA study (see later), which found that normal fear is extraordinarily common in the general population. Sixty percent of the 20 000 people interviewed had experienced at least one 'unreasonable fear' in at least one situation at some point in their lives (Table 4.3).

Table 4.3 Prevalence of fears in the normal population (ECA study, Easton & Kessler, 1985)

Object feared	*Prevalence (%)*
Bugs, mice, snakes, bats, etc.	22.4
Heights	18.2
Water	12.5
Public transport	10.5
Storms	9.3
Closed spaces	8.0
Animals	3.9

Although it is generally accepted that fear develops through the interaction of innate and learned elements, there is no single theory that satisfactorily integrates all known data.

Abnormal fear

Abnormal fear responses feature prominently in many psychiatric disorders. The example par excellence of abnormal fear is phobic disorders, but fear is an important component in other disorders such as post-traumatic stress disorder and panic disorder, where it forms the core subjective experience of the patient's symptoms.

Phobias

Phobias are fears that are excessive to the situation, difficult to explain rationally, and often lead to subjective distress and vulnerable disability. Marks (1969) characterises phobia as a special kind of fear which:

1. Is out of proportion to the demands of the situation.
2. Cannot be explained or reasoned away.
3. Is beyond voluntary control.
4. Leads to avoidance of the feared situation.

The object of the fear, i.e. the content of the phobia, is usually a real situation or event.

Epidemiology of phobias

Population studies of the prevalence rates of phobias have shown wide variation because of the problems of definition of threshold and severity. One of the largest surveys ever carried out was the *epidemiological catchments area study* (ECA) involving five centres in the USA. More than 20 000 subjects were interviewed and DSM-III criteria were employed. Of all the subjects interviewed, 18.5% met the criteria for at least one phobic disorder during their lifetime (unfortunately this includes subjects who would be characterised as panic disorder with agoraphobia by DSM-IV standards) (Easton & Kessler, 1985). Lifetime prevalence of various phobias is shown in Table 4.4. Simple phobia was the commonest phobic disorder (15%) and almost half of this group was formed by those who reported abnormal fear of mice, bugs, snakes (creepy crawlies). The second largest group reported agoraphobia (7.6%), one of the most common phobias among adults, and the most disabling.

Our understanding of the mechanisms and processes that underlie the acquisition of phobias have undergone considerable change over the last two decades. It is now believed that different phobias may have quite *different* aetiological mechanisms. Whereas some phobias such as dog phobia and dental phobia do appear to be acquired as a result of specific traumatic experiences, such specific events are rarely found in the development of other phobias like height phobia or blood injury phobia. The other major factor that has contributed to the better grasp of the mechanisms involved in the acquisition of

Table 4.4 Lifetime prevalence of phobias (ECA study, Easton & Kessler, 1985)

Object feared	*Lifetime prevalence (%)*
Simple phobia	15.1
Bugs, mice, snakes, bats	6.1
Heights	4.7
Animals	1.1
Water	3.3
Agoraphobia	7.6
Social phobia	3.2
All phobias	18.5

phobias is the appreciation of the important role of cognitive factors in phobic disorders. The two-factor theory (see Chapter 1) has been replaced by more cognitively orientated theories. More recently, Davey (1997) has put forward a model of phobia that uniquely combines cognitive factors and classical conditioning.

Anxiety

Normal anxiety

Anxiety is regarded as a key emotion but there have been considerable difficulties in 'placing' it in the range of normal emotions. It is usually grouped together with the family of emotions associated with fear. Undoubtedly there are features that are common to both and sometimes the term anxiety has been used to denote mild fear. For example, separation anxiety in children is thought to be due to fear of separation from an attachment figure.

The antecedents or situations that produce normal anxiety are not life threatening. Facing an examination or interview may be important for one's career but it hardly endangers life, compared to meeting with an accident. The former produces anxiety whereas the latter results in fear. Normal anxiety is usually situational. Like fear, normal anxiety is often associated with an identifiable source, as in the case of an interview or examination. The difference between the two emotions, in terms of the person–environment interaction, lies in the fact that in anxiety the action tendency, avoidance/flight, is blocked. Ambivalence, entertaining both positive and negative feelings and attitudes towards the situation, is a characteristic feature of normal anxiety. The physiological responses are similar to those of fear but mild in nature. Motor restlessness, fidgeting, inability to relax, muscle tension and apprehension are typical features of anxiety. Phenomenologically, anxiety consists of a sense of apprehension and dread together with a feeling of tension.

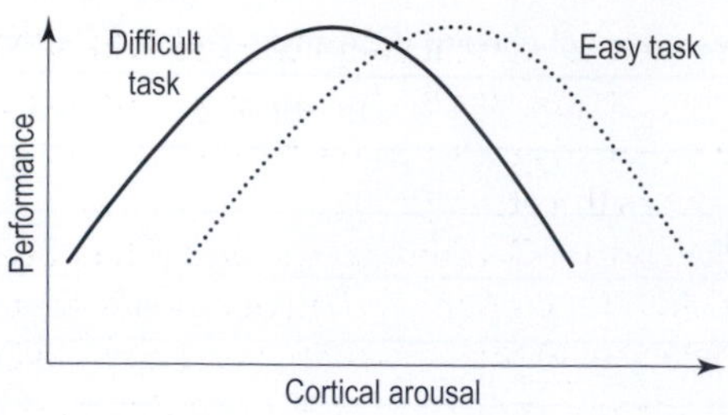

Fig. 4.6 Yerkes–Dodson Law. Performance in two different conditions of task difficulty

The Yerkes–Dodson law

Anxiety serves a useful function under normal circumstances. A certain amount of anxiety is almost a prerequisite for normal functioning in that it helps prepare the individual for the impending event. The relationship between anxiety and performance has been a longstanding subject of study. One of the best known 'laws' in psychology, the Yerkes–Dodson law (1908), states that there is an inverted-U relationship between arousal and performance such that moderate levels of arousal increase task performance up to an optimum level and any further increase in levels of arousal produces a marked decrease in performance. In addition, there is a systematic relationship between task difficulty and performance. Performance on easy tasks is best when arousal is relatively high, whereas a lower level of anxiety is more favourable for difficult tasks (Broadhurst, 1957). This is illustrated in Figure 4.6.

Abnormal anxiety – anxiety disorders

Anxiety disorders form an important group within the psychiatric classification system but anxiety is also a feature of a number of psychiatric disorders including depression and schizophrenia. Abnormal anxiety forms the core of three important conditions: generalised anxiety disorder (GAD); panic disorder; and post-traumatic stress disorder (PTSD). Other disorders included under the umbrella of anxiety disorders are phobic disorders, obsessive-compulsive disorders, adjustment disorder, and dissociative disorder. In each of these conditions high anxiety may be a feature. Because comorbidity is common in anxiety disorders, some authors have made a case for a *general anxiety syndrome*.

Generalised anxiety disorder (GAD)

The key feature of GAD is the persistent and pervasive anxiety, which is not related to any particular situation or environmental circumstances (hence called 'free-floating anxiety'). Features of sympathetic over activity and restlessness are evident together with the subjective feeling of apprehension and dread but the individual is usually unable to identify any event or situation that provoked the state.

Studies using various experimental tasks have consistently shown that in GAD the person shows a distinct predilection or bias in favour of threat-related stimuli.

In other words, compared to normal subjects those with GAD exhibit distorted information processing of potentially threatening situations, as evidenced by selective attention to threatening stimuli, high vigilance and a propensity to interpret ambiguous stimuli as threatening.

Psychological theories of GAD are few. Worry has been implicated as a central feature of GAD. One cognitive theory holds that it is worry about worry (known as metaworry) that produces the vicious cycle that leads to the perpetuation of the anxiety process. For a cognitive perspective on anxiety disorders see Beck and Emery (1985).

Abnormal anxiety – panic disorder

Panic refers to sudden, severe, discrete and short-lived episodes of severe anxiety that are unrelated to a particular situation or the presence of potential danger. When the attacks of panic are frequent and disabling, the syndrome is said to qualify to be called a disorder. Attacks are usually unpredictable. During attacks the individual experiences extreme psychological and physiological distress, but is free of anxiety in-between them. The best-known cognitive theory of panic disorder is that put forward by Clark (1986). Studies on patients with panic disorders (McNally & Foa, 1987) have demonstrated that they show two distinctive features: (1) they tend to interpret ambiguous stimuli of bodily sensations as threatening; and (2) they are more introceptive (perceptive of bodily sensations) than controls.

Sadness

In spite of its obvious relevance to abnormal states like depression and grief, very little is known about sadness. Sadness is unique among emotions in that it does not satisfy an important criterion in the definition of emotions: there is no specific action tendency associated with sadness. In fact, the action tendency in sadness is inaction (Lazarus, 1991). The adaptive value of sadness is also unclear. The antecedent to sadness is usually loss of some sort, for example loss of a loved one from death or separation. However, the loss may be intangible, as in loss of role, power, control or self-esteem. It could also be extended to include disappointment and failure.

The intensity of sadness may vary from mild (apathy, sorrow) to severe (misery, despair, grief, melancholy). Sadness is associated with feelings of helplessness, that nothing can be done and that the situation is beyond one's control. The downcast face and stooping bodily posture is characteristic of sadness. A surprising finding from available research is that sadness and joy are two distinct and discrete emotions, not polar opposites of the same emotional spectrum.

Worry

An emotion close in resemblance to anxiety and sadness is worry. In common with anxiety, feeling worried about day-to-day issues such as relationships, work and health is functional to the extent that it motivates people to get things done. Normal worry has been considered as a mental process aimed at problem solving and as a signal system that warns the individual of impending threat such as a deadline for submission of a piece of work. The key feature of worry is the particular intrusion into one's consciousness of negative thoughts and images, which can be preoccupying and self-absorbing and take the form of ruminations. Excessive worry is often maladaptive and leads to dysfunction and is a central feature of pathological conditions such as anxiety, depression and post-traumatic stress disorder. Interestingly, worry is an area that has been the subject of much study and scrutiny. For an interesting account of this common emotion the reader is referred to the textbook edited by Davey and Tallis (1994).

Depression

Psychology has consistently failed to define the relationship between sadness and depression. It is not at all clear whether depression represents pervasive and serious sadness, i.e. malignant sadness, or an abnormality of the emotion of sadness. It is generally accepted that depression is a complex emotion involving a constellation of emotions such as anger, despair, guilt and anxiety. Helplessness, pessimism and hopelessness are predominant in the mental state of depressed patients, as are loss of enjoyment (anhedonia) and loss of interest.

The two popular psychological theories of depression are Seligman's (modified) theory of learned helplessness (Seligman, 1975) and Beck's model of depression (Beck, 1976). Both are cognitive theories in which learning is purported to play an important part. Both theories, especially Beck's theory, have provided useful working hypotheses that have formed the basis of interventions like cognitive therapy. The concept of learned helplessness was discussed in Chapter 1; Beck's theory of depression is outlined in Chapter 6.

Jealousy

Jealousy is a complex emotion comprising a mixture of fear, anger and sadness. It is unique among emotions in that it involves a third person who is perceived to compete for affection. Jealousy is a powerful emotion that often involves high arousal and occasionally results in violence, and even murder. Jealousy is seen both in males and females and in all cultures. Curiously it is more prevalent in high masculine cultures where freedom for women is highly restricted (Hofstede, 1981).

Jealousy is generated by the perception of a real or potential romantic attraction between one's partner and a rival, either real or imagined (White & Mullen, 1989). It necessarily involves three people, the subject, the object whom the subject loves and a third party (the love triangle), and is therefore situated within interpersonal relationships.

An emotion that is closely related to jealousy is envy. One is envious of the other person's possessions. Unlike jealousy, it is a phenomenon involving only two people.

The antecedents to jealous emotional reactions involve a perception of threat at the possibility of losing one's partner. The situational factors that provoke jealousy are:

- Sexual infidelity. The most intense and destructive reactions are brought about by sexual involvement of the partner with a perceived rival (for example one partner finding the other in bed with the rival). Sexual jealousy is characterised by anger rather than sadness.
- Emotional threat. Jealous reactions are more often elicited by the person 'sensing' that the partner is attracted by another person or is having an affair with them. This may take the form of intense scrutiny of the time that the partner spends with the potential rival.

Primary appraisal involves assessments of the existence of, and degree of threat posed by, the rival. Secondary appraisal processes pertain to coping strategies and the intense search for meaning. White and Mullen (1989) have described the four types of secondary appraisal:

1. Motive assessment. Why the partner finds the rival attractive.
2. Social comparison to rival. Is the rival more desirable than oneself?
3. Alternatives assessment. The options open to oneself.
4. Loss assessment. The effects to self of losing a partner; usually involves emotions such as fear and depression.

Jealousy is an intense experience, involving a number of different emotions. Research indicates that jealous individuals report feelings of hurt, betrayal, rejection, helplessness and confusion, but the three emotions central to jealousy are fear, sadness and anger. These may be accompanied by guilt, shame and embarrassment. The general behaviour responses are varied and numerous (Guerrero et al., 1995):

- Surveillance. Repeated checking up on the partner, looking for 'evidence' of infidelity, e.g. checking handbags, pockets and clothes, spying, following and employing a detective agency.
- Compensatory behaviour. Behaviour intended to improve relationship, e.g. buying presents, etc.
- Restrictions and prohibitions. Limiting or stopping contact of partner with the rival.
- Emotional manipulation. Behaviour aimed at making partner feel guilty, using infidelity threats.
- Contact with the rival in an attempt to stop the relationship.
- Violent behaviour towards partner or rival.

Morbid or pathological jealousy (also called Othello syndrome) may be associated with a number of psychiatric conditions such as dementia, alcohol and substance misuse, depression, paranoid schizophrenia and personality disorders. Morbid jealousy is associated with potential for violence and it is one of the few disorders where there is a real risk of murder.

Anger

Anger has been considered a basic and intense emotion, which carries with it a degree of spontaneity or uncontrollability. No specific anger disorder as such has been described in psychiatry but anger may be a feature of a number of psychiatric conditions. Anger is often a feature of conduct disorder in adolescents and antisocial personality disorder in adults (see Chapter 10 on aggression). The intensity of anger may range from annoyance, hostility and anger to fury and rage. The situations that provoke anger responses are usually interpersonal interactions. The general theme common to all anger-producing situations appears to be personal offence caused by another person. The common clusters of instigation to anger are (Canary, Spitzberg & Semi, 1998):

- Identity threats: insults, blame, rejection, teasing.
- Aggression by other: physical, verbal or sexual.
- Frustration: obstruction of goal, powerlessness.
- Unfairness, unfaithfulness and betrayal.

An interesting finding is that once provoked, the experience of anger is intensified by other factors such as the reaction of the victim or the presence of a weapon ('weapon effect'). The behavioural responses or action tendencies in anger have been grouped into several clusters (Shaver et al., 1987):

- Verbal attacks, including shouting and yelling.
- Physical attacks, including clenched fists and threatening gestures.
- Non-verbal display of protest, frowning, stamping, and slamming doors.
- Uneasiness, crying, discomfort.
- Internal withdrawal, brooding.
- Avoidance, suppression.

Communicating that one is angered by another person's actions is an important aspect of assertive behaviour in day-to-day interactions and a necessary skill to make others reflect on their behaviour. One of the instruments used to assess anger is Spielberger's *state-trait anger scale* (Spielberger, 2004) (see also Chapter 10).

REFERENCES

Beck AT (1976) Cognitive Therapy and Emotional Disorders. New York: Meridian.

Beck A, Emery G (1985) Anxiety Disorders and Phobias: a cognitive perspective. New York: Basic Books.

Broadhurst PL (1957) Emotionality and the Yerkes–Dodson law. Journal of Experimental Psychology, 54, 345–352.

Cacioppo JT, Bernteson GG, Larsen J, Poehlmann KM, Ito TA (2000) The psychophysiology of emotions. In M Lewis & JM Haviland (eds), Handbook of Emotions (2nd ed., pp. 173–191). New York: Guilford Press.

Canary DJ, Spitzberg BH, Semi BA (1998) The experience and expression of anger in interpersonal settings. In PA Anderson & LK Guerrero (eds), Handbook of Communication and Emotion: research theory application and context. San Diego, CA: Academic Press.

Cannon WB (1929) Organisation for physiological homeostatics. Physiological Review, 9, 280–289.

Clark DM (1986) A cognitive approach to panic. Behaviour Research and Therapy, 24, 261–470.

Clark DM, Teasdale JD (1982) Variation in clinical depression and accessibility of memory to positive and negative experiences. Journal of Normal Psychology, 91, 87–95.

Davey GCL (1997) Phobias (Ch. 15, pp. 302–322). Chichester, UK: Wiley.

Davey GCL, Tallis L (eds) (1994) Worrying: perspectives on theory assessment and treatment. Chichester, UK: Wiley.
Easton WW, Kessler LG (eds) (1985) Epidemiologic Field Methods in Psychiatry: the NNIMH epidemiologic catchment area program. Orlando, FL: Academic Press.
Ekman P (1982) Emotions in the Human Face (2nd ed.). New York: Cambridge University Press.
Ekman P (1992) An argument for basic emotions. Cognition and Emotion, 6, 169–20.
Ekman P (2003) Emotions Revealed. New York: Time Books.
Ekman P, Friesen WV (1975) Unmasking the face. Englewood Cliffs, NJ: Prentice Hall.
Fehr B, Russell JA (1984) Concepts of emotion from a prototype perspective. Journal of Experimental Psychology, 113, 464–486.
Fish FJ (1967) Clinical Psychopathology. Bristol, UK: John Wright.
George MS, Ketter TA, Parekh PI, Horowitz B, Herscovitch P, Post RM (1995) Brain activity during transient sadness and happiness in healthy women. American Journal of Psychiatry, 152(3), 341–349.
Guerrero LK, Anderson PA, Jorgensen P, Spitzberg PH, Eloy SV (1995) Coping with the green eyed monster: conceptualising and measuring communicative responses to romantic jealousy. Western Journal of Communication, 59, 270–304.
Hofstede G (1981) Cultures Consequences. International differences in work related values. Beverley Hills, CA: Sage.
Hohman GW (1966) Some effects of spinal cord lesions on experienced emotional feelings. Psychophysiology, 3, 143–156.
James W (1884) What is an emotion? Mind, 9, 188–205.
James W (1890) Principles of Psychology. New York: Holt.
Kendall PC, Finch AJ Jr, Auerbach SM, Hooke JF, Mikulka PJ (1976) The state–trait anxiety inventory: a systematic evaluation. Journal of Consulting and Clinical Psychology, 44, 406–412.
Laird JD (1974) Self attribution of emotion: the affect of facial expression on the quality of emotional experience. Journal of Personality and Social Psychology, 29, 475–486.
Lazarus RS (1991) Emotion and Adaptation. New York: Oxford University Press.
Marks IM (1969) Fears and Phobias. London, UK: Heinemann.
McNally RJ, Foa EB (eds) (1987) Cognition and agoraphobia. Bias in the interpretation of threat. Cognitive Therapy and Research, 1, 567–585.
Rachman S (1997) The evolution of cognitive behaviour therapy. In DM Clarke & CG Fairburn (eds), Science And Practice Of Cognitive Behaviour Therapy. Oxford, UK: Oxford University Press.
Schachter S, Singer JE (1962) Cognitive social and psychological determinants of emotional state. Physiological Review, 69, 379–399.
Seligman M (1971) Phobias and preparedness. Behaviour Therapy, 2, 307–320.
Seligman MEP (1975) Helplessness. San Francisco, CA: Freeman.
Shaver P, Schwarz D, Kirkson D, O'Connor C (1987) Emotional knowledge: future explorations of a prototype approach. Journal of Personality and Social Psychology, 52, 1061–1086.
Spielberger CD (1983) State–Trait Anxiety Inventory Manual. Palo Alto, CA: Consulting Psychologists Press.
Spielberger CD (2004) State–Trait Anger Expression Inventory-2 (STAXI-2). Odessa, FL: Psychological Assessment Resources.
Strongman KT (1996) The Psychology of Emotions: theories of emotion in perspective (4th ed.). Chichester, UK: Wiley.
Teasdale JD, Barnard P (1993) Affect, cognition and change. Mahwah, NJ: Erlbaum.
Teasdale JD (1983) Negative thinking in depression: cause effect or reciprocal relationship? Advances in Behaviour Research and Therapy, 5, 3–25.
White GL, Mullen PE (1989) Jealousy: theory research and clinical strategies. New York: Guilford Press.
Yerkes RM, Dodson JD (1908) The relation of strength of stimulus to rapidity of habit formation. Journal of Comparative Neurology and Psychology, 18, 459–482.
Zajonc RB (1980) Feelings and thinking. Preferences need no inferences. American Psychologist, 35, 151–175.

FURTHER READING

Davey GCL (ed.) (1997) Phobias. Chichester, UK: Wiley.

- A formidable but highly readable account of the contemporary view phobias.

Dobson KS (ed.) (1988) Handbook of Cognitive Behaviour Therapies. London, UK: Hutchinson.

- A good overview of CBT.

Lewis M, Haviland JM (eds) (2000) Handbook of Emotions (2nd ed.). New York: Guilford Press.

- The standard textbook on the subject, with useful chapters on various aspects of emotion.

Oatley K, Jenkins JM (1996). Understanding Emotions. Oxford, UK: Blackwell.

- A readable and up-to-date account of various aspects of emotion.

William JMG, Watts FN, MacLeod C, Mathew A (1997) Cognitive Psychology and Emotional Disorders (2nd ed.). Chichester, UK: Wiley.

- An impressive book that includes normal and abnormal emotional processes.

Motivation

5

'Victory belongs to the most persevering.'
Napoleon Bonaparte

Motivation refers to the processes involved in initiation, direction and persistence of purposeful behaviours. The study of motivation aims to look for the purposes that underlie people's goal-directed behaviour. It seeks to answer the question *why* people choose to think and behave in particular ways. Why do individuals strive for excellence at work or sports at great cost to themselves? Why do people starve themselves to attain a perceived ideal weight? The scope for the study of motivational factors covers almost the entire domain of human behaviour, ranging from biological functions, such as eating, drinking and sexual behaviour, to what people do in social situations, such as work, education, and public life.

It is useful, at the very beginning, to distinguish between two types of motivating forces: homeostatic and non-homeostatic:

- *Homeostatic motives* refer to those motives that arise from physiological needs, such as hunger, thirst and temperature control, that are concerned with basic survival. An example of a homeostatic motive, hunger, is considered in the second part of this chapter.
- *Non-homeostatic motives* are psychological drives that underpin activities aimed at satisfying such phenomena as curiosity, adventure or achievement. Some believe that there are several non-homeostatic motivational systems that direct human behaviour.

Motives may be internal or external, innate or learned, conscious or unconscious. An understanding of the motivational influences that underlie health-harming behaviours such as smoking and drinking are central to designing preventative programmes. In clinical work, motivating people to seek help when necessary and encouraging them to adhere to treatment programmes requires an understanding of the motivational principles that underpin such health-harming behaviours.

THEORIES OF MOTIVATION

In psychology, there have been three distinct traditions relating to the study of motivation (Box 5.1).

1. The *biopsychological* perspective examines the physiological motives in humans and animals, such as hunger, thirst, sexual drive and aggression.

Based on homeostatic and drive theories, these motives are biological and behavioural in their orientation. They are dependant on obtaining something extrinsic to the organism and are therefore also called *extrinsic motivational theories*. The homeostatic drive theory (Cannon, 1929), drive reduction theory (Hull, 1943) and the arousal reduction theory (Hebb, 1949) are examples of this approach.

2. The *sociopsychological* approach addresses the cognitive motives behind people's complex behaviour in the context of their social situations such as work, learning, family and society. The motivational properties are not in the external environment; rather the activities themselves are intrinsically satisfying and rewarding. These theories are hence also called *intrinsic motivational theories*. They include the needs theory (McClelland, 1985) and goal theories (Locke et al., 1981).

NB. Intrinsic and extrinsic *theories* of motivation should not be confused with intrinsic and extrinsic *motivation*. Intrinsic motivation is the desire to do something because one wants to (for pleasure, satisfaction or amusement) whereas extrinsic motivation is behaviour aimed at obtaining rewards or avoiding punishments.

3. *Humanistic theories of motivation* are a third group of motivational theories that attempt to account for why people strive to achieve higher and higher goals in an attempt to attain self-fulfilment. The best-known humanistic theory of motivation is that of Maslow (1943).

Motives as drives: drive theories

Over the past century, two broadly different conceptions of motivation emerged: drive reduction and goal achievement. At the turn of the twentieth century motivation was viewed as a drive, i.e. an internal state, need or condition that impels individuals towards an action. In this tradition needs were thought to reside largely within the individual. These drive theories evolved from the *homeostatic theory* of Cannon (1929). Humans and animals have an overwhelming need to maintain a relatively constant environment (homeostasis). Such physiological needs energise the organism (motivate) to produce goal-directed behaviours. Physiological needs that are concerned with basic

Box 5.1 Theories of motivation

The biopsychological approach
- Homeostatic drive theory (Cannon, 1929)
- Drive reduction theory (Hull, 1943)
- Arousal reduction theory (Hebb, 1949)

The sociopsychological approach
- Needs theory (McClelland, 1985)
- Goal theories (e.g. Locke, 1981)

The humanistic approach
- Maslow's hierarchy of needs (Maslow, 1943)

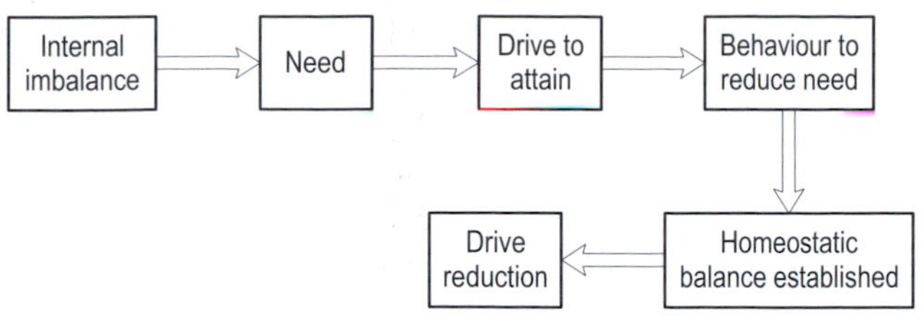

Fig. 5.1 Homeostatic Drive Theory (Cannon, 1929)

survival are often described as 'tissue needs'. Dehydration, for example, is a tissue need that produces thirst, which motivates the organism to seek for water. Tissue needs are said to give rise to psychological states known as *drives*, which motivate the animal to behave in ways that reduce the drives, as shown in Figure 5.1 (Cannon 1929).

Hull, a behaviourist, combined the learning theory with the homeostatic drive theory. For Hull (1943) motivated behaviour was the result of reinforcement. According to him, positive and negative reinforcement were fundamental to drive reduction. Reduction of tissue need (e.g. thirst) by drinking (goal-directed behaviour) reduces the distressing state (negative reinforcement). At the same time, drive reduction produces a positive reinforcement effect. This is shown in Figure 5.2.

Hull produced a series of equations to show that his theory was testable. The basic hypothesis was stated as the equation:

$$\text{Likelihood of learned behaviour} = \text{Drive motivation} \times \text{Habit strength}$$

He later added incentive and other factors to the equation but his basic assumption was that behaviour was the product of drive (motivation) and learning (habit). Drive-reduction theories provide a reasonable explanation as to how primary biological needs, such as hunger, thirst, air, rest, sleep and pain avoidance, are fulfilled but are less satisfactory in accounting for complex behaviours such as curiosity and exploration.

Other workers have attempted to explain motivated behaviour on the basis of a postulated need to maintain arousal at an optimum level, known as the *arousal reduction theory* (Hebb, 1949). Arousal refers to a state of activation of the nervous system mediated via the reticular activation system. People are said to strive to maintain an optimum level of arousal. Individuals who are hypothesised to have low levels of arousal seek out strong stimuli to attain

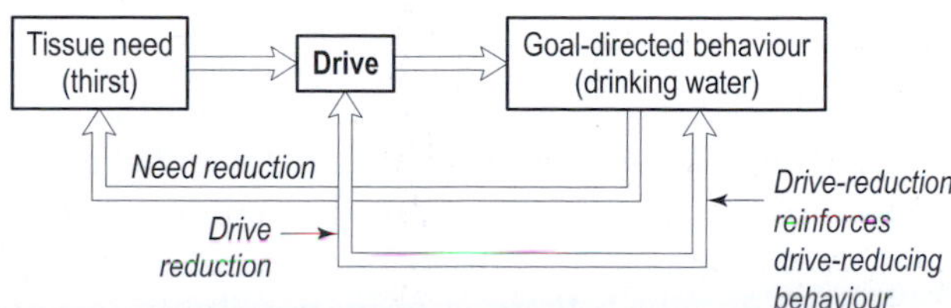

Fig. 5.2 Hull's Drive-Reduction Theory (Hull, 1943)

optimum levels of stimulation ('augmenters') and thrive on stimulation. Those having high basal levels of arousal ('reducers') indulge in calming activities. The concept of arousal has been used to imply a number of different meanings and is somewhat out of fashion in psychology now.

Motives as goals

An alternative view to motives-as-drives is the view that achievement of goals is a powerful motivator of individuals towards action. Goals are what individuals aspire to achieve. The goal/drive distinction is evidently arbitrary. The same achievement behaviour can often be construed as either satisfying a need or achieving a goal. For example, getting a good job is both a need and an achievement. Nevertheless, the choice of goals, actions and strategies and mobilisation effort are crucial manifestations of motivation for achievement. Two general kinds of goals have been described:

1. Mastery or learning goals: seeking to increase one's competency, understanding or mastery of something new.
2. Performance goals: seeking favourable judgements from others.

Two fields in which goal theory has been influential are educational and management. Goal-setting improves performance only when certain conditions are met. Commitment to the goal, feedback about one's performance, rewards for attainment and support from others are necessary for successful task performance (Locke et al., 1981).

'Needs' as motivators

One line of approach to the study of motives is the concept of needs. Needs were conceptualised by Henry Murray (1938) as internal determinants that direct and organise feelings, thoughts and behaviours. He distinguished between primary (viscerogenic) needs, which are physiological (e.g., water, food), and secondary (psychogenic) needs, which are not primarily associated with biological processes. While primary needs are universal to all human beings, secondary needs show marked individual variation from person to person and, according to Murray, constitute an important facet of personality.

Murray identified thirty needs together with a list of environmental factors called 'presses', which influenced their expression. Of these, three needs were held to be of overriding importance: achievement motive; affiliative motive; and power motive. The need for achievement has received the most attention.

Need for achievement

The need for achievement (*nAch*) is defined as the need to do things better than others and achieve a level of excellence (McClelland et al., 1953). Those with a high need for achievement derive satisfaction and pleasure from striving for and achieving goals that they value. People with high *nAch* are attracted to situations in which there is some possibility of improvement. They undertake challenging and realistic ventures and constantly look for competition so that they can prove themselves to be successful. They usually avoid tasks that are too difficult or too easy, the former because failure is certain and the latter because of a lack of the risk of failure. For these people fear of failure is an important consideration in the choice of tasks. They choose tasks that are sufficiently challenging but in which the chances of success are high. They thrive on positive feedback and improvement in performance is their main incentive. They prefer tasks that carry personal responsibility for the outcome so that they get feedback on their achievement.

In contrast, people with a low need for achievement tend to choose very easy or very difficult tasks so that success is assured (in the former case) or because failure is the expected outcome (in the latter) and thus they cannot be blamed. The main components of *nAch* are the belief that work is a good thing, the search for excellence, the wish to dominate others, competitiveness (against predetermined standards, rather than against people), acquisitiveness (desire for money) and mastery.

Achievement need is usually assessed by projective tests rather than by self-report questionnaires because the latter is usually a reflection of the conscious value that people place on achievement. The most commonly used measurement tool is the *Thematic Apperception Test* (TAT) originally developed by Murray (1938). In the assessment of *nAch* the subject is shown pictures associated with the motive. For example, they are shown a picture of an employee knocking at his boss's door and are asked to describe what happens in the picture, the possible antecedents, what the person thinks and the possible outcome.

Achievement motivation has been shown to be an enduring attribute that is learned early in life, mainly from parents who set high standards of performance for their children. Measures of *nAch* have obvious implications in performance, efficiency and attitude towards work in organisations and is hence a hot topic in business management.

The need for affiliation

Social relatedness is a fundamental characteristic of all human beings. The need for affiliation is the need to establish and maintain relationships with other people. The incentive for affiliative motives include:

- Comparing oneself against others as a point of reference (self-referencing) and thus reducing uncertainty.
- Receiving attention from others.
- Being stimulated by social interaction.
- Establishing intimacy.

Those with a high need for affiliation seek out friendships, care for others and value friendships and personal relationships.

The need for power

Exercising power over others is a potent motivational factor seen at all levels of society. The need for power is closely associated with the desire to control

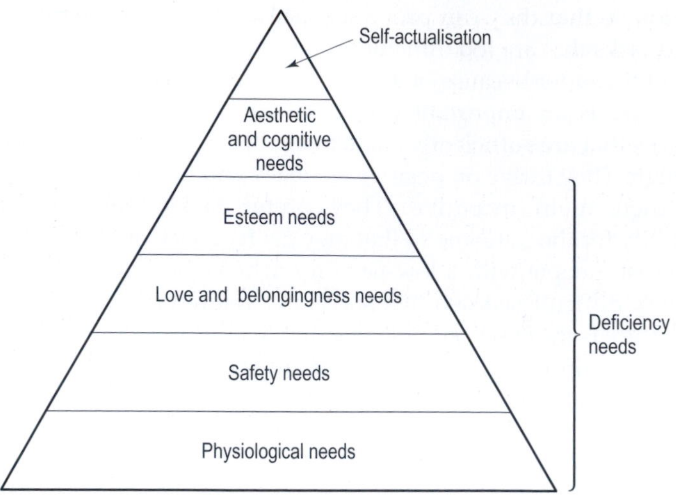

Fig. 5.3 Maslow's hierarchy of needs (Maslow, 1970)

and influence others. Individuals with a high need for power choose careers that allow them to control others and exercise authority over them, such as teaching, management, business and politics.

Maslow's hierarchy of needs

Abraham Maslow (1943, 1970) took a humanistic approach to human motivation by focusing more on the positive side of human nature. For Maslow, self-actualisation – 'becoming everything one is capable of becoming' – is the ultimate goal of all human beings. Maslow ordered the needs along a hierarchy, in which those lower in the hierarchy must be satisfied before the next category of need can be pursued. He delineated six sets, often represented by a pyramid (Fig. 5.3), with physiological needs at the bottom and self-actualisation needs at the apex; the lower four needs are referred to as deficiency needs (Maslow, 1970).

1. *Physiological needs*. Needs for food, water, sleep, activity and sex.
2. *Safety needs*. Needs for safety, security, freedom from pain.
3. *Love and belonging needs*. The need to give and receive affection and love. Also included here is the need for affiliation and membership of groups.
4. *Esteem needs*. The need to develop a sense of personal worth and competence and the need for recognition by others.
5. *Aesthetic and cognitive needs*. These are growth needs involving knowledge, understanding, beauty, justice, order and symmetry.
6. *Self-actualisation needs*. The need to attain one's highest potential in one's own unique way. The motivation is not to meet deficits, as in other needs, but to enrich one's life.

Although self-actualisation as a motive exists in all people, not all people are self-actualisers. Maslow considered people such as Albert Einstein, Abraham Lincoln and Ghandi to have reached the stage of self-actualisation. According to Maslow, some features of self-actualisers are:

- They show greater acceptance of themselves.
- They have a fresh outlook.
- They have peak experiences.
- They are ethical and creative.
- They are not easily seduced by society.

Maslow's vision of self-actualisers became the philosophy of the humanist movement and the rallying point for Carl Rogers and other humanistic psychologists. He has been criticised by others for being overly optimistic about human nature and justifying selfish individualism. The merit of Maslow's hierarchy of needs lies in the fact that it emphasises the fact that until certain basic needs are met, people will not engage in achieving higher-order needs. An unemployed lone parent struggling to bring up children would need material and social assistance before pursuing self-knowledge and self-advancement, a fact that middle-class professionals need to be aware of. The hierarchy of needs serves as a useful framework for viewing people's needs and priorities in a systematic and ordered way. It is a particularly useful construct when dealing with adults and children who experience social and emotional deprivation.

Case example

A 13-year-old boy was referred to child mental health services as an emergency because of extreme erratic behaviour at school. He had run out of the class in a very disturbed emotional state and, according to the teachers, his speech was incoherent and he was shaking uncontrollably. According to the head teacher, he had never seen such behaviour in his 20 years as a teacher. The teachers and the GP were convinced that the boy was experiencing a 'psychotic break down'. When seen in the clinic, it became evident that the family had been homeless for a month and had been living in a car. Apart from the practical difficulties, he had been subject to ridicule by his mates who made remarks like, 'Where is your toilet?' He was, understandably, extremely upset and angry about the situation. In this case, the teachers could only see his behaviour and not the fact that basic needs were not fulfilled. (It is not uncommon for some professionals to assign behaviour that they find difficult to understand to mental illnesses.)

Motivation in clinical practice

Research on motivation has important implications in clinical practice, where more effective ways are needed to encourage and sustain changes in maladaptive behaviours. Getting people to take up healthy behaviours such as adopting a healthy lifestyle (e.g. exercising and using safe sex practices) have important public health significance.

Two recent developments in motivation in clinical work are the systematic study of how people go through the process of change and an interview technique aimed at motivating people who are unsure about changing their behaviour. These are mentioned briefly here, the reader may find the original works rewarding to study (see further reading).

Stages of change

Recent advances in motivation research emphasise the importance of internal factors in the maintenance of positive behaviours, such as stopping smoking or drinking and participation in therapeutic programmes. One helpful model of how change occurs is that of Prochaska and DiClemente (1984). According to their *stages of change model*, change in behaviour, especially health-related behaviour, is thought to follow five key stages:

1. *Pre-contemplation*. The individual has not considered the possibility of change.
2. *Contemplation*. The individual is ambivalent about change, being aware of both reasons to change and reasons to stay the same.
3. *Preparation*. The individual is prepared to take action.
4. *Action*. The individual is currently engaged in attempts to change.
5. *Maintenance*. The individual has been successful in achieving a change in behaviour. However, some patients may withdraw (relapse phase).

The authors have developed interview methods and measures to identify the current stage of motivation of the client.

Motivational interviewing

An innovative method of motivating people to change is the technique of *motivational interviewing*. Miller, the pioneer of the method, defines motivational interviewing as 'a client-centred, directive method for enhancing intrinsic motivation to change by exploring and resolving ambivalence' (Miller & Rollnick, 2002). According to the model, motivation is not a trait that resides in the client; it arises from an interpersonal process. Motivational interviewing is essentially a method of communicating with the person in a way that elicits the person's own reasons for, and advantages of, change rather than advising, prescribing or advocating change. Motivational interviewing is based on the assumption that most individuals are still ambivalent about changing their behaviour, such as drinking, drug taking or dieting, when they consult for treatment. Therefore, attempts to get the patient to confront the problem by challenging, advising or instructing often leads to 'defensive reactions' rather than change. Motivational interviewing is a particular way of helping people recognise and do something about their present or potential problem. The interview model is described as 'confrontational in purpose but not in style'.

It is particularly helpful with people who are reluctant to change or ambivalent about changing. Motivational interviewing techniques are most useful during the pre-contemplation and contemplation stages of change. It has been shown to be effective in dealing with alcohol and other addictive behaviours and, more recently, eating disorders. The technique is based on four guiding principles (Miller & Rollnick, 2002):

1. *Express empathy* without judging, criticising or blaming.
2. *Develop discrepancy* by creating and amplifying the inconsistency between present behaviour and the person's broader goals and values. The client rather than the clinician should present the arguments for change.

3. *Roll with resistance* in order to turn the resistance that the client offers into new momentum for change. It goes without saying that confrontation has to be avoided.
4. *Support self-efficacy* in the person's belief in the possibility of change and place the responsibility for choosing and enforcing change on the client.

Treatment compliance, adherence and concordance

Another area of study is treatment compliance and motivation to adhere to treatment programmes including adherence to drug treatment and psychotherapy. Studies on treatment compliance show that about half the patients with chronic illnesses, such as diabetes and hypertension, are non-compliant with their medication regimens. Non-compliance with medication in patients with chronic mental illnesses is recognised as a serious problem. In a study of 200 patients with first episodes of psychosis, for example, almost 40% had stopped taking the medication within the first year (Coldham, Addington & Addington, 2002). Although the reasons for non-adherence to medication are many, including the side effects of medication and the effect of the illness on the individual's general and social functioning, lack of motivation is an important factor.

The concept of compliance has been criticised as a concept that devalues the patient's autonomy and dignity while fostering the power and authoritarianism of doctors. In order to bridge the gap between the agendas of doctors and patients, a more robust model called *concordance* has been proposed as a way of moving to a more collaborative way of working (Royal Pharmaceutical Society of Great Britain, 1997). Concordance describes the process whereby patients and professionals exchange their views on treatment and come to an agreement about the need (or not) for a particular treatment.

Every clinical encounter is concerned with two sets of contrasting and equally cogent health beliefs – those of the client or patient and those of the clinician. The client's health beliefs may or may not be congruent with those of the clinician although the latter is professionally more informed. The intention is to form a therapeutic alliance to help the client make as informed a choice as possible. For doctors it means a change in values from the ethos of 'doctor knows best' to one of partnership; for the patient this implies active involvement in the processes and taking responsibility.

Enlightened views hold that prescribing medication and treatment regimes involve four important tasks (Elwyn, Edwards & Britten, 2003):

- Eliciting patients' views about having to take medicines.
- Exploring those views with the patient.
- Informing the patient of the advantages and disadvantages of taking and not taking medicine.
- Involving the patient in treatment decisions (and deferring decisions, if necessary).

In general, treatment programmes that vest control in the patient (internal control) rather than in the service system (external control) are more effective in producing long-term compliance. The critical factor appears to be how the procedure is communicated (framed) to the patient.

HUNGER AND APPETITE

Having discussed non-homeostatic needs, we next turn to homeostatic needs. Hunger and eating have been considered prototypical motivational forces that involve fundamental biological and physiological factors. Questions such as what causes us to start eating, what makes us stop eating, why it is easier to gain weight than to lose weight may seem basic but the answers are not simple. Our knowledge of the regulation of hunger and appetite, eating behaviour and regulation of body weight are incomplete and fragmentary. An understanding of the factors and mechanisms that determine eating is important because, in Western societies, around one third of the population is obese and about 2% of females have serious eating disorders. Moreover, disturbance of appetite and eating is common in other psychiatric disorders such as depression.

It is tempting to suggest that biological factors play a powerful role in eating behaviour because of its obvious relevance to our survival. It is now clear from various lines of research that eating is rarely begun or ended by physiological signals alone and the motivations for food intake are not exclusively physiological – social and psychological factors play a more powerful role. In fact, the mechanism that controls appetite, hunger and eating is a typical example of interaction of bio–psycho–social factors in human and animal behaviour.

Our understanding of the processes involved in the intake of food has undergone remarkable change over the last two decades and some traditional theories have been shown to be outdated. In the past, a distinction was made between hunger and appetite. The former was thought to be a biologically based sensation and the latter to stem from psychological factors. Recent work shows this assumption to be false. Another erroneous belief is that energy balance is intimately connected to hunger and food intake. This too has been proved to be wrong, and current studies focus on determinants of meal frequency and meal size. Before considering factors that control initiation and cessation of eating, it is worth reviewing the phases involved in food intake.

Phases of a meal

Each meal consists of three phases – initiation, maintenance and cessation – with each phase separated from the next by an inter-meal period (Figure 5.4).

In physiological terms these correspond to the four phases of digestion:

1. Pre-ingestion or cephalic phase (part of inter-meal period).
2. Ingestion or oral phase (initiation).
3. Post-ingestion (gastric and intestinal) phase (inter-meal period).
4. Post-absorptive phase (inter-meal phase).

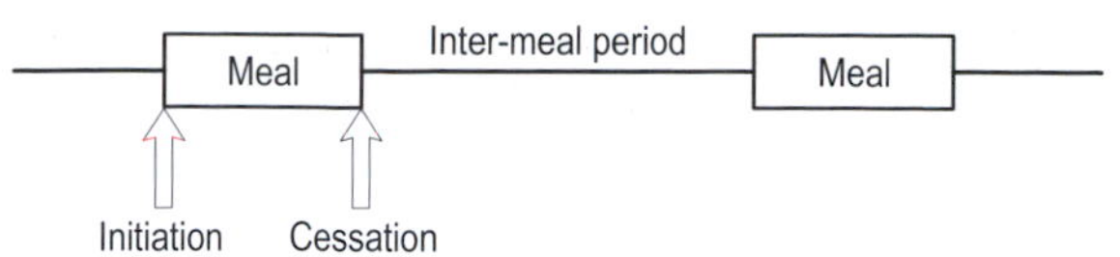

Fig. 5.4 Phases of a meal

The traditional view that eating behaviour is controlled by a feedback loop consisting of hunger that initiates eating and satiety signals that terminate eating are only partially true. Eating may occur without hunger (the extra dessert!) and, in spite of severe hunger, one may deny oneself of food (due to famine or extreme poverty or in hunger-strike). Bio-psycho-social factors are closely involved in both the initiation and cessation of eating and interact with each other in numerous ways. They are considered separately for the sake of clarity.

Initiation of eating

The beginning of the eating process is brought about by a combination of signals. The main stimuli involved are as follows:

Psychological factors. The thought, smell and sight of food are the most potent stimuli for the initiation of eating. These involve conditioned reflexes that are learned on the basis of past experiences leading to conditioned preferences and aversions. Pre-ingestive signals, such as anticipation of food and the smell and flavour of food, are powerful determinants of food intake, while during the ingestive phase palatability of food is by far the most effective drive. Palatability of food acts as a strong reinforcer, producing an incentive to eat. Sweet-tasting foods, like sweetened drinks, produce a 'craving' for similar foods. (This finding has been exploited by the food industry. On the one hand, adding sweeteners like saccharine to drinks increases 'craving', but, on the other hand it doesn't provide calories, thus hunger for the product is increased. Similarly, the high salt content of 'pop' drinks induces thirst, which results in drinking more of the same.)

Foods that involve a variety of flavours and tastes are more satisfying than a single palatable food and result in more eating and larger meal sizes in both man and animals. Similar-tasting food produces satiety relatively rapidly in both rats and humans. Conditioned hunger is common. From infancy the timing of food intake plays an important part in establishing a pattern of eating as certain 'meal times' become associated with eating. Feeding and eating are linked with care giving and provision of comfort from infancy onwards. The distressed infant crying in hunger is comforted and fed by the mother, this establishing a strong link between food on one hand and care and comfort on the other. Psychoanalytic theories emphasis the feeding relationship and the meaning of food or what it stands for. It is thought to symbolise the mother–child relationship whether the parent is real (in childhood and adolescence) or internalised and symbolic.

Biological factors. Contrary to the common belief that contraction of the stomach produces hunger, experiments have shown that an empty stomach is not necessary for initiation of eating. Indeed, it has been demonstrated that involvement of the stomach is not necessary to produce the sensation of hunger – patients who have had a total gastrectomy still report hunger. A number of metabolic signals trigger food intake. Chemical stimuli arising from the blood level of nutrients appear to influence food intake to a degree. A transient decline in blood glucose has been shown to have an effect on initiation of eating, but this is considered to be a weak signal compared to psychosocial and environmental stimuli, especially those that have been learned as part of daily routine. The hypothalamus and liver appear to be sites of glucoreceptors, neurones sensitive to local glucose levels. They appear to provide the signals that trigger feeding. Similar neuroreceptors sensitive to fatty acids (liporeceptors) also appear to be involved in generating feeding signals. It must be emphasised that these feedback mechanisms (previously called glucostatic and lipostatic theories), once hypothesised to be highly significant determinants of eating, play only a minor part in generating feeding signals.

Social factors. It is a common experience that we tend to eat more when eating in the company of others. This appears to be true of rats as well. Rats fed in groups eat more food than those eating in isolation. Cultural attitudes to food are by far the most important social factors that determine the quantity and pattern of eating in man. In Western societies females are under enormous pressure to strive for an idealised body shape and weight. It has been estimated that, at any given time, about half of all teenage girls and young women are on a 'diet'. This trend is fast spreading to men and to the 'developing' countries.

Cessation of eating

Cessation of eating is usually brought about by satiety. Satiety is the inhibition of hunger produced by ingestion of food. Several factors appear to act in concert to determine satiety.

Psychological factors. As in initiation of eating, pre-ingestive and preabsorptive factors play a crucial role in inducing satiety, and include both unconditioned and conditioned learning.

Biological factors. Two sets of overlapping negative feedback signals have been shown to operate together to produce satiety. The neural mechanism, which consist of reflexes that have the overall effect of inhibiting eating, and the chemoreceptive mechanism, which is responsible for secretion of inhibitory gut hormones.

Neural mechanisms:

- Sequential stimulation of receptors in the mouth and small intestine release peptides from the stomach and small intestine that inhibit feeding.
- Distension of the stomach and intestine stimulates mechanoreceptors, which activate vagal afferents that produce cessation of eating. It is likely that these visceral afferents produce their effect via gastrin-releasing peptide.

Gut hormones. Several gut hormones released in response to food in the small intestine are considered to be important satiety signals. There are two well-known gut 'satiety hormones': (1) Cholecystokinin (CCK), a peptide produced by the small intestine; and (2) Pancreatic glucagon, another hormone identified in both animals and humans, which inhibits food ingestion. More recently, it has been discovered that CCK is also released in the brain. CCK appears to act on receptors in the brain to induce satiety. Two important features of gut peptides deserve to be emphasised. First, the satiety-inducing effect of gut hormones take place before the absorption of food and digested material, i.e. in the pre-absorptive phase. In experimental situations, when intraduodenal and intravenous infusions of glucose are administered that produce identical blood glucose levels, the former decreases hunger and meal size, the latter does not. Second, the effect of the neural and hormonal satiety effects are not just additive, they act synergistically to produce exponential effects.

Brain mechanisms and eating

It used to be believed that the hypothalamus regulated food intake, that the lateral hypothalamus (LH) was the 'hunger centre' and that the ventromedial hypothalamus (VMH) was the 'satiety centre'. This 'hypothalamic hypothesis' was based on experimental findings that damage to the LH reduces feeding and electrical stimulation of it causes increased eating (hyperphagia). Ablation and stimulation of the VMH resulted in correspondingly opposite effects. Recent research has disproved this hypothesis, and the hypothalamus, though thought to play an important part in eating, is no longer believed to be the seat of feeding regulation. Ablation and stimulation of the hypothalamic areas appears to have involved the other tracts and neurones as well. Current brain models of feeding motivation are based on neural networks distributed in various parts of the brain (Leeg, 1994).

The brain structures implicated in the central control of eating are now understood to occur at three interconnected levels (Figure 5.5). Brain-stem networks are responsible for basic physiological control of eating. Palatability of food is thought to provide the signal to eat or reject the food. Decerebrate cats (whose hindbrains are disconnected from the diencephalons and forebrain) are capable of ingesting and rejecting food (consummator behaviour) but will not search for food (appetitive behaviour). The decerebrate cat cannot learn taste-aversion association, indicating that neurones at a higher level are necessary for conditioning. The hypothalamus integrates the internal and external information as well as organising neural signals from higher areas (especially prefrontal region) and the lower brain-stem networks. Hypothalamic neurones respond to the taste and smell of food. Conditioned learning appears to occur at a hypothalamic level. The cortex is responsible for integration of input from memory, sight and smell of food.

The neurotransmitters dopamine and serotonin, and also opioids, have been shown to play an important part in the regulation of eating. Dopamine plays an important role in the promotion of eating by its effect on reinforcement and enjoyment of food. Serotonin has an inhibitory effect on eating.

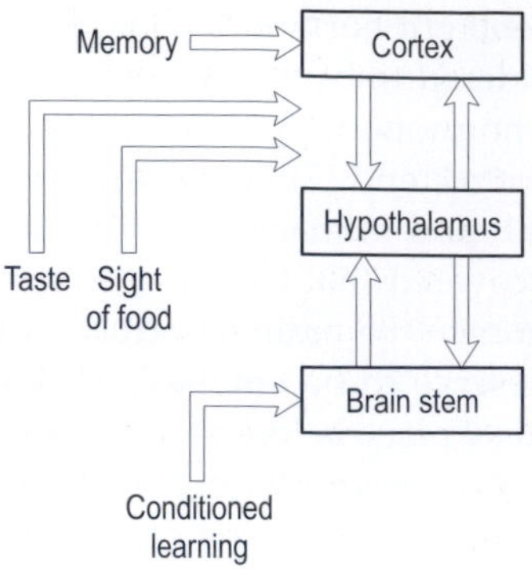

Fig. 5.5 Brain mechanisms involved in satiety and ingestion

On the one hand, endogenous opioids appear to have a specific role in enhancing palatability, while, on the other hand, palatable foods, such as sweet or high-fat foods, increase endogenous opioid secretion and prolong meals.

In man, the mechanisms for the production of the sensation of hunger are strong and more highly developed than those for satiety. While the signals indicating the lack of food are strong and powerful, the feedback from increasing food intake is weak and often overridden by other factors. The homeostatic control of food intake is thus incomplete and skewed in the direction of intake. Therefore the propensity of human beings to over eat, and hence the tendency to become obese, is quite marked.

Psychological effects of starvation

One of the most significant findings from research into eating disorders is that severe starvation produces psychological effects that are not dissimilar to the clinical features of anorexia nervosa; many of the symptoms of anorexia nervosa, which were once regarded as primary features of the illness, are in fact symptoms of starvation.

One of the most revealing studies into the effects of food restriction and weight loss was 'the starvation study' carried out by Keys and colleagues at the University of Minnesota over half a century ago (Keys et al., 1950). They carefully selected 36 physically and psychologically healthy volunteers who, during the first three months, were observed and tested for their eating pattern and personality. After this period of baseline assessment, their food intake was restricted to half their normal intake. During the following six months they lost an average of 25% of their weight. They showed a number of striking changes in their behaviours, cognitions and feelings. All the men showed an extreme preoccupation with food. Their minds were constantly occupied with thoughts of food and eating, and food became their main topic of conversation. They smuggled food, became interested in cookbooks and menus, and collected recipes and cooking utensils. Hoarding objects unrelated to eating (e.g. old books) was observed in a few. Their eating habits showed remarkable change. They spent most of their time planning how they would eat their allocated rations. They ate their food slowly and took hours to finish eating. Binge eating was common and they broke the rules of the experiment to eat large quantities of food. Interestingly some of them hid their rations without eating.

Emotional and personality changes too were prominent. In spite of their psychological robustness at the beginning of the experiment, most experienced significant depression, extreme emotional distress and, in a few cases, periods of elation. Irritability and anger outbursts were common and two subjects developed psychotic-like symptoms. Bizarre behaviours, like shoplifting of items like trinkets, occurred, and self-harming behaviour was witnessed in one subject. Cognitive changes such as impaired concentration, poor judgement and lack of alertness was common. They reported a drastic reduction in sexual interest and a lack of sexual desire.

At the end of the experiment, when they were rehabilitated by refeeding, most of their abnormal attitudes and behaviours regarding food persisted for the next three months. Some complained of feeling fat and flabby. What made the Minnesota starvation experiment remarkable was that it clearly demonstrated that semi-starvation by itself produced clinical features that are characteristic of anorexia nervosa. It follows from this that weight restoration alone could be expected to reverse some of the features of the illness. An accurate assessment of psychological functioning could only be made after the weight was restored to near-normal levels.

REFERENCES

Cannon WB (1929) Bodily Changes in Pain, Hunger, Fear and Rage (2nd ed.). New York: Appleton.

Coldham EL, Addington J, Addington D (2002) Medication adherence of individuals with first episode of psychosis. Acta Psychiatrica Scandinavia, 106, 286–290.

Elwyn G, Edwards A, Britten N (2003) 'Doing Prescribing': how doctors can be more effective. British Medical Journal, 327, 864–867.

Hebb DO (1949) The Organization of Behaviour: a neuropsychological theory. New York: Wiley.

Hull CL (1943) Principles of Behaviour. New York: Appleton-Century-Crofts.

Keys A, Brozek J, Henschel A, Mickelsen O, Taylor HL (1950) The Biology of Human Starvation (2 Vols). Minneapolis, MN: University of Minnesota Press.

Leeg CR (1994) Appetite: neural and behavioural bases. London, UK: Oxford University Press.

Locke EA (1982) A New Look at Work Motivation: theory V (Technical Report GS-12). Arlington, VA: Office of Naval Research.

Locke EA, Shaw KN, Saari LM, Latham GP (1981) Goal-setting and task performance: 1969–1980. Psychological Bulletin, 90, 125–152.

Maslow AH (1943) Dynamics of personality organisation, I and II. Psychological Review, 50, 514–558.

Maslow AH (1970) Motivation and Personality (2nd ed.). New York: Harper & Row.

McClelland DC (1985) Human Motivation. Glenview, IL: Scott, Foresman & Co.

McClelland DC, Atkinson MW, Clark RA, Lowell EL (1953) The Achievement Motive. New York: Appleton-Century-Crofts.

Miller WR, Rollnick S (2002) Motivational Interviewing: preparing people for change (2nd ed.). New York: Guilford Press.

Murray HA (1938) Explorations in Personality. New York: Oxford University Press.

Prochaska JO, DiClemente CC (1984) The Transtheoretical Approach: crossing the traditional boundaries of therapy. Malabar, FL: Krieger.

Royal Pharmaceutical Society of Great Britain (1997) From Compliance to Concordance: achieving shared goals in medicine taking. London, UK: RPS.

FURTHER READING

Miller WR, Rollnick S (2002) Motivational Interviewing: preparing people for change (2nd ed.). New York: Guilford Press.

- The definitive book on motivational interviewing.

An introduction to cognitive psychology

6

'Our normal waking consciousness, rational consciousness as we call it, is but one type of consciousness, whilst all about it, parted from it by filmiest of screens, there lie potential forms of consciousness entirely different. We may go through life without suspecting their existence; but apply the requisite stimulus, and at a touch they are there in all their completeness.'
William James, 1960, pioneer American psychologist

Historically, psychology has always considered that its subject matter, the study of the mind, could be divided into three parts – cognition, affection and conation, called the trilogy of mind. Cognition, broadly defined, is concerned with the processes involved in how we come to know the world. Affection, or affect, is a general term used to describe emotions, feelings and mood. Conation is the term used to describe mental processes associated with volition, striving, activity and behaviour. This tripartite classification of mental activities has been helpful in describing the entire universe of psychology as it is studied, researched and experienced (Box 6.1).

During the various phases of the trilogy's historical development one or other of its components – cognition, affect or behaviour – gained temporary dominance, resulting in the relative subordination of the other two fields. During the era of behaviourism that lasted until the 1960s, the study of cognition and emotions were neglected, and even derided. In contemporary psychology it is cognitive psychology that is on the ascendancy. Yet the old trilogy is a useful frame of reference because it helps to remind us of aspects that are neglected in study and application and re-engages us with the global sweep of the subject matter of psychological science (Hilgard, 1980).

Cognition is defined as the act, or processes, of knowing. Cognitive psychology is concerned with how human beings come to know the world and the processes involved in acquiring this knowledge. Thus, the term cognition refers to the highest levels of mental processes, such as perception, memory, abstract thinking, reasoning and problem solving, as well as the more integrative control processes subsumed under the name *executive functions*. The most striking difference between the approach adopted by cognitive psychologists and behaviourists is that the former are interested in what happens between the stimulus and response.

The cognitive revolution. Cognitions depend on the information-processing systems. In the 1950s, the information-processing theory proposed the notion of the human mind as an information processor, together with the associated concept of feedback and control. This approach was further enhanced by the invention of the computer. The computer as a metaphor for the mind was intuitively appealing because complex outcomes were shown to be produced by simple instructions. The mind was conceptualised not as 'a thing' but as 'a system of procedures operating on symbols'.

Box 6.1 The tripartite division of mind

- *Cognition*. Perception, thinking, memory, reasoning, problem solving
- *Conation*. Volition, will, activity, behaviour
- *Affect(ion)*. Feeling, sentiment, emotion

These advances coincided with the intellectual challenge to behaviourism that came from Naom Chomsky and others, whose all-out attack on Burrhus Skinner shook the very foundations of behaviourism. According to the radical behaviourist school, language was nothing more than verbal behaviour learned through trial and error involving conditioning principles. In a well-argued article Chomsky challenged Skinner's view about the acquisition of language by children (Chomsky, 1959). Children acquire language within two years of birth and for it to be learned through reinforcement, argued Chomsky, was an impossibility. He proposed that aspects of language production are innate. These and other findings that came out around this time brought about the downfall of behaviourism and ushered in the cognitive revolution in psychology.

The mind, according to the cognitive model, was a sort of central processing unit, the centre of operations and computations. Hence, what proponents of the theory meant by cognition was 'all the processes by which sensory input is transformed, reduced, elaborated, stored, recovered and used' (Neisser, 1967, p. 4). Cognitive psychology places information processing at the centre of our mental processes. Thus the S–R paradigm of behaviourism is replaced by the stimulus–information processing–response paradigm. Cognitive activities play a pivotal role in information processing. They are usually abstract in nature, involving representation, beliefs, expectancy, intentionality, and so forth. The rest of this chapter provides an outline of the general process involved in cognition, followed by a brief description of some very selected aspects of cognition. Although important, thinking and speech are not dealt with in this book.

The Information Processing Model. The information model provides a structure containing four components: input; integration; storage; and output. Information flowing from stimuli (input) are selected, attended to and analysed, transformed and retrieved, i.e. processed. The output takes the form of actions, behaviour, speech, and so on (Figure 6.1).

Automatic and conscious (controlled) processes

Often most cognitive processes, such as perception, attention and thinking, are assumed to be conscious processes operating within one's awareness. As the 'cognitive revolution' swept through the field of psychology and the information-processing paradigm became established, the emphasis was placed mostly, if not exclusively, on conscious cognitive processes. Research carried out on perception, attention and thinking were almost entirely involved with conscious processes and goal-directed activities. Do we perceive stimuli before we become aware of them? Do past memories that are not retrievable influence our behaviour? These are some of the questions that experimental psychologists have grappled with in the recent past.

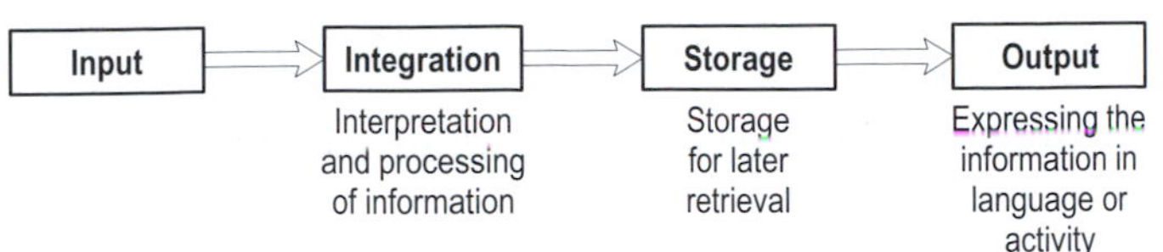

Fig. 6.1 The information processing model

Experimental psychology has always recognised that certain cognitive phenomena are not available to conscious awareness and these were variously referred to as 'pre-conscious', 'pre-attentive' and 'implicit' processes. There is now extensive evidence for non-conscious attention, non-conscious perception, non-conscious learning and non-conscious memory (Shevrin & Dickman, 1980).

Non-conscious attention. There is now general agreement that the part of cognition related to attention takes place outside of awareness. Automatic and non-conscious selective attention to some stimuli and the exclusion of others from the field of attention has been demonstrated in a number of experiments on auditory perception on dichotic listening tasks (see later).

Non-conscious perception. An example of non-conscious visual perception is *subliminal perception*. Subliminal stimuli are those stimuli that do not become conscious simply because they are weak in intensity, even though they may be highly pertinent. In experiments, these stimuli are presented so quickly that they remain undetectable and hence do not enter awareness. Nevertheless, they have been shown to have detectable effects on conscious processes, both immediately and, in some cases, after an interval of time (and in dreams). In one typical experiment the subliminal stimuli were interspersed with conscious stimuli. The subliminal stimulus was either the word *angry* or the word *happy*, while the conscious stimulus was faced with an ambiguous expression that could be judged either way. The subjects were shown to report the face as angry or happy depending on the subliminal exposure to the angry/happy word stimulus (Bach & Klein, 1957).

Non-conscious learning. There is substantial experimental support, too much to be recounted here, for the existence of non-conscious or implicit learning.

Non-conscious memory. Over the last two decades there has been a general acceptance that certain aspects of memory may function without awareness. A striking example of unconscious memory process is implicit or non-declarative memory (see Chapter 7).

Almost one hundred years after Freud spoke of mental unconscious processes, scientific psychology has come to accept (albeit with certain reservations) that unconscious cognitive processes exert a powerful influence on our psychological processes. There is now compelling evidence to support the following conclusions (Shevrin & Dickman, 1980):

- The conscious cognitive processes that we know as perception, memory, thought, learning, and so forth, involve corresponding non-conscious processes. The initial stages of all conscious processes occur outside consciousness. Non-conscious processes influence and affect processing of information at every stage.

- Non-conscious processes are active in that they affect ongoing behaviour and experience, even though the person may be unaware of these influences
- The rules governing conscious and non-conscious mental operations are fundamentally different. Non-conscious cognition has almost unlimited capacity, involves parallel processing and is insensitive to strategic manipulations. In contrast, conscious cognitive processes are of limited capacity and more flexible.

The clinical implications of automatic cognitive processes are far reaching indeed, especially so for cognitive behaviour therapies (see later).

PERCEPTION

Our sense organs – eyes, ears, skin, nose and proprioceptors – are bombarded with an array of stimuli from the environment every minute of our lifetime. Sensing and perceiving the environment and the stimuli that impinge on us effectively and accurately is fundamental to our daily life and, indeed, to our survival. Sometimes a distinction is made between sensation and perception. *Sensation* refers to the registration and encoding of sensory data from the sense organs. It involves the transformation of physical energy, such as sound or light, into neural signals. *Perception* refers to the process by which we make sense of the sensory data, interpreting them and transforming them into experiences of sight, sounds, taste, and so on. Conscious awareness or the outcome of the perceptual process is known as a *percept*. The boundary between sensation and perception is blurred for we cannot experience a sensation without elaboration and interpretation. For example, what is written on this page is a collection of lines and shapes (sensations) that are made out to be letters and words (percepts). Perception is thus an active process involving comparison with past experience, filling in missing information and making sense of sensory data.

Perception is the access point to all other forms of cognition. It serves the purpose of generating a faithful internal representation of meaningful events from the external world, which are often, but not invariably, used for higher cognitive performance. Each modality of perception (for example, visual or auditory) has its unique features. Most research has focused on visual perception, perhaps because it lends itself to study better than other perceptual systems. The following account refers mainly to visual perception.

Perception may be seen to be occurring in two stages:

1. *Perceptual organisation*. This involves the establishment of the features of an object, such as colour, size, movement and form (feature description).
2. *Object recognition*. This entails the matching of the pattern to existing representations of that object (object identification). Thus a voice is perceived not only as sounds but as words articulated by the owner of the voice. A more sophisticated form of visual recognition is face recognition.

During the process of visual perception, sensory stimuli are held briefly (for about 250 to 500 milliseconds) in *sensory memory* as iconic images. During this time perceptual processes analyse, interpret and recognise the object. It is then transferred to *working memory* to be encoded. Thus, working memory is based not on sensory stimuli but on the perception of those stimuli. Herein lies a possible source of perceptual abnormalities such as illusions (errors of perception) and hallucinations (false perceptions).

Perceptual organisation

Visual processing is an active process that provides information about the colour, form, position, movement and other attributes of an object. But in order to make a coherent picture out of these fragments of information the perceptual system is thought to employ different strategies. The pioneering work of Gestalt psychologists – a group of German psychologists who studied patterns – has been influential in understanding some of the fundamental principles of the organisation of visual stimuli. *Gestalt principles* hold that mental experiences can only be understood if they are viewed as organised whole structures; they are not revealed by simply analysing the several parts that make them up. The main Gestaltist principle is summarised by their slogan, 'the whole (the Gestalt) is greater than the sum of its parts'. Gestalt psychologists argued that perception, learning and other cognitive functions could not be understood by studying their discrete components or by treating them as a simple combination of elements, rather they should each be seen as an organised whole.

Gestalt principles

One of the earliest findings of the Gestalt psychologists was the phenomenon of 'apparent perception'. This refers to the phenomenon whereby two lights flashed in succession produce the illusion of continuous motion, which is the principle underlying cinema and television images. Well known among these principles are the *Gestalt laws of organisation*. These refer to the tendency to group stimuli together such that we tend to see meaningful whole objects even when viewing the simplest collection of visual objects. Among the most well known are the laws involving *proximity* (objects that are close together are seen as forming a group), *similarity* (elements that are similar are seen as a group), *closure* (the tendency to fill in missing parts or areas to create a whole), *continuity* (the tendency to see continuous forms such as lines and disregard other possibilities), *texture* (the tendency to group together items with a similar texture), *simplicity* (grouping items together in the simplest way) and *common fate* (grouping together sets of objects moving in the same direction at the same speed) (Figure 6.2).

Another well-known Gestalt concept is *figure–ground perception*. This describes the relationship between the object of focus and the rest of the perceptual field (background). In perceiving an object we tend to single out the features of that object and disregard those in the background. The diagram

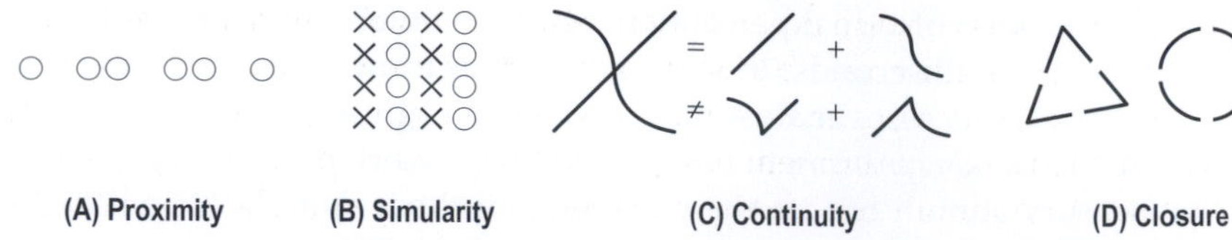

Fig. 6.2 Gestalt principles of perceptual grouping: **(A)** We tend to perceive groups of two circles plus two single circles, rather than as three groups of two circles or some other arrangement; **(B)** we see two columns of Os, not four rows of XOXO; **(C)** we see the X as being made up of two continuous lines, not as the odd forms shown; **(D)** we perceive the disconnected segments as a triangle and a circle

that best represents this phenomenon is the Rubin's face–vase figure (Figure 6.3). In this, one can see two faces against a white background or a white vase against a black background. It is an example of two possible perceptions but, at any given time, only one object can be perceived.

In the area of vision, several perceptual phenomena have been identified and studied by psychologists: perceptual constancy; depth perception; and perceptual set.

Perceptual constancy. The perception of the size, shape and colour of objects in the physical world tends to remain the same despite changes in the sensory input originating from them. For example, objects are perceived as having the same size (size constancy) even when at a distance in spite of the fact that distant objects produce smaller retinal images. Shape constancy is evident when a book, for example, lying on the table is perceived as a rectangle even though the retinal image may be trapezoid. The general tendency to assume constancies in size, shape, colour and brightness of objects is a striking feature of our perceptual system.

Depth perception. Although the images that are projected on to the retina are two dimensional and flat, we see the world around us as three

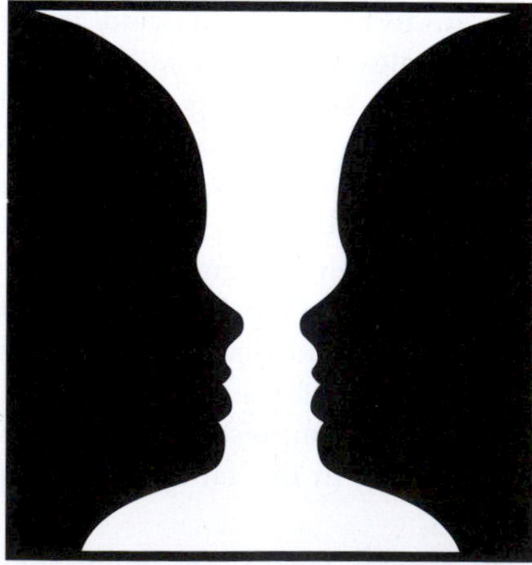

Fig. 6.3 Figure and ground. The image can be perceived as two people facing each other; the space between their faces is the background, but it can also be viewed as a vase or candle holder; the spaces around the figure now becomes the (back) ground.

dimensional. This is made possible partly by the way the eyes are positioned and partly by visual cues available in the environment. Each eye receives slightly different images (binocular disparity), which are integrated by the brain, and the slightly different perspectives so produced allow the brain to gauge the distance of the object from the eyes (stereopsis). The accommodation reflex and the convergence of eyes when shifting focus provide cues as to the distance. Other visual cues such as the relative size, linear perspective (apparent closeness of distant objects compared to those in the foreground) and reduced clarity of distant objects help us to estimate distance and three-dimensional perception irrespective of whether the vision is binocular or monocular.

Perceptual set. The general tendency or predisposition to experience events in a particular way is called *set*. In perception this refers to the readiness to perceive particular features of a stimulus. For example, the readiness with which an incomplete form of a letter of the alphabet is perceived as the complete one and the ease with which we are able to 'fill in' the missing words from sentences testify to the power of perceptual set. In such situations we selectively interpret the material on the basis of previous experience, memory, probabilities and learning. Thus, perception is an active process involving both top-down and bottom-up processing (see later). Similar sets operate in other spheres of cognition, emotion and motivation.

Object recognition

Establishment of the properties of an object leads on to the recognition of the object. Recognition of objects is a complex process involving access to different kinds of stored information that goes beyond perception. At the most basic level it involves pattern recognition. For example, a pen is recognised as a pen regardless of its orientation, size, shape and colour. Likewise, a sound may be recognised as a word spoken by a particular person. What makes this possible? Several different ways of understanding the processes involved in object identification have been put forward:

- *Templates*. A pattern is thought to be recognised by matching it with a template stored in memory.
- *Feature analysis*. A set of attributes is thought to constitute a pattern. For example, a face is made up of a nose, a mouth, two eyes, and so on. The individual features are recognised first, followed by integration of the information and comparison with memory stores.
- *Recognition by components*. According to this theory, objects are thought to consist of basic shapes (known as 'geons') such as cylinders, spheres, arcs, and so on (Biederman, 1987). Different combinations of geons are said to enable us to recognise objects in the same way that we recognise words from a combination of phonemes (speech sounds).

Although numerous explanatory theories have been advanced, and a great deal of research has been carried out into it, our understanding of the phenomenon of object recognition is rather rudimentary.

Theories of perception

The cognitive system is thought to be hierarchically organised. The lower-level systems, such as perception, are said to be located at the bottom of the hierarchy while more complex cognitive processes, such as memory and thinking, are situated towards the apex of the hierarchy. The process involved when information flows from bottom towards the top of the system is called *bottom-up processing*. The perceptual system gathers and organises incoming information. In the visual system this involves the analysis and organisation of stimuli such as edges, lines, contours and other physical features. Thus, the process is guided by individual elements and is said to be data driven. In *top-down processing*, information flows from the top of the system to the lower levels. Top-down processing involves the higher cognitive functions, and information coming into the system from perceptual processes is interpreted on the basis of existing thoughts, knowledge, experiences and expectations. For instance, when we fill in a word missing from a sentence, we are actively constructing percepts using previous knowledge, context and hypotheses. A similar effect is evident in the recognition of letters. It has been shown that individuals recognise a letter more readily when it forms part of a word rather than when it is presented in isolation (word-superiority effect). For example, the *c* in cat is recognised more quickly than when presented as *c* alone. This involves top-down processing.

Face recognition

Recognising faces is a unique and special form of perception. Face recognition deserves special mention because it is immensely more complicated than object recognition and, moreover, it plays an important part in social interactions and human emotional development (especially attachment). Development of face recognition occurs as early in infancy as three months and is a prime example of the interaction of biological, or inborn, capacities and the environment (see Chapter 12). There is evidence that the parts of the brain concerned with face recognition are different from those involved in object recognition. In patients who have an inability to recognise faces (prosopagnosia) the capacity to identify objects and recognise people by their voices is unaffected. Available evidence indicates that face recognition involves at least three interactive components (Burton, Bruce & Johnson, 1990):

1. Face recognition units consisting of a pool of information about known faces.
2. Person identity nodes or units that identify familiar faces.
3. Semantic information units that hold names and other information about the person.

Illusions

In the realms of vision, when there is conflicting information about depth, form and organisation the result is a visual illusion. Such perceptual failures are also known as *optical illusions*. Please note that the word illusion as used

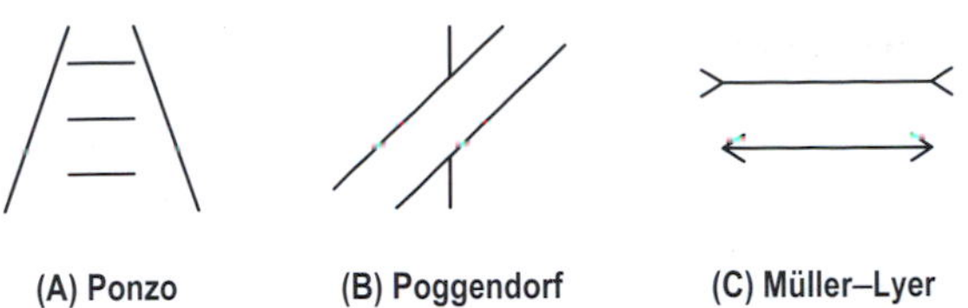

Fig. 6.4 Perceptual illusions: **(A)** the three horizontal lines are in fact the same length; **(B)** the vertical line appears offset but is, in fact, aligned; **(C)** the Müller–Lyer illusion, the convergence of arrow heads in the second figure makes the shaft appear shorter

here is different from the psychiatric usage of the term. (In phenomenology illusions refer to false or mistaken perceptions.) The better known illusions are (Figure 6.4):

- *Ponzo illusion*. Horizontal lines between two converging lines appear to be of different lengths.
- *Moon illusion*. The moon appears larger when lower in the sky than when viewed overhead.
- *Poggendorff illusion*. A vertical line crossing two oblique parallel lines appears offset.
- *Müller–Lyer illusion*. The perceived length of a line depends on the shape and position of the lines that enclose it.

Abnormalities of perception

Abnormalities of perception are generally divided into: (1) sensory distortions, where a real perceptual object is perceived in a distorted way (e.g. hyperacusis, i.e. intensity of sound is perceived to be high); and (2) sensory deceptions. The latter are subdivided into illusions (misinterpretation of stimuli) and hallucinations (perceptions in the absence of appropriate stimuli). The reader is referred to a text book on descriptive psychopathology for details of these phenomena (e.g. Sims, 2002).

ATTENTION

Attention is one of the less-well-understood cognitive functions. It cannot be captured in a single definition, nor can it be measured by a single test. Very little is known about the cerebral structures responsible for attention. What is generally referred to as attention is really a composite of several cognitive functions. Attention implies one's ability to focus on certain stimuli or sensations while, at the same time, excluding other stimuli from conscious experience. It also involves keeping one's attention fixed or sustained for a period of time without being distracted from the task. Curiously, it also necessitates the capacity to shift attention from one set of stimuli to another at will. For example, reading this paragraph may involve concentrating on the sentences, ignoring distractions provided by the television or a colleague, keeping one's attention focused on the task long enough to make sense of the material and being able to shift one's attention long enough to take down notes when necessary. It should be clear from the preceding account that attention really consists of several independent and overlapping cognitive activities. The main components of attention that have been studied are:

- Selective (focused) attention.
- Sustained attention (also called vigilance).
- Attentional shifting or switching.

Several other cognitive functions are closely related to attention. Inhibition of attention, or lack of it (impulsivity), is an important phenomenon, not least because it is a salient feature of hyperkinetic disorder in children. Working memory is considered by some to be a part of the attentional process.

Selective (focused) attention. Selective attention is directing attention to specific stimuli from among a myriad of potentially available stimuli. Selectivity also implies excluding irrelevant or extraneous stimuli. An example of this is the well-known phenomenon of mothers' selective attention to their babies' cries in a maternity ward. Another well-documented observable fact is the *cocktail party phenomenon*. This refers to our ability selectively to attend to a single person's speech in the presence of many others. Selectivity involves not only directing attention to one set of stimuli but also the suppression of attention to other, irrelevant stimuli, that is the prevention of distraction.

Selective attention may be tested by:

1. *Dichotic listening tasks*. Two different messages are fed by earphones simultaneously into both ears of the subject, usually in the form of word lists. The subject is instructed to ignore the set of information provided to one ear (distractor) while focusing on the other (target). The subject is asked to repeat or shadow the target message. The task can be made more difficult by making the target and distractor words resemble one another.
2. *Visual search tasks*. The subject is presented with an array of stimuli from which he or she is asked to detect the target stimuli. A well-known example of this group of tests is the *letter cancellation task* (Lezak, 1983). This consists of rows of letters in which the target letter is randomly distributed. The subject is asked to cancel the target letters one by one and the time taken to complete the test is noted.
3. *The Stroop colour–word test*. In this test (Stroop, 1935) the subject is presented with stimuli consisting of contradictory information. The test consists of a list of colour names printed in non-matching colours and the subject is asked to name the colour (not read the word). For example, the word GREEN is printed in red ink and the respondent is asked to name the colour. It is a timed test, which requires the subject to name as many colours as possible within a fixed time. Norms are available for various age groups. The subjects' task is difficult because they have to focus on the colour in which the word is printed and ignore the meaning.

   The test is based on the observation that individuals can read words faster (through automatic processing) than they can identify and name colours. The task requires two strategies: selective attention to the primary stimulus (colour); and inhibition of the dominant tendency to name the word or distractor stimulus. It is thought to measure interference control and requires the inhibition of an over-learned automatic response. The cognitive domains tapped by the Stroop task are many. In addition to selective attention it reflects cognitive flexibility and resistance to interference from outside stimuli. It has been argued that the Stroop task is a measure of inhibitory control, considered to be a component of executive functions rather than of focused attention. Patients with schizophrenia have been shown to find the Stroop task particularly difficult (Cohen & Servan-Schreiber, 1992).

4. *Clinical tests of focused attention.* A number of bedside tests of focused attention may be carried out rather quickly and efficiently. The digit span test (Chapter 7), especially the backward digit span, is thought to reflect focused attentional capacity. Recitation of the months of the year and the days of the week in reverse order gives an approximate measure of attention span and is useful in subjects with moderate to severe impairment of attention. Another test that is popular with clinicians is serial subtraction tests (e.g. taking away sevens from 100).

It is doubtful whether these test are 'pure' tests of selective attention. Many other processes appear to be involved in some of the above tasks. For example, digit span tests involve working memory and the Stroop test involves executive functions.

Sustained attention. This refers to the ability to keep one's attention fixed on a task or stimulus over a considerable period of time. Early work in this area was carried out during the Second World War on radar operators whose job involved paying concentrated attention to radar screens for possible enemy aircraft. Sustained attention requires that task performance continues to be accurate over extended periods of time. Sustained attention for low-frequency events, such as in radar detections, is known as vigilance while detection of high-frequency stimuli is sometimes termed monitoring.

The most commonly used tests of sustained attention are *Continuous Performance Tests* (CPTs), of which there are many forms. The most widely used CPT is the one devised by Rosvold and colleagues (1956). In this test, the subject is presented with a random series of letters on a visual display at a regular rate. The participant has to press a button when the target stimulus (for example, the letter X) appears on the screen. In a second condition, called the successive discrimination task, the subject is instructed to respond to the designated target (e.g. the letter X) only if preceded by a warning signal (e.g. the letter A). In performing the CPT two types of errors could occur: (1) errors of omission, i.e. not responding to the target stimulus; and (2) errors of commission, i.e. faulty responding.

It is generally held that *omission errors* measure lapses in sustained attention (vigilance) and *commission errors* those of poor inhibition control or impulsivity. There is considerable dispute as to what is measured by CPT. Attention as measured by CPT includes other cognitive processes such as behaviour inhibition, self control, and even executive functions.

Disorders of attention

Disordered attention is common in many psychiatric conditions. It is commonly associated with acute confusional states (delirium) where disorientation in time, place and person occur in conjunction with impaired attention. Hyperkinetic disorder (HKD, ICD-10) or attention deficit hyperkinetic disorder (ADHD, DSM-IV) is a condition seen in children and considered to consist of three primary groups of symptoms: (1) poor sustained attention; (2) hyperactivity; and (3) impulsiveness, that begin before the age of seven years and are evident in more than one situation (e.g. home and school). The diagnosis is made on the basis of clinical signs and symptoms and to date there is no objective test for the condition. Several forms of CPT have been studied on populations of children with ADHD but the results have been unconvincing.

Despite the extensive research on the use of CPT in this group of children, it has been shown to be of no use in discriminating children with ADHD or HKD from controls (Corkum & Siegal, 1995). In part this is due to the lack of standardisation of task variables, such as length of task and interval between stimulus presentations. More importantly, there is little evidence to show that children with ADHD have impaired CPT accuracy over time, that is, they are not poorer at sustaining attention (van der Meere, Wekking & Sergeant, 1991). The name attention deficit disorder thus appears to be a misnomer because there has been no convincing evidence presented so far to demonstrate either impairments or deficits in attention in spite of extensive research in this field. The emerging view is that children with ADHD show difficulties in behaviour inhibition and self-regulation rather than attentional difficulties.

In summary, it should be clear from the above discussion on attention that: (1) attention is a broad multidimensional concept and includes several overlapping phenomena and constructs and cannot be thought of as a single process (for example, focused attention if prolonged over time becomes sustained attention); (2) important aspects of attention such as divided attention and attentional capacity have received little scrutiny; (3) most, if not all, tests of attention, index more than attention and may include other cognitive domains such as some aspects of executive functions; and (4) in children with ADHD, or HKD, contrary to popular belief, there is little convincing evidence of demonstrable attention deficit.

SCHEMAS

How 'objective' are our cognitive processes? As mentioned above, Gestalt psychologists made the observation that we contribute something to all perceptual inputs from our past experiences. In making sense of perceptions they are analysed and interpreted by comparing them with those that we are already familiar with. In short, perceptual inputs are not simply recorded in the mind in the way that a tape recorder records sound. Thus, a flower that we had never seen before is nevertheless recognised as a flower. Bartlett

(1932), a British psychologist, was the first to demonstrate that a similar process operates for other cognitive modalities as well, most notably, memory (see Chapter 7). He called the hypothesised mental structures responsible for these processes *schemas* (or *schemata*).

In simple terms, the schema theory suggests that perceptions, memories and thoughts are powerfully influenced by what we already know or expect to happen. Thus, based on their past experience, people carry in their minds general ideas about events, objects, people and situations. These schemas play an important role in making sense of the world and the events that occur around us. Schemas are helpful short cuts so that one does not have to learn again and again.

All of us have schemas about what a flower looks like, what happened in our last interview, and about aspects of ourselves. Schemas provide a framework in which information is encoded and interpreted. Because schemas are knowledge organisations that already exist, our perceptions, thinking and memories are prone to errors and distortions caused by existing schemas. Since schemas are based on our past knowledge and personal experience they can be expected to differ from person to person. Thus, the same event may mean different things to different people.

There are several schema theories and related concepts (e.g. the internal working models described by Bowlby, and the schemas in children's cognitive development described by Piaget; see Chapter 12). Most schema theories hold that schemas are not fixed but are active dynamic structures. Thus, the incorporation of new knowledge into schemas then renders them liable to modification. The best-known schema theory in the clinical field is Beck's cognitive theory of emotional disorders (see Chapter 5). This theory is, in fact, an offshoot of a form of therapy called cognitive behaviour therapy.

COGNITIVE BEHAVIOUR THERAPY

One of the outstanding achievements in psychology and psychiatry over the last few decades has been the acknowledgement of the central role of cognitions in emotional disorders such as depression and anxiety. This realisation arose not from academic cognitive psychology or the 'cognitive revolution' in psychology, but from clinical observation, experimentation and theoretical formulations. It heralded a comparable 'cognitive' revolution in psychiatry and clinical psychology. The best-known form of cognitive intervention is cognitive behaviour therapy, commonly known as CBT.

Cognitive behaviour therapy is the term used to describe psychotherapeutic interventions that aim to reduce psychological distress and maladaptive behaviour by altering cognitive processes. CBT is based on the underlying assumption that emotions, moods and behaviour are largely products of cognitions and, as such, cognitive interventions can bring about changes in thinking, feeling and behaviour. CBT therefore embraces the core elements of both cognitive and learning theories. The most popular cognitive theory of emotional and behavioural disorders is that of Aaron Beck.

Beck is a psychiatrist who had received psychoanalytic training. In studying the contents of cognition in patients with depression he found that the Freudian formulation of depression as motivational phenomena ('anger turned inward' and grieving for losses) were not valid in most patients. According to Beck, emotional disorders are the result of distorted thinking or unrealistic cognitive appraisal of one's life events. In essence it means that cognitions, to a large extent, determine a person's emotional state, especially in abnormal emotional conditions, such as depression. Emotions and cognitions are thought to reinforce each other resulting in a vicious circle of emotional and cognitive impairment. The publication of his book *Depression: Causes and treatment* in 1976 was a landmark in psychotherapy. Subsequently, he has extended his newly gained insights to the treatment of many other psychiatric conditions, such as anxiety disorders (Beck & Emery, 1985), personality disorders (Beck & Freeman, 1990), and substance abuse (Beck et al., 1993). As yet, there is no unified psychological theory of schizophrenia. CBT for delusions and hallucinations (in schizophrenia), based on psychological theories, has gained prominence in the recent past; these therapies are beyond the scope of this book and may be found elsewhere (e.g. Birchwood & Tarrier, 1994).

Beck's Cognitive theory of emotional disorders rests on three basic concepts:

1. Dysfunctional schemas.
2. Negative automatic thoughts.
3. Systemic errors in logic (cognitive distortions or biases).

For Beck, the term *schemas* refers to hypothetical cognitive structures in the mind. However, in the schema theory of emotional disorders, it is the content of these structures that is given most consideration. Beck has described two types of content: core beliefs; and assumptions.

1. *Core beliefs* are constructs that are usually global, over-generalised and unconditional in nature and taken as truths about the self and the world (e.g. 'I am a failure').
2. *Assumptions* are conditional, less firmly held and relate to contingencies and self-appraisal (e.g. 'If I faint I will make a fool of myself').

Schemas screen, organise and evaluate experiences and information and are crucial in producing attitudes, emotional responses and behaviours. In well-adapted individuals they help the person to predict and make sense of their experiences. In the maladapted person they become counterproductive and dysfunctional. Schemas are thought to develop early in life and remain dormant until triggered by stressful life events.

Negative automatic thoughts are produced when such dysfunctional schemas are activated. They are automatic in that they arise from nowhere, unprompted by events or reflection. They are negative because they are self-defeating, self-critical and often self-depreciating. These thoughts might be about the past, present or future. Beck described a *cognitive triad* that is characteristic of depressed individuals consisting of negative thoughts about oneself (that one is inadequate, worthless, etc.), the current experience (interpretation of the present situation as insurmountable) and the future

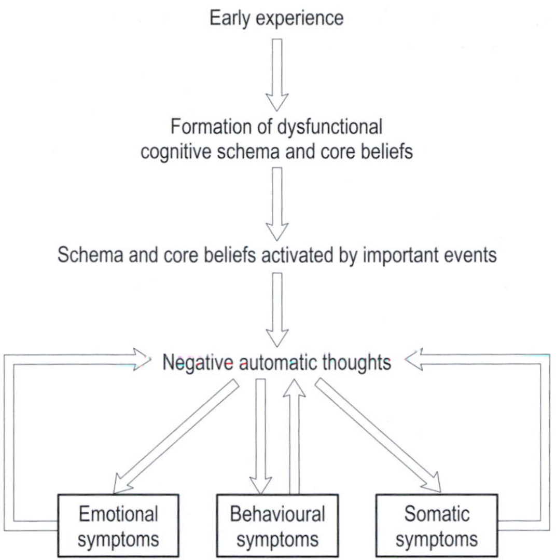

Fig. 6.5 The cognitive model of emotional disorders

(bleak, dark and without hope). These, in turn, lead to the constellation of symptoms of depression in the following domains:

- *Emotional symptoms* – anxiety, guilt, lack of enjoyment.
- *Cognitive symptoms* – hopelessness, helplessness, pessimism.
- *Behavioural symptoms* – withdrawal, impaired activity, retardation.
- *Motivational symptoms* – passivity, inertia, lack of interest.
- *Physical symptoms* – diminished sleep, appetite, impaired libido.

According to Beck the depressed person's cognitions are characterised by systematic *logical errors* or *cognitive distortions* in thinking. Common cognitive errors or distortions include the following:

- *Arbitrary inference* – drawing inferences in the absence of sufficient evidence.
- *Selective abstraction* – focusing one aspect of the situation while ignoring the more important features.
- *Overgeneralisation* – applying conclusions to a wide range of situations based on experiences of isolated incidents.
- *Magnification and minimisation* – exaggerating or reducing the importance of events.
- *Personalisation* – relating external events to oneself when there is no obvious reason to do so.
- *Dichotomous thinking* – 'black and white' thinking.
- *Catastrophising* – dwelling on the worst possible outcome of a situation.
- *Mind reading* – assuming people are reacting negatively to you when there is no evidence for it.

The cognitive model is summarised in Figure 6.5. The identification and modification of core beliefs is the central task in CBT. The automatic thoughts, together with the assumptions on which they are based, are systematically challenged using various cognitive and behavioural strategies.

Although research has provided some support for biases in information processing as proposed by the theory, the issue of causality in the relationship between cognition and pathological emotional states remain uncertain.

EXECUTIVE FUNCTIONS

The term executive function (EF) is an umbrella term used for various complex cognitive processes and subprocesses. It has been described as 'a product of the coordinated operations of various processes to accomplish a particular goal in a flexible manner' (Funahashi, 2001). Executive function is, therefore, inherent in all coordinated and controlled goal-directed behaviour. Thus the domain of executive function is distinctive in cognitive domains such as perception, memory and language. It overlaps with attention, reasoning and problem solving, but not perfectly. A typical list of executive functions includes:

- Organisation of behaviour, especially goal-directed, purposeful actions (planning).
- Novel problem solving.
- Modifying behaviour in the light of new information (set shifting and set maintenance).
- Ability to plan strategies and derive solutions on tasks that need hypothesis testing.
- Capacity for self-control and response inhibition (behaviour inhibition).

In short, the flexible coordination of various cognitive processes to achieve a specific goal is the function of the executive system. Naturally, much complex human behaviour requires executive function. When these systems are impaired, behaviour becomes poorly controlled and disinhibited

Executive functions are thought to be predominantly dependant on, but not identical to, frontal-lobe functions. Although the terms frontal-lobe function and executive function are often used interchangeably, it would be more accurate to infer that frontal lobes contribute to a number of components of executive functions. Patients with frontal-lobe damage typically show deficient executive functions in the form of impaired judgement, organisation, planning and decision-making. Recent findings suggest that not only do executive functions depend on the prefrontal cortex but also that the basal ganglia are intimately involved. Executive functions have been shown to be impaired in Parkinson's disease and Huntington's syndrome. Executive dysfunction is associated with a range of psychiatric and developmental disorders including schizophrenia, Alzheimer's disease and childhood autism. The nature of the dysfunctions in these disorders is unclear. Because executive functions are impaired in a variety of conditions these malfunctions have sometimes been called the *dysexecutive syndrome.*

A number of varied tests are used to measure the different domains subsumed under the umbrella of executive function. Clinical tests of executive functions, which are essentially crude tests of frontal-lobe functioning, are

Box 6.2 Some clinical tests of executive functions (in addition to performance on the test, look also for perseveration, imitation, intrusion, lack of spontaneity and disinhibited behaviour)

- *Word fluency*. Generating as many words beginning with a given letter, or naming as many animals or items in a supermarket as possible in one minute. The letters most commonly used in tests are F, A and S. Normal adults are able to produce about 15 words in one minute for each letter. Subjects with executive function deficits tend to perseverate, or shift set
- *Motor sequencing*. Three hand movements are demonstrated (e.g. fist–edge–palm) and the subject is asked to repeat them (Lauria test)
- *Abstraction*. The subject is asked to interpret common proverbs
- *Cognitive estimations*. The subject is asked to estimate the height of an average man or woman, the largest object in the room or the height of a building
- *Grasp reflex*. Stroke lightly and simultaneously both palms of the patient's hands from root to fingers with both your hands palms up. Look for grasping action in patient's fingers

listed in Box 6.2. Neuropsychological tests of EF are many and varied. Computerised versions of most these tests are now available. The most commonly used individual tests are as follows:

1. *Trail making test*. The basic task of the trail making test is to connect a series of stimuli (numbers or letters) in a specific order as quickly as possible. The subject is presented with a page in which circles numbered from 1 to 25 are randomly arranged (Form A). The subject's task is to join the circles in numerical order as quickly as possible. In the second part of the test a page contains both numbers and letters displayed randomly (Form B). The subject's task is to connect consecutively numbered and lettered circles (i.e. 1, A, 2, B, and so on). The trail making test is heavily influenced by selective attention, resistance to distraction and cognitive flexibility (set shifting). It is extremely sensitive to many types of neurological deficits. Disproportionately poor performance on Trail B is taken as an index of poor set shifting and is thought to reflect defective executive functioning.
2. *The Wisconsin card sorting test (WCST; Heaton et al., 1993)*. This is a widely used measure that, in part, assesses aspects of inhibitory control and flexibility in problem solving. In this task, subjects are asked to match cards according to three categories (colour, shape and number) The examiner tells the subject if the cards have been placed correctly or incorrectly, but does not reveal the sorting strategy (e.g. match by colour). Once 10 consecutive cards have been categorised correctly, the sorting principle is changed without warning or comment from the examiner. All sorts according to the previous strategy now receive negative feed back and subjects are expected to shift eventually to a new categorization principle. As with the Stroop task, the dominant response – in this case, a recently learned rule – will have to be inhibited for accurate performance. The procedure is repeated a number of times. The most widely used and sensitive variable derived from the WCST is errors of perseveration, obtained by the number of times the subject sorts according to a previously correct principle despite negative feedback from the examiner (reflecting inflexibility in set shifting). Raw scores are standardised to normalised standard, percentile and *T*-scores. Although the WCST has long been thought of

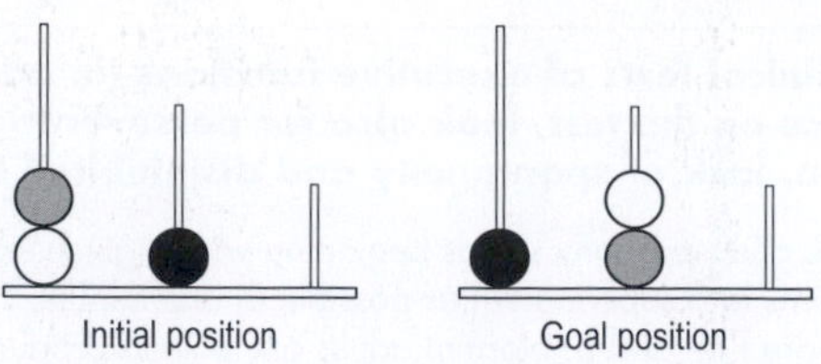

Fig. 6.6 An example of the Tower of London test (Shallice, 1982). The subject is shown the goal position and must duplicate the arrangement on a second apparatus where the starting position is determined by the examiner while obeying the following rules: (1) only one bead may be moved at a time; (2) beads cannot be placed on the table. The illustration shows a four-move problem

as a test of frontal-lobe functions, most studies have shown that the test is not specific to frontal-lobe damage and may be impaired in diffuse brain damage. Moreover, in some instances of demonstrable frontal-lobe dysfunction (as shown by neuroimaging), WCST scores are within normal limits.

3. *Tower of Hanoi (ToH) test*. The ability to plan ahead to solve a problem is an executive function that may be assessed by the Tower of Hanoi test. This test consists of an apparatus consisting of three vertical posts, and three doughnut-like discs, of different colour and size, that fit over the pegs. The testee is shown the model and must duplicate an arrangement on a second apparatus in the minimum number of moves, while obeying the following rules: (1) only one disc may be moved at a time; (2) a larger disc must not be placed on top of a smaller one; and (3) discs may not be placed on the table. A simplified form of the test is the Tower of London puzzle devised by Shallice (1982). It involves similar reasoning but is easier in format. Rather than discs of different size, perforated balls of different colours are used, and the pegs are of different lengths. The illustration (Figure 6.6) shows a four-move problem. The number of moves needed to complete the task is commonly taken as an index of executive function. Patients with frontal-lobe problems show pronounced impairments in the task. Impaired functioning on the tower tasks has been found in various clinical groups, including people with autism.

Since executive function is a composite of several cognitive processes, no single test could be expected to measure them all. It is usually tested by a battery of subtests. An example of such a battery is the *Delis–Kaplan executive function system* (D–KEFS; Delis, Kaplan & Kraemer, 2001), which is shown in Table 6.1. It claims to provide a comprehensive assessment of the key components of the executive functions believed to be mediated primarily by the frontal lobes.

The various executive function domains and the tests for them are summarised in Table 6.2 and the common clinical tests of executive functions are enumerated in Box 6.2. When carrying out the tests the clinician looks out for the following pathological behaviours:

- *Perseveration*. Patient responds with the requested behaviour but repeats it over and over, inappropriately.
- *Imitation*. Patient repeats the interviewer's words (echolalia) or behaviours (echopraxia).
- *Intrusion*. Patient includes items from a previous task inappropriately.

Table 6.1 The Delis–Kaplan executive function system (D-KEFS; Delis, Kaplan & Kraemer, 2001)

Test	*Executive function assessed*
Sorting test	Problem solving flexibility in thinking
Trail making test	Flexibility in thinking in visual–motor task
Design fluency test	Fluent production in special domain
Verbal fluency test	Fluent verbal production of words
Twenty question test	Hypothesis testing
Word context test	Deductive reasoning
Proverb test	Metaphorical thinking
Colour–word interference test	Verbal inhibition
Tower test	Planning and reasoning in special modality

- *Lack of spontaneity*. Patient takes a long time to respond (long latency) and the examiner has to encourage the patient again and again to respond.
- *Disinhibition*. Patient responds to the task as requested but speaks and behaves in an inappropriate and flippant way.

Cognitive deficits in schizophrenia

There is now mounting evidence that neurocognitive deficits are central to the difficulties that patients with schizophrenia experience. These impairments form an integral part of the clinical picture and are independent of medication effects. Although neuroleptic medication improves some of the deficits, some significant deficits remain and present considerable problems in patients' daily living. The main deficits are as follows:

1. *Deficits in executive functions*. Poor planning abilities, lack of inhibition and avolition are characteristic of schizophrenia. Patients with schizophrenia perform poorly on the Wisconsin card sorting test; they tend to perseverate on their responses and tend not to shift set when the 'rules' are changed. It has been observed that the cerebral blood flow, as indexed by PET, was lowered during the performance of this task (Weinberger, Berman & Zec, 1986). Thus reduced frontal-brain metabolism (hypofrontality) during activation appears to be characteristic of schizophrenia.
2. *Memory deficits*: Patients with schizophrenia show subtle memory deficits. Pooled data from various studies suggests that in schizophrenia the specific memory dysfunction is a degree of anterograde deficit, including difficulties in encoding and rapid forgetting.

THE PLACEBO EFFECT

The term placebo effect refers to beneficial physiological or psychological changes associated with the use of inert medications, sham procedures, or in

Table 6.2 Summary of the domains and tests of executive functions

Set shifting	Wisconsin card sorting test Trail making test, part B
Planning	Tower of Hanoi test Tower of London test
Inhibition	Stroop colour word test Continuous performance test Matching familiar figures test
Working memory	Digit span
Fluency	Thurstone word fluency test

response to therapeutic encounters. It has been estimated that placebo effects are seen in about 30% of subjects. The mechanism through which its effects are mediated is poorly understood and its potential remains unexploited.

In practice, placebo treatment consists of administering pharmacologically inert medication or an intervention, which ranges from surgery to forms of verbal interaction such as psychotherapy, listening or history taking. Placebo responses have been demonstrated in sham surgical procedures for patients suffering from angina and osteoarthritis.

In the past it had been believed that there were placebo 'responders' and 'non-responders' and much energy has been expended in trying to identify personality factors that may render individuals more prone to respond to placebos. But research has consistently failed to demonstrate any personality trait related to the placebo reaction. Other variables like gender, suggestibility, IQ and lower social class do not affect responsiveness to placebos. So selecting those patients who are most likely to benefit from placebo is therefore difficult. It is believed that the capacity to elicit a placebo response is inherent in everyone.

The placebo effect depends largely on the interactions between the clinician, the treatment process and the subject. Often, however, neither the clinician nor the patient is aware of the placebo effect.

Characteristics of the clinician. A placebo response is more likely to occur in the clinic when the patient regards the clinician as competent, experienced and optimistic. The clinician's enthusiasm and expectation of a good treatment response are, by far, the most important physician variables that are known to produce good responses. The subtle communication of the clinician's outcome expectations to the patient is well illustrated by a double-blind dental pain study that involved two sets of patients. All patients were told that they might receive one of the following: a narcotic analgesic; a narcotic antagonist; or a placebo. They were also told that the treatment might decrease their pain, increase their pain, or have no effect. The doctors administering the drugs were themselves allocated to one of two conditions. Half the doctors were told that patients might receive an analgesic and experience pain relief, whereas the other half believed that there was no chance of the patients receiving the analgesic. In fact all the subjects were given a placebo. The results showed that only the patients in the first set (i.e. the group in whom the doctors thought there was a chance of receiving an analgesic) showed positive pain relief to the placebo. Thus the clinician's knowledge, and expectations of treatment effects influenced the placebo effects (Gracely et al., 1985).

Outcome expectations. These include the plausibility of the treatment regimen and the likelihood that treatment will produce the response expected. In an experiment one group of subjects was treated in a double-blind fashion so that neither they nor the experimenters knew which type of coffee they would be served in the trial. However, a second group was told that they would be given regular coffee when in fact they were given a decaffeinated brew. Results showed that those in the second group had higher pulse rates and systolic blood pressure and reported more alertness (Kirch & Weixel, 1998).

It has been noted that what matters most in a placebo response is the physiological or psychological effects of meaning in the treatment of illness. This has been termed *meaning response* (Moerman, 2002) and refers to the process in which patients and clinicians ascribe meaning to the various occurrences in the course of their encounters. These include contextual factors such as the setting (e.g. clinic, office), procedures (what is done and said) and how the information is integrated into the personal and cultural beliefs of the person. In one study, two groups of medical students were given packets each containing one or two pink or blue capsules. The pills were inert but they were told that one capsule was a stimulant and that the other one was a sedative. Results indicated that the red capsules acted like stimulants while the blue ones acted like sedatives, and two capsules had more effect than one. Obviously red capsules were associated with heat and danger, blue with cool or calm and the greater the number of tablets taken the more potent they were thought to be.

Classical conditioning. Classical conditioning theory had been used to explain *some* placebo effects. Conditioning is common in subjects habitually using caffeine, nicotine, alcohol, illicit drugs and medications.

Little is known about the intermediary neurophysiological and immunological mechanisms involved in the placebo response. What is clear is that it involves several pathways from conditioning to outcome expectations and anxiety reduction.

REFERENCES

Bach S, Klein GS (1957) The effects of prolonged subliminal exposure to words. American Psychologist, 12, 336–345.

Bartlett FC (1932) Remembering. Cambridge, UK: Cambridge University Press.

Beck AT (1967) Depression: Causes and treatment. Philadelphia, PA: University of Pennsylvania Press.

Beck AT, Emery G (1985) Anxiety Disorders and Phobias: a cognitive perspective. New York: Basic Books.

Beck AT, Freeman A (1990) Cognitive Therapy for Personality Disorders. New York: Guilford Press.

Beck AT, Wright FD, Newman CF, Liese BS (1993) Cognitive Therapy of Substance Misuse. New York: Guilford Press.

Biederman I (1987) Recognition-by-components: a theory of human image understanding. Psychological Review, 94, 115–147.

Birchwood M, Tarrier N (1994) Psychological Management of Schizophrenia. Chichester, UK: Wiley.
Burton AM, Bruce N, Johnson RA (1990) Understanding face recognition with an interactive activation model. British Journal of Psychology, 81, 361–380.
Chomsky N (1959) Review of Skinner's verbal behaviour. Language, 35, 26–58.
Cohen JD, Servan-Schreiber D (1992) Context, cortex and dopamine: a connectionist approach to behaviour and biology in schizophrenia. Psychological Review, 99, 45–75.
Corkum P, Siegal L (1995) Debate and argument. Reply to Dr Kolega: is continuous performance test useful in research with ADHD children? Comments on a review. Journal of Child Psychology and Psychiatry, 36, 1487–1493.
Delis DC, Kaplan E, Kraemer JH (2001) Delis–Kaplan Executive Function System (D–KEFS). San Antonio, CA: Psychological Corporation.
Funahashi (2001) Neuronal mechanism of executive control by prefrontal cortex. Neuroscience Research, 39, 147–165.
Gracely RH, Dubner R, Deeter WR, Wolskee PJ. (1985) Clinician's expectations influence placebo analgesia. Lancet, 1, 43.
Heaton RK, Cheline GJ, Talley JL, Kay GG, Curtiss G (1993) Wisconsin Card Sorting Test Manual – Revised and Updated. Odessa, FL: Psychological Assessment.
Hilgard ER (1980) The trilogy of mind: cognition, affection and conation. Journal of the History of Behavioural Sciences, 4, 107–117.
James W (1960) The Varieties of Religious Experience. London, UK: Fontana.
Kirch I, Weixel LJ (1998) Double blind versus deceptive administration of a placebo. Biomedical Therapy, XVI(3), 242–246.
Lezak MD (1983) Neuropsychological Assessment. New York: Oxford University Press.
Moerman DE (2002) Explanatory mechanisms for placebo effects: cultural influences and the meaning response. In HA Guess, A Klineman, JW Kusek, & LW Engel (eds), The Science of the Placebo: towards an interdisciplinary research agenda (Ch.4). London, UK: BMJ Books.
Neisser U (1967) Cognitive Psychology (p. 4). New York: Appleton-Century-Crofts.
Rosvold HE, Mirsky AF, Sarason I, Bransome ED Jr, Beck LH (1956) A continuous performance test of brain damage. Journal of Consulting Psychology, 20, 343–353.
Shallice T (1982) Specific impairments in planning. Philosophical Transactions of the Royal Society of London, B298, 199–209.
Shevrin H, Dickman S (1980) The psychological unconscious: a necessary assumption for all psychological theory. American psychologist, 35(5), 421–434.
Sims A (2002) Symptoms in the Mind: an introduction to descriptive psychopathology (3rd ed.). London, UK: Baillière Tindall.
Stroop JR (1935) Studies on interference in serial and verbal reactions. Journal of Experimental Psychology, 18, 643–662.
van der Meere J, Wekking E, Sergeant J (1991) Sustained attention and pervasive hyperactivity. Journal of Child Psychology and Psychiatry, 32, 275–284.
Weinberger DR, Berman KF, Zec RF (1986) Physiologic dysfunction of dorsolateral frontal cortex in schizophrenia: I. Regional blood flow evidence. Archives of General Psychiatry, 43, 114–124.

FURTHER READING

Beck JS (1995) Cognitive Therapy: basics and beyond. New York: Guilford Press.

- A remarkable book, by the master's daughter, that provides a solid basic foundation for the practice of CBT. Highly recommended.

Williams JMG, Watts FN, MacLeod C, Mathews A (1997) Cognitive Psychology and Emotional Disorders (2nd ed.). Chichester, UK: Wiley.

- A scholarly piece of work that summarises the evidence for the psychological processes involved in emotional disorders. Chapters 9 and 10 on Schemata and Non-conscious processing make interesting reading

Memory and disorders of memory

7

'What matters in life is not what happens to you but what you remember and how you remember it.'
Gabriel Garcia Marquez, from his autobiography

Retention of information over time and the ability to recall events, places, faces and other information is a vital cognitive function that is essential for everyday life and, indeed, our survival. Other psychological functions such as thinking, learning and social interactions, to name but three, are inextricably linked to and dependent upon memory. The singularity of the term 'memory' is misleading – there is no single store or system that governs all memory-related experiences. Rather, as research has amply demonstrated, there are many memory systems, which are separate and operate independently of one another. There have been considerable advances made in our understanding of the structure, organisation and the processes that underlie memory functions over the last two decades. In this chapter four main aspects of memory are outlined: memory processes, forgetting and retrieval, disorders of memory, and models of memory, together with a brief mention of tests of memory.

MEMORY PROCESSES

Three different processes are thought to occur sequentially in all operations involving memory (Figure 7.1):

1. *Encoding*. The input process that receives information from the outside – it leads to the formation of initial memory traces.
2. *Storage*. Retention of information and its maintenance.
3. *Retrieval*. Accessing and recovering information from memory stores.

Memory failure, or forgetting, can be due to failure or faulty functioning at each of these stages – deficient encoding at the time of acquisition (as in not paying attention), poor storage of information and inadequate retrieval – may all result in forgetting (see later).

Encoding. Encoding is dependant on the modality in which material is presented, the common forms of encoding are:

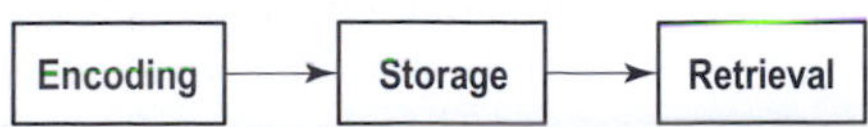

Fig. 7.1 The three memory processes

- Visual representations, such as written words, objects and images.
- Acoustic representation, as in speech, sounds and music.
- Semantic representation, referring to abstract meaning (e.g. animal, food).
- Motor representation, such as motor skills (cycling, writing).
- Sensory representations, like pain, smell, emotions and taste.

In real life, memory representations are complex and involve a number of modalities. For instance, an item of food is remembered by its taste, colour, shape and size.

Storage and components of memory systems. There is considerable evidence to support the division of memory into short-term and long-term memory systems. The most compelling evidence comes from the demonstration of 'double dissociation' in groups of amnesic patients. Some patients with brain damage show impaired short-term memory but intact long-term memory while others exhibit poor long-term memory and normal short-term memory. In general three memory systems have been delineated:

1. Sensory stores.
2. Short-term memory (also called primary memory) – memory that is conscious and current.
3. Long-term memory (also called secondary memory) – memory that stores information over a very long period of time.

Sensory memory

Information from the environment is initially received by the sensory stores. These stores are modality specific; visual stimuli are held in iconic stores and auditory stimuli in echoic stores, and so on. Information from the environment is held in the sensory stores for very short periods, usually a few milliseconds. Information that is attended to is transferred to short-term memory store and information that is not selected for processing is rapidly lost.

Short-term memory

The term short-term memory (STM) is used to refer to memory for events that occurred in the immediate past, where the delay between presentation of the information and its recall is measured in seconds rather than in minutes.

It is unfortunate that the terms STM and long-term memory (LTM) are used somewhat differently in psychology and psychiatry and this is likely to lead to some confusion. In psychology STM refers to immediate memory as tested by the recall of digits immediately after their presentation (digit span). In psychiatry the term STM is sometimes (erroneously) used to refer to the component of memory as evidenced by the recollection of a name and address (or, in memory-impaired subjects, the names of three items) five to ten minutes after their presentation. This is really a test of LTM and should not be considered as a test of STM. In psychiatry it is seen as a test of recent memory (which, in fact, is a part of LTM). In scientific terms, digit span is the test of STM; in psychiatry this is often referred to as a test of immediate

Table 7.1 Different usages of the terms short-term and long-term memory

Term used in psychology	*Term used in psychiatry*	*Common clinical test*
Short-term memory	Immediate memory	Digit span
Long-term memory	Recent memory (minutes hours days)	Recall of items after five minutes Recall of last meal Recall of recent topics in news
	Remote memory (weeks to years)	Recall of distant personal events

memory. Thus, what is called STM in psychology is sometimes called immediate memory in clinical practice and is usually tested by the digit span test. Both recent and remote memory are parts of LTM. This is summarised in Table 7.1.

STM is a temporary memory store from which information is lost very rapidly. It acts as a temporary but active working space receiving encoded data from the sensory store and transferring them to LTM. Information is held in STM for very short periods indeed, usually up to 20 seconds. The main features of STM are:

- *Limited capacity*. It holds small amounts of information. The average capacity of STM has been shown to be about seven items plus or minus two, thus the magic number is 7 ± 2 whether it is numbers, letters or words. STM is usually measured by the *digit span test*. However, the contents of STM are increased by holding 7 ± 2 'chunks' in STM. Chunks are bits of information coordinated together with the help of LTM. Thus, one is able to recall 28 digits or letters as long as they are arranged in meaningful chunks. For example, the letters 'yromemmrettrohs' are difficult to remember; but when made into three chunks in 'short-term memory' all 15 letters are easily recalled.
- *Temporary storage*. The duration for which information is held in STM is very short indeed and under normal situations is usually 15 to 20 seconds. STM is very fragile and information is lost easily. One way in which this has been tested was by providing a distraction task (such as counting a three-digit number backwards) immediately after the digit span test in order to prevent rehearsal. This procedure, known as the Brown–Patterson task has shown that by 15 seconds the original material is completely forgotten.
- *Encoding*. STM relies heavily on acoustic coding; visual encoding fades quickly.
- *Retrieval*. Recall of information is effortless and usually error free. Items are searched for one at a time up to the last one (serial exhaustive search).
- *Rehearsal*. Information is held in STM by the process of rehearsal. Rehearsal refers to the repetition of items in one's mind (and occasionally by verbal repetition), as we do, for example, in trying to remember a telephone number. This form of rehearsal is referred to as maintenance rehearsal (to distinguish it from rehearsal that involves more extensive understanding of the meaning of the material, called elaborative rehearsal, a process

involving LTM). The process of maintenance rehearsal not only maintains information in STM stores but also helps the transfer of mnemonic information to LTM.

- *Forgetting*. Loss of information from STM occur mainly through displacement. New or recently acquired items entering STM displace existing material. Decay (recently acquired material in the store has a higher trace strength than older items) may also play a part. Forgetting by displacement is item dependent, whereas forgetting by decay is time dependent.
- *Recency and primacy effects*. In free recall experiments items that are presented towards the end of the list are more likely to be remembered (recency effect) than those in the middle of the list. Also, material that was presented first is better recalled than items in the middle (primacy effect).

- Studies in cognitive neuropsychology and brain imaging provide convergent evidence that the brain areas mediating performances in STM are principally the prefrontal lobes.

This information is summarised in Box 7.1.

Working memory

In the 1970s STM was reformulated by Baddeley and co-workers as 'working memory' (Baddeley & Hitch, 1974). The concept of working memory is much broader than the traditional notion of STM, which typically refers to temporary retention of words, letters and numbers. Working memory is conceptualised as a limited-capacity mental work-space, and involves both the short-term storage of information and the manipulation of the contents of the store by executive processes. It helps to keep track of what we are doing or where we are from moment to moment, holding information just long enough to make a decision, for example, to dial a telephone number or repeat what we have just heard.

A key feature of working memory is that it is not simply a passive recipient of sensory input (as the concept of STM suggests) but an active store used to hold information while it is being analysed and worked upon. It is also interactive, in that current information is integrated with previous knowledge (from LTM) to help learning and plan actions. There is no pure measure of working memory, although tasks could be designed to make high demands on it.

Box 7.1 Features of short-term memory

- Limited capacity – 5 to 9 digits, items or chunks
- Fragile – information is lost easily
- Very short duration – about 20 seconds
- Retention of information is by maintenance rehearsal
- Mainly echoic or visual modality
- Tested by digit span
- Forgetting occurs mainly by displacement and decay
- Prefrontal brain regions are involved
- Now reformulated as 'working memory'

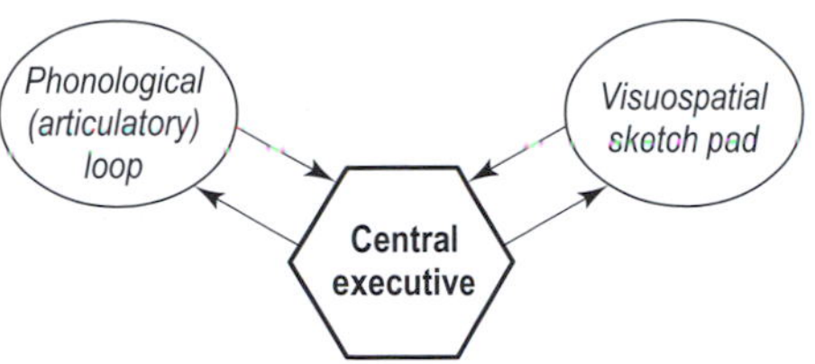

Fig. 7.2 Model of working memory (Baddeley & Hitch, 1974)

STM performance is not supported by a unitary system but is subserved by a suite of distinct systems (Baddeley, 1986). According to this model (Figure 7.2), working memory is comprised of three components, a central executive and two 'slave systems': (1) a central control system (the central executive); (2) a phonological STM system (the articulatory loop); and (3) a visuospatial STM system called the (visuospatial scratch pad). Material is thought to be stored in the phonological loop in terms of sound-based phonological qualities, whereas the sketch pad has the capacity to maintain visual information. The central executive performs a range of high-level functions, including retrieval of information from LTM stores and coordination of the flow of information through working memory. Its operations are not restricted to any particular input, so it is said to be 'modality free'.

The tripartite working memory model has received considerable support from experimental studies and brain imaging. In the case of the phonological STM system the left hemisphere regions of Broca's area and the prefrontal cortex are implicated, whereas the visuospatial STM appears to be mediated by parietal and prefrontal areas of the right hemisphere. Working memory is important because of the role it plays in thinking, problem solving and language processing.

Long-term memory

The term long-term memory (LTM) refers to memory for events that occurred minutes, hours, days, months or years ago. LTM has no known limits on capacity or duration of storage and can potentially hold enormous quantities of information over one's life time. It differs from STM in that it uses semantic coding (encoding meaning) and different forms of organisation. The information held in LTM is characterised by great diversity, for example it stores

Box 7.2 Features of long-term memory

- Large capacity
- Duration – days, weeks, years to decades
- Encoding mainly semantic, but also acoustic and imagery
- Stable but liable to revision and modification
- Tested by delayed recall, recollection of personal information and public events
- Forgetting is mainly due to retrieval failure; storage failure may be due to proactive inhibition, retroactive inhibition and decay
- Limbic structures involved
- Now reformulated and subdivided into explicit/implicit memory and further subtypes

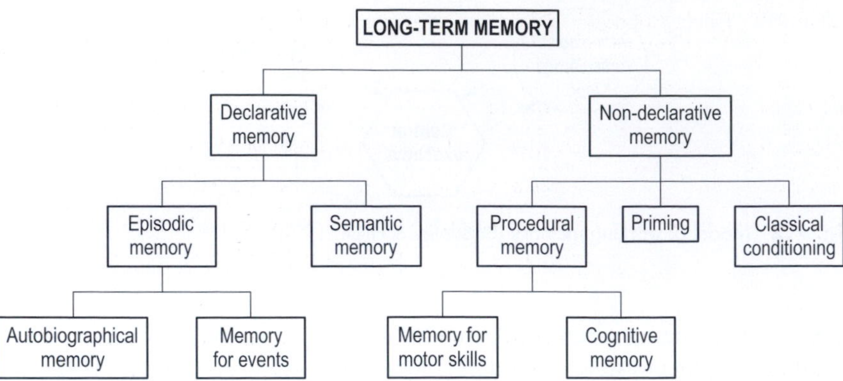

Fig. 7.3 Components of long-term memory

knowledge, language, music, events, people, places, smell, skills, and so on. Many long-term memories are not accessible to conscious recollection and may be brought into awareness by providing cues, elaboration, hypnosis or by psychoanalysis. LTM is dynamic, it is constantly modified, revised and reconstructed in the light of new information or experiences. The brain structures responsible for LTM are located in the regions of the limbic system, especially the hippocampus and entorhinal cortex of the medial temporal lobe. LTM is usually tested by delayed recall of words, figures, addresses and personal events in the recent and distant past. A number of distinct memory systems and processes appear to support LTM (Box 7.2). The realisation that LTM is not a singular, stand-alone entity but consists of several different systems is one of the main findings of recent memory research.

Declarative (explicit) and non-declarative (implicit) memory

An important advance in our understanding of LTM has been the distinction made between its two forms: declarative (explicit); and non-declarative (implicit) memory, and their subdivisions (Fig. 7.3).

Declarative memory

Declarative memory refers to the recollection of events, facts and information. It is tested by clinical tests of recall and recognition. Declarative memory is dependent on the integrity of the hippocampus and related structures. It is divided into two subcomponents – episodic and semantic memory (Tulving, 1972).

Episodic memory. This refers to memories for events and personal experience from the past. Often the recall of information is more than mere recollections from the past – they are usually embedded in the context of time and space as well as emotions associated with the events. Episodic memory is actively remembered. What one had for breakfast and what happened on the first day in work or school belong to episodic memory. It also includes impersonal events such as political events (e.g. 11 September 2001). An important component of episodic memory is memory for events in one's life known as *autobiographical memory*. Autobiographical details of events that happened

Table 7.2 Features of declarative and non-declarative memory

	Declarative memory	*Non-declarative memory*
Information	Facts, events	Motor skills, conditioning, priming
State of awareness	Conscious recollection	No-conscious
Operation involved	Remembering (what?)	Knowing (how?)
Brain structures involved	Temporal lobe and diencephalic structures	Different brain structures depending on the task

years and decades ago endure over long periods of time but are always incomplete. The memory is frequently accompanied by personal interpretations, and encompasses three important aspects: specific event (e.g. getting injured), general class of event (e.g. accident) and life-time period (e.g. while working in Derby) (Conway, 1996). Autobiographical memories for events that occur in one's lifetime show a particular pattern (Rubin, Wetzler & Nebes, 1986). In a study of a group of 70 year olds it was shown that memory for personal events fall along the following lines:

- Infantile amnesia – there is a total lack of memories for events that occur during the first few years of life. Usually there is amnesia for events that occurred in the first 2 to 5 years. However, the average age of the earliest retrieved memory is 3.5 years.
- A relatively good retention of memories for events occurring up to the age of 20 years.
- Increasingly better memories for recent material (60 to 70 years)

An interesting area of study has been around vivid and enduring memories that people have for certain dramatic events such as the suicide bombing of the twin towers on 11 September 2001. These memories have been termed *flashbulb memories*. Usually subjects are able to remember details such as where they were, what they were doing and other details of the time that they heard the news (Brown & Kulik, 1977).

Semantic memory. This is an important part of declarative memory, and is concerned with remembering facts, ideas and concepts. It refers to what is *known* rather than when and how the knowledge was acquired. For example, in answering the question 'What is the capital of Egypt?' one is using semantic memory. Most abstract knowledge consists of material drawn from semantic memory.

Non-declarative memory

Whereas episodic and semantic memories are available to conscious access, other forms of learning occur to which we do not have conscious access. These have been named *non-declarative memory*. This refers to a collection of abilities and skills that has been acquired previously. The distinguishing feature of non-declarative memory is that it does not involve conscious recollection of previous experience. Unlike declarative memory, non-declarative memory cannot be considered a system. It is a collection of memory for a variety of tasks. A key observation has been that in amnesic patients with damage to the hippocampus and associated structures these skills are spared. Non-declarative memory is more enduring than declarative memory. Three groups of tasks associated with non-declarative memory have been described:

1. *Procedural memory*. This refers to memory for motor, perceptual and intuitive cognitive skills. Driving a car and playing the piano are examples of procedural memory. It is about 'knowing how' as opposed to declarative memory's 'knowing that' (Cohen & Squire, 1980).
2. *Conditioning*. Memory for conditioned responses is a part of non-declarative memory.
3. *Priming*. This refers to the enhancement of the efficiency of identification through previous experience. The main features of declarative and non-declarative memory are summarised in Table 7.2.

FORGETTING

Memory for events and facts declines over time – in minutes, hours, months and years. This long-term forgetting with the passage of time was objectively demonstrated more than 100 years ago by Hermann Ebbinghaus (1885). He attempted to memorise nonsense syllables (e.g. FIW, BOEZ) and recall them at various time intervals over a period of 31 days. By plotting the proportion of words retained in memory against time, he was able to plot the forgetting curve. The curve, as seen in Figure 7.4, shows a sharp drop over the first nine hours, and particularly during the first hour. After nine hours, the rate of forgetting slows and declines little thereafter, even after the lapse of 31 days.

Ebbinghaus tested his own memory under laboratory conditions. Subsequent researchers have carried out studies on everyday memory and their findings have largely confirmed those of Ebbinghaus (Linton, 1986). The main findings from these and other studies are:

- Forgetting is maximum in the first few hours and the rate of forgetting gets less with time.
- Forgetting is never complete, some information is retained over long periods of time, even for life.
- Recalling the material during the test period increases the probability of remembering items or events.

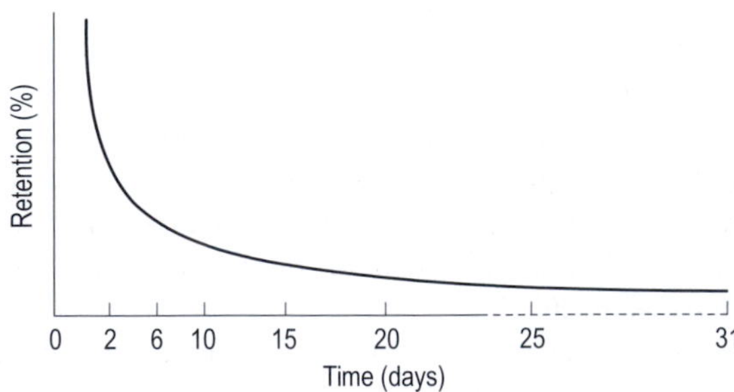

Fig. 7.4 The forgetting curve (Ebbinghaus, 1885)

- Continuous motor skills, such as cycling, show no forgetting at all. Discrete motor skills, like typing, are lost more quickly.
- Learned skills like cardiac resuscitation (CPR) are lost quite rapidly in the first year (hence the need for frequent retraining).

A number of cases where memories as old as 50 years have been recalled have been recorded. Stimulation of the temporal lobe under anaesthesia has been shown to produce memories that have been long lost. It appears that memory traces remain in long-term stores indefinitely and that forgetting is mainly due to retrieval failure. The cause of long-term forgetting may be attributed to failure in one or more memory processes: failure in encoding at the time of input; failure of transfer of information from short-term memory to long-term memory; or, more commonly, retrieval failure.

Encoding failure

Forgetting over time may be due to defective or impaired initial encoding of information into memory. Both neuroimaging and cognitive studies have shown that a significant proportion of forgetting is likely to occur when insufficient attention is paid to the material at the time of encoding. It may also be due to 'shallow' processing of information (see depth of processing theory, below).

Retrieval failure

The commonest cause of failure to access long-term memory is failure of retrieval. The memory trace is 'there' but the route to retrieving appears to be 'blocked'. Retrieval is facilitated by cues. Retrieval cues are stimuli associated with stored information. Hearing an old tune, for example, brings the memories of the words of a long-forgotten song. It appears that in some forms of memory failure information is still present in LTM but no suitable retrieval cue is available to trigger off the recall process (*cue-dependent forgetting*). Research into retrieval process has produced a number of findings and associated theories.

- *Encoding specificity principle*. It has been suggested (Tulving, 1972) that when information is encoded the target item as well as the context, are both incorporated into the memory trace. That contextual information available at the time of retrieval has a strong influence on the retrieval process was convincingly demonstrated in a study where subjects learned a list of words under two conditions, either on land or twenty feet under the sea. When they were subsequently tested, recall of the word list was approximately 50% higher when the context of the learning and recall were the same. That is, memory was better in those who learned on land and recalled on land, than those who learned and recalled under water (Godden & Baddeley, 1975).
- The phenomenon of *context-dependent memory* for recall has been replicated in a number of studies. The fact that contextual and environmental cues are effective in activating recall of information has been utilised in

crime detection. Television programmes that reconstruct the crime scene and visits to scenes of crime by witnesses have been found to be effective in triggering recall of details of the crime.

- *State-dependent memory*. A similar phenomenon is state-dependent memory (or state-dependent learning) in which the retrieval cue at the time of encoding information is one's 'internal' mental state, rather than the external context. Thus, subjects who learn the information while under the influence of alcohol, amphetamines or marijuana remember the items better when under similar intoxicated states (Goodwin et al., 1969).
- *Blocking*. This is said to occur when the subjects are unable to access information that they know exists in their memory despite great efforts at recalling, even in the presence of retrieval cues. A typical example is when one 'knows' but cannot remember the name of a person or the author of an article. Blocking may occur both in the case of episodic memory (name, incident) or semantic memory (information, general knowledge). Blocking is particularly pronounced in older adults, particularly in remembering names. A well-investigated example of blocking is the *tip-of-the-tongue state* (TOT). TOT refers to an experience when one is unable to retrieve a word, despite the strong conviction that the item is present in one's memory. TOT states may last for a few seconds (e.g. forgetting the right word or name in the course of a lecture) or for a few days (e.g. as when one remembers a colleague's name a few days later). A striking feature of the TOT state is that although the word eludes the subject, semantic memory for it is quite intact, that is, one is able to describe or provide the meaning of it although unable to remember the word (Brown & McNeill, 1966).
- *Failure of prospective memory*. Remembering to carry out particular actions or perform planned actions is known as prospective memory. Failure of prospective memory is a common cause of absent-mindedness. Failure to take medication or keep appointments are examples of lapses in prospective memory, which can be potentially damaging, or even disastrous. Prospective memory is related to action plans that we make and appears to involve the prefrontal lobes of the brain.

Schema

As Ebbinghaus' experiments with word lists suggest, recall and memory for information is not a simple process of regurgitation of stored memories. Scholarship and research in psychology has tended to follow two distinct traditions. The first views the study of human cognitions as 'pure science' akin to physics and attempts to discover universal laws and truths that underlie all psychological phenomena. Typically, these researchers carry out experiments in the laboratory, usually under artificial conditions, so that the data is not 'contaminated' by pre-existing knowledge. The second group seeks to study cognitions in the context of the individual's previous knowledge, beliefs and experiences. They tend to study subjects under ordinary social conditions and the study design includes beliefs and experiences. Ebbinghaus was a proponent of the first method and his studies on forgetting exemplify the 'pure science' approach. One of the pioneers of the second approach was the British psychologist Frederick Bartlett (1932). He made a radical departure from the Ebbinghaus tradition by testing people in their natural social environment rather than in the laboratory. His work received little attention from psychologists of the day but he is now accepted as one of the pioneers of the cognitive revolution that was to shape psychology in the 1960s.

One of Bartlett's experiments was his famous study on memory for a story about American Indians called 'the war of ghosts'. The story made little sense to western subjects because it included magic and ghosts unfamiliar to the experimental subjects. When they tried to recall the story it was found that, in an attempt to reconstruct the story so that it was meaningful to them, they had incorporated their own views into the narrative. For Bartlett, this was a clear demonstration of the reconstructive nature of memory. When presented with material for recall, people do not simply reproduce stored memory traces, rather they actively reconstruct information using past experiences, prior beliefs, values and knowledge. He referred to this process as 'effort after meaning'. He was responsible for introducing into psychology the term *schema*, which he borrowed from the neurologist Henry Head.

Accuracy of memory

How accurate are memories? In addition to total or partial failure to remember past events, memory is susceptible to various forms of distortions, revisions, omissions, modifications and reconstructions. These 'sins' of memory have important applications for both day-to-day living and clinical practice (Schacter, 1999). False recall of information as evidenced by the controversy over recovered memories of child sexual abuse and false recognition in instances of eye witness misidentification in criminal cases have been the subject of intense debate and recent scientific, clinical and media discussions. The three main processes involved in producing potential inaccuracies and distortions in memory in normal subjects are suggestibility, bias and misattribution. A fourth factor that increases the chances of discrepancies, omissions and distortions in memory is the emotional state of the subject at the time of recall. Moreover, psychiatric disorders, especially depression and post-traumatic stress disorders, can affect the quality of episodic and autobiographical material that people remember.

RETRIEVAL

Retrieval refers to the process of extraction of relevant memories from long-term memory stores. There are two components of retrieval: (1) involuntary or automatic retrieval; and (2) voluntary retrieval.

Involuntary retrieval

A certain amount of recall is automatic, non-conscious and involuntary. This is especially true of recognition memory. The difference between recall and recognition is striking. While individuals may be able to *remember* items that have been learned, they are able to recognise many more.

Voluntary retrieval

Conscious retrieval is an active process that involves attempts by the subject to recall previous incidents, events or experiences. This has been studied most often in the case of autobiographical memory. Some of the features of retrieval from autobiographical memory are of clinical importance:

- Studies have shown that unpleasant memories are recalled less readily than pleasant ones.
- People remember events and incidents that are personally salient better than non-important ones. Changes of employment or residence or past illnesses are better recalled than the meal that one had a month ago.
- Rehearsal of past events facilitates subsequent retrieval. Family experiences are told and retold so often that they become part of family narratives.
- Cueing is a powerful method of recalling autobiographical memories.
- Memories that carry a personal, emotional component are retrieved better than other episodes. Events involving fear, anger and disgust are better recalled than neutral ones. A study carried out in Japan showed that patients with Alzheimer's disease recalled the 1995 earthquake in Kobe district in Japan better than a subsequent MRI scan that they had undergone (Ikeda et al., 1998).
- Memory distortions may occur, and are indeed common. Retrieval is an active process in which memories for events and incidents are constantly reconstructed. During reconstruction the memories may undergo distortion, elaboration or falsification. Gaps may be filled with new material or information may be lost. This is particularly relevant in 'false-memory syndrome'. Material recalled under hypnosis is particularly prone to distortion because of the element of suggestibility.
- Recall is accurate so far as the broad generality of the incident or the event is concerned but not for its details. Thus retrieval errors are common but the account of the main experience is by far true, although they may not be accurate.

Repressed memories, recovered memories and false-memory syndrome

In the 1990s there was a series of court cases in which young women, most of whom were undergoing psychotherapy, allegedly 'remembered' childhood sexual abuse for the first time. Ostensibly they had forgotten or repressed memories of abuse until they were 'recovered' during therapy. Some of the alleged abusers were initially convicted but many were found not guilty on appeal. In the USA, some therapists were ordered to pay large sum of money as damages to those accused as abusers. What are the true facts that we know about recovered memories, repressions and the false-memory syndrome?

The following is a summary of the available evidence (Brewin, 1996):

1. There is evidence that people sometimes forget unpleasant experiences, but memories of such events may be recalled later.
2. Up to a quarter of women who have been sexually abused report severe memory loss for the events. Such memory deficits are common in those who have suffered violent abuse.
3. The concept of repression, enunciated by Freud in his early writing, as an active process in which painful thoughts and memories are pushed to the inaccessible corners of the mind has received little experimental support.
4. The past is constantly remembered and forgotten. Retrieval is not the same as the play-back function of a video or tape recorder. It is an active process, which involves reconstruction, elaboration and modification of memories. Memories can, therefore, be distorted and false memories do occur.
5. False memories may arise during psychological therapies, particularly with hypnosis, abreaction, guided recall and suggestion.
6. Report of long-forgotten abuse should neither be accepted uncritically nor rejected outright. Each case needs to be dealt with individually.
7. External collaboration for evidence of abuse should always be sought.
8. Practitioners should be extremely careful not to suggest past memories of sexual abuse while treating or interviewing patients.

Both the Royal College of Psychiatrists and the British Psychological Association have provided guidelines to practitioners on the subject of recovered memories of childhood sexual abuse (Brandon et al., 1998).

MODELS OF MEMORY

A number of models of memory have been described. The two well-known examples are processing theories and the multi-store model.

Processing theories

Processing theories are general psychological models based on the assumption that the mind is composed of different processes or procedures (not systems) that can function in a variety of ways. Cognitive processes such as attention, perception, thinking and remembering are seen to interact with one another rather than having dedicated systems in the brain.

In the case of memory, the *levels of processing theory* (Craik & Lockhart, 1972), has been the most popular model. The main proposition of this theory is that the degree or depth of analysis at the time of encoding determines how well the memory is retained. When processing information at the time of input is shallow, material is less well remembered than when there is deep processing involving extraction of meaning (semantic processing). Several experiments have confirmed that elaborative processes carried out at the time of encoding lead to long-term retention. Although there is some evidence to support the levels of processing theory it fails to explain why deep processing leads to better long-term memory.

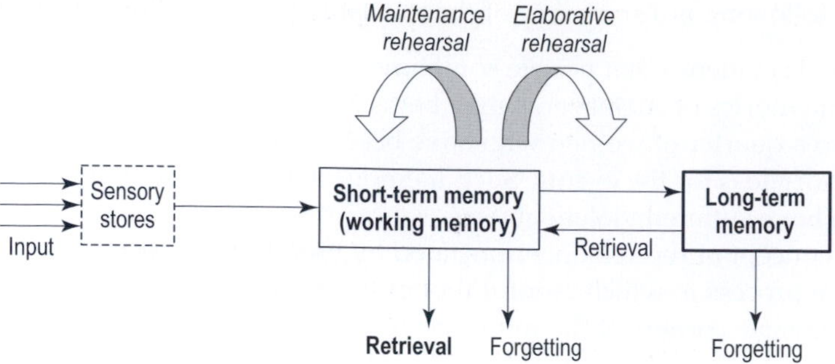

Fig. 7.5 Multi-store model of memory (Atkinson & Shiffrin, 1968)

The multi-store model

Multi-store models of memory hold that memory is not a singular entity but is composed of several memory systems that can operate independently of one another, although they are interconnected and interrelated. The best-known multi-store model is the one proposed by Atkinson and Shiffrin (1968). According to their theory, memory is characterised as the flow of information between three interrelated stores: sensory store; short-term store; and long-term store (Figure 7.5).

The existence of two forms of memory stores, LTM and STM, had been known and studied long before Atkinson and Shiffrin proposed their model. In their model, information input from the environment is received by the sensory stores, some of it is transferred on to the STM and a proportion of that held in the STM is passed on to the LTM. STM plays a pivotal role in the organisation of memory because not only does it temporarily hold information coming from the sensory stores but it also receives information from LTM by the process of retrieval. Information can be held in STM for longer periods by a process of (maintenance) rehearsal.

DISORDERS OF MEMORY

Although 'normal' forgetting is a feature of everyday life and aging, severe forgetfulness and memory deficits are features of a variety of clinical conditions. A classification of memory impairment is provided in Figure 7.6.

Age-associated memory impairment

It is not uncommon for older adults to complain of declining memory. Forgetting names and appointments and misplacing everyday items, such as keys, is a common subjective complaint in the elderly. Studies comparing the objective memory performance in people between the ages of 35 and 44 years and those between the ages of 70 and 74 years has shown that the younger age group had scores up to 50% higher than those in the older group. Tests have also demonstrated that memory for non-verbal material seems to be more affected by aging than memory for verbal material, and delayed recall is affected more than

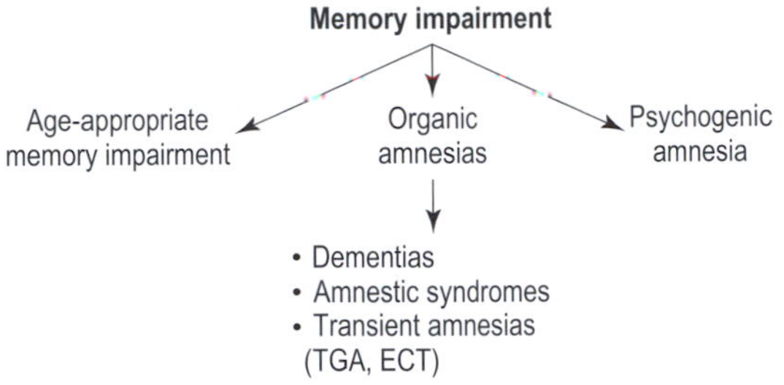

Fig. 7.6 A classification of the causes of memory loss

immediate recall. This demonstrable loss of memory with increasing age has been termed *age-associated memory impairment* (AAMI). AAMI has been strictly defined (Crook et al., 1986) and the criteria for its diagnosis laid down:

1. Perception by the subject of memory loss (e.g. misplacing articles such as keys, spectacles, etc.).
2. Objective evidence of impairment of memory on standardised tests of delayed recall for verbal information.
3. A score of one standard deviation below that of a young adult on tests of memory.
4. Absence of other conditions that may affect memory, including depression and dementia.

Approximately 40% of individuals aged 65 and over show AAMI. A common bedside test is to give a list of 20 words to the subject to study and then ask him or her to recall as many as possible 20 minutes later (delayed recall). The score is compared with standardised scores for the given age. There is considerable individual variation in the memory impairment in this group and there appears to be a subgroup of elderly individuals whose memory and cognitive functions are well preserved. Although the declining memory increases with increasing age, it does not appear to have any particular prognostic significance (Small, 2002).

Dementia

The term dementia has been used in two different ways. It has been used to describe a symptom, the gradual, and usually progressive, decline in memory. In the second usage the term dementia is employed to describe a clinical syndrome (as defined in DSM-IV and ICD-10) in which there is marked loss of memory, deterioration in adaptive functioning and, at least one other additional sign of major cognitive deficit (aphasia, agnosia or loss of executive functions). The syndrome of dementia is therefore similar to anaemia or renal failure in that it may be caused by numerous pathological processes. Thus, the syndrome consists of a collection of symptoms that imply widespread cerebral damage. The most common cause of this syndrome in individuals over 65 is Alzheimer's disease (AD), which accounts for approximately two-thirds of all cases of dementia.

The pattern and progression of cognitive impairments in AD are selective and follows a predictable course over the duration of the disease. The earliest sign of AD is loss of memory and the major memory system affected is episodic memory. The impairment of episodic memory is evident early in the course of AD and is best demonstrated by tests of delayed recall such as remembering a name and address after 5 to 10 minutes. Loss of remote memory becomes evident next. It begins with difficulties in recall of recent events and proceeds, according to Ribot's law, to extend to more distant memories. Semantic memory also shows deterioration early in the course of AD but may not be apparent to the subject or the clinician unless specific tests are carried out. In comparison with marked deficits in LTM, working memory remains remarkably intact even in the later stages of the disease; implicit memory is spared until very late stages of the disease.

In addition to AD, various other disorders can give rise to the syndrome of dementia, most notably vascular and other degenerative pathologies. For more details the reader is referred to a textbook on organic psychiatry (e.g. Lishman, 1997).

The *mini-mental state examination* (MMSE; Folstein, Folstein & McHugh, 1975) is a popular screening and rating tool for dementia. In addition to memory it assesses orientation, praxis and other functions. The *Cambridge cognitive function examination* (CAMCOG) is a well-established research instrument for the assessment of dementia in elderly people. It assesses a wider range of cognitive functions than memory (attention, abstraction, language, and so on). It is part of a standardised psychiatric assessment schedule for the elderly, the CAMDEX (Roth et al., 1986).

Amnesic syndromes

The *amnesic syndrome* has been defined as 'an abnormal mental state in which memory and learning are affected out of all proportion to other cognitive functions in an otherwise alert and responsive patient' (Victor, Adams & Collins, 1971). In the typical amnesic syndrome, the memory deficit is circumscribed and dense but intelligence, speech and reasoning are well preserved.

Various disorders can give rise to an amnesic syndrome, including herpes encephalitis, severe cerebral hypoxia and thiamine deficiency. The characteristic features of memory loss in the amnesic syndrome are:

1. Intact short-term memory. Immediate memory is unimpaired. Thus performances on digit span test and other measures of primary memory (requiring the recall of information within a few seconds) are remarkably intact and within normal range. However, performances on these short-term memory tests are sensitive to proactive interference. If, for example, patients are given a second distractive exercise (such as repeating three digits backwards) before recalling the test items, the patients are unable to recall the original items.
2. Anterograde amnesia (AA). This refers to the inability to acquire new information. The acquisition (learning), retention and recall (retrieval) of verbal

and non-verbal material are key elements in the assessment of anterograde memory. The classical pattern of anterograde amnesia consists of normal immediate recall as indicated above (e.g. digit span) and impaired delayed recall (e.g. recall three items or an address after five minutes). Because of the inability to learn and retain new information, most patients experience difficulties in remembering recent events such as the ingredients of their last meal, the name of the hospital or, even, the date.

3. Retrograde amnesia (RA). Retrograde amnesia is the inability to retrieve information that had been stored prior to the onset of amnesia. While in amnesic syndrome AA is typical and characteristic and invariably present, RA shows considerable variability both in extent and severity. The degree of RA depends to a large extent on the locus of damage and the extent of brain damage. Generally, RA tends to show a temporal gradient, i.e. remote events are better remembered than more recent events (Ribot's law)
4. Preserved global intellectual abilities.
5. Preserved implicit memory.

Two subtypes of the amnesic syndrome have been described based on neuroanatomical distinctions:

1. Medial temporal lobe amnesia (MTL) resulting from bilateral damage to the medial temporal lobe and the hippocampal system following anoxia, encephalitis or head injury. Typically patients with MTL amnesia have been described as having:
   - preserved insight;
   - increased rate of forgetting (severe AA);
   - limited RA; and
   - lack of confabulation (falsification of memories).
2. Diencephalic amnesia is characterised by extensive retrograde amnesia covering many decades, with a pattern of relative preservation of more distant memories (temporal gradient). In addition to the memory deficits, patients show confabulation (falsification of memory) and a lack of insight in to the memory disturbance. Impairment in memory in this patient group has been attributed to damage to medial thalamic structures, mammillary bodies and hypothalamic regions. Damage needs to be bilateral in order to produce memory deficits. The diencephalic form of the amnesic syndrome is best exemplified by Korsakoff's syndrome.

Recent work has cast doubts on whether or not the pattern of deficits across patients with mediotemporal or diencephalic pathology actually show significant difference (Kopelman & Stanhope, 1997).

Korsakoff's syndrome. This is a specific form of the amnesic syndrome resulting from nutritional depletion, notably thiamine deficiency. The most common cause of the syndrome is alcohol abuse. The pattern of memory deficit in Korsakoff's syndrome involves a severe impairment of new learning (anterograde amnesia) and extensive retrograde loss. This retrograde memory loss extends back at least 25 to 30 years and includes loss of memory for remote information and autobiographical memory for incidents or events from the patient's past. These aspects of retrograde memory show a temporal gradient, with relative sparing of the most distant memories and the gradient is significantly steeper than that seen in dementing disorders such as Alzheimer's disease. Working memory, priming and procedural memory are well preserved. Neuroanatomical lesions are thought to involve the limbic–diencephalic circuits. The characteristic pathological features of the disorder are found in the paraventricular and periaqueductal grey matter. There is consensus that the lesion is either in the thalamus or the mammillary bodies or both. More recent studies emphasised the importance of the circuit comprising the mammillary bodies, the mammillothalamic tract and the anterior thalamus (Kopelman, 1995).

Memory loss in head injuries

Immediately following head injury many patients (after recovering consciousness) show an impairment of memory for events that occurred previously. This amnesic gap is known as post-traumatic amnesia (PTA) or post-concussion amnesia. PTA is the time between the injury and recovery of normal continuous memory. PTA is the result of transient disruption of neurological function following concussion. The length of PTA is considered to be more accurate than the length of coma in predicting recovery of function. The longer the period of PTA the more severe the brain damage and poorer the prognosis for the recovery of functions. A typical PTA grading system is as follows:

- PTA less than 1 hour – mild head injury.
- PTA from 1 to 24 hours – moderate head injury.
- PTA longer than 24 hours – severe injury.

During the period of PTA the patient, however, can acquire new skills indicating that non-declarative memory is intact. Post-concussion amnesia is thought to result from the inability of the patient to consolidate memory from short-term working memory to the long-term store.

In addition to PTA, in severe head injuries, subjects show impairment in learning of new material (as tested by learning word lists or remembering an address five minutes after its presentation) in the period immediately following the accident, but their short-term memory as tested by digit span remains intact (similar to those observed in organic amnesic syndromes). In such patients, the anterograde amnesia may persist long after the termination of

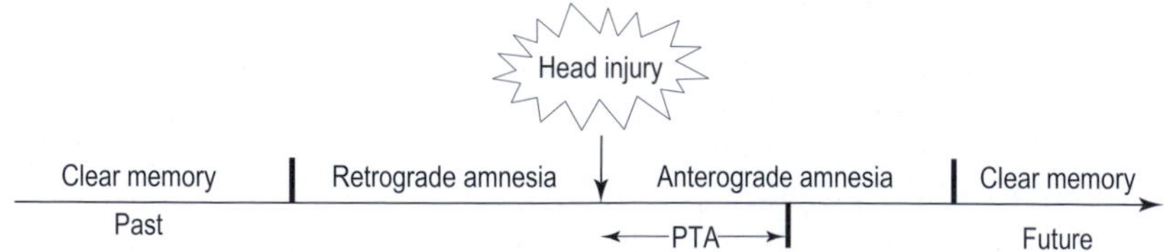

Fig. 7.7 Schematic diagram of memory loss following head injury (the lengths of amnesia are not to scale)

PTA (Figure 7.7). The point is that, in head injury, PTA and AA do not refer to the same thing and this has been a source of confusion in the literature.

Retrograde amnesia is also common after head injury. RA is the time between the injury and the last clear memory before the injury. It refers to loss of memory for events occurring before the time of injury. Amnesia extends backward in time for a variable period. As memory is regained, RA shows shrinkage and the most remote memories return first. In most cases the amnesic gap is very short, usually lasting one minute or less. It is not a good indicator of prognosis.

Memory loss following electroconvulsive therapy (ECT)

In most patients, the impairment of memory following ECT (given usually for the treatment of severe depressive disorder) is temporary and follow-up studies have demonstrated that there is no lasting memory impairment (Warren & Groome, 1984). Immediately after the administration of ECT some patients show impairment in memory similar to that seen in concussion. Research studies suggest that there may be both anterograde and retrograde amnesia, both of which shrink rapidly and the patient is left with amnesia for the treatment itself and a few hours preceding it (Squire, Slater & Miller, 1981). A systemic review of patients' experience found that approximately a third *describe* persistent loss of memory following ECT (Rose et al., 2003). Most trials did not measure memory, especially autobiographical memory, over the long term. It has been suggested that high-quality collaborative trials are necessary to overcome the inherent bias in research done by consumers for consumers and clinicians for clinicians (Carney & Geddes, 2003). Memory impairment is less pronounced in unilateral ECT.

Transient organic amnesias

Short-lived and temporary amnesia is common in a number of organic conditions ranging from epilepsy to head injuries. A specific syndrome termed *transient global amnesia* (TGA) describes a condition occurring in middle-aged or elderly men in whom there is profound but temporary failure of memory lasting several hours. During the attack the subject is unable to acquire new lasting memories (AA) and, therefore, continues to have a permanent memory gap for the period of attack. The general consensus is that TGA results from transient dysfunction of the limbic–hippocampal circuits.

Psychogenic amnesias

Psychogenic amnesias are thought to be caused by psychological factors, especially traumatic events, which are unacceptable to the person. There is no actual brain damage and the amnesia recovers over a period of time. In clinical practice two types of psychogenic amnesia have been recognised: 'global' and 'situation-specific'. In the former, sometimes known as fugue state, there is sudden loss of all autobiographical memories and knowledge of self and personal identity. This is usually associated with wandering, for which there is an amnesic gap upon recovery. Global amnesia usually follows exposure to some form of psychological trauma. Often such patients report having made trips over a period of hours but do not recall what happened during that time. Patients are usually unaware of the memory disturbance. Usually memory recovery is complete after few hours or days. Situation-specific amnesia may arise in states of extreme arousal including committing an offence, being the victim of an offence or of child sexual abuse. It may also occur in post-traumatic disorder.

TESTS OF MEMORY

Tests of short-term memory

Immediate or STM is tested by recall of information seconds after its presentation. *Digit span* is the commonest test of auditory, verbal short-term or working memory. In clinical practice, both the forward digit span and the backward digit span are measured. The subject is given a string of digits beginning with two digits and asked to repeat it immediately. The score is the longest series correctly repeated. For reverse digit span, exactly the same method is used except that the subject is asked to repeat the digits in the reverse order. The normal range of digits forwards is 6 ± 1 and for reverse digit span it is 5 ± 1. An example is as follows: 4–9, 6–3–2, 6–4–3–9, 7–2–6–8, 4–2–7–3–1, 7–5–8–3–6, 6–1–9–4–7–3, 5–9–1–7–4–2–3, 5–8–1–9–2–6–4–7–8.

Tests of recent memory

Recent memory can be tested informally by asking patients to recall very recent events such as how they came to the clinic or hospital, their last meal, or events that may have happened that day.

Recent memory, as indicated before, is a part of LTM. More formal tests of recent memory may be carried out in a series of tests beginning with recall of three items and progressing on to more complex material. These are tests of anterograde amnesia and new learning. The *three word learning test*, where the subject is read out (and shown) three items (e.g. watch, pen, desk) and asked to recall them five minutes later, is used with patients with severe memory loss. The commonest test of recent memory is the *name and address recall test*. This consists of seven items such as 'Peter Marshall, 43 Market Street, Stockport, Merseyside' and the subject is asked to recall as many items, without prompts, in five to ten minutes. Where the memory impairment is less severe, the test could be made more demanding by asking the patient to recall a short piece of narrative. Here the subject is read a short story from the *Wechsler memory scale* (WMS) containing 25 elements and both immediate and delayed recall (after an interval of 30 minutes) is tested. Word list learning tasks is another method used to test recent memory. Here the subject is given a list of about 15 nouns and asked to recall them in a series of trials.

Non-verbal memory may be tested by the getting subjects to reproduce a geometric shape. One such test is the *Rey–Osterrieth complex figure test*. This

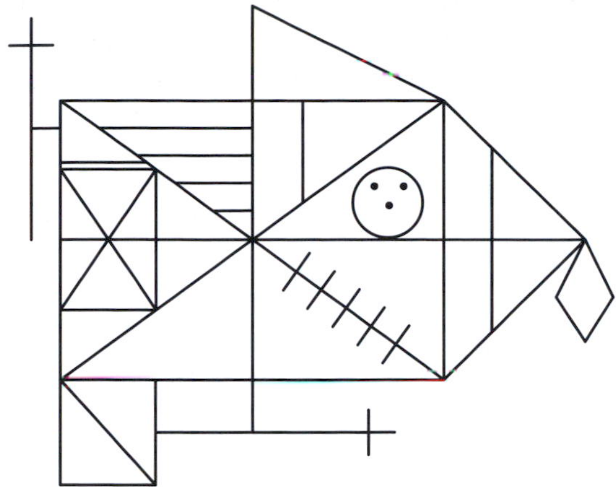

Fig. 7.8 The Rey–Osterrieth complex figure test. Patients are first asked to copy the figure freehand and then to reproduce it from memory after 20 to 30 minutes. The test can be scored according to a standardised scoring system. In addition to providing a measure of nonverbal memory it tests constructional abilities (Osterrieth, 1944)

consists of a complex geometric figure (Figure 7.8) that the subject is first asked to copy and then to draw from memory after an interval of 30 minutes. Recall is impaired in patients with amnesic syndrome, selective right temporal damage and those with mild AD. Normative data are available from the test manufacturer. Remote or retrograde memory may be assessed from questioning the person about a variety of past events from the preceding months, years or decades. It is usual to ask about public events, news items and famous events from various past eras.

Autobiographical memory can be assessed by asking for memory of personal events starting from recent events such as the last birthday to more distal events like the schools attended. Often independent confirmation may be necessary. A formal test of autobiographical memory is the *autobiographical memory interview* (AMI). It is a structured interview, which probes for personal facts and episodes from three life periods: school, early adult and recent. A typical example is the AMI designed by Kopelman, Wilson and Baddeley (1990) to test personal remote (retrograde) memory. Normative data, with cut offs for probable and definitive impairment, are available.

Wechsler memory scale

Several neuropsychological test batteries, which provide a comprehensive assessment of most aspects of memory, are commercially available. One of the best-known is the Wechsler memory scale (WMS). The most recent edition, WMS–III^{UK} (Wechsler, 1987), consists of a number of tests grouped under two domains, verbal and non-verbal memory. These can be subdivided into verbal and non-verbal memory tests, all of which have immediate and delayed recall and/or recognition components. A third group of tests involve 'mental control' tasks. A brief description of the subtests are given in Box 7.3. The WMS may be applied in its entirety or specific subtests may be used in

Box 7.3 Subtests in the Wechsler memory scale-III (Wechsler, 1987)

Verbal subtests

1. Stories (logical memory). Two paragraph-length stories consisting of about 25 'elements' are read out separately and tested for recall immediately and after 30 minutes
2. Verbal paired associates. Pairs of words (e.g. baby–cries, crush–dark) are presented and the subject is read the first word of the pair and asked to recall the second word, immediately and after 30 minutes
3. Word list. A list of about a dozen words is read out followed by a second word list. Subject is asked to recall the first list (second list is the interfering list), immediately and after 30 minutes

Non-verbal subtests

1. Faces. Twenty-four photos of faces of various people are shown and the subject tested for immediate recognition and delayed recognition using decoys as well as the photos
2. Family pictures. A drawing of a family with grandparents, two children, parents and a dog engaged in four activity scenes is shown. Questions are asked about each scene for immediate and delayed recall
3. Drawings (visual designs). Five designs of increasing complexity are shown one at a time and the subject asked to draw them. They are asked to draw as many designs as they can after 30 minutes

Mental control subtests

1. Mental control. Involves rapid serial counting, alphabet recitation and reverse counting
2. Digit span. Repetition of strings of numbers
3. Spatial span. The visual equivalent of digit span. Involves tapping on a series of blocks
4. Letter–number sequencing. The subject is read increasingly large strings of letters and numbers and asked to mentally rearrange these strings, and say them with all of the numbers listed first, in order (1–9) and all the letters in the string, in alphabetical order (e.g. 4–Q–2–H–7–V would have to be resequenced as 2–4–7–H–Q–V). This task is thought to make demands on working memory

accordance with clinical need. Extensive normative data for various age bands are available and the scale has been validated on a national UK sample.

The commonly used tests of memory are summarised in Box 7.4.

Box 7.4 Common tests of memory

Bedside tests

- Digit span
- Recall of three objects
- Recall of seven item address
- Recall of recent incidents and events
- Recall of famous names
- Recall of remote personal memory

Specialised tests

- Rey–Osterrieth complex figure test
- Story recall
- Autobiographical memory interview

Neuropsychological batteries

- Wechsler memory scale
- Rivermead behavioural memory test

REFERENCES

Atkinson RC, Shiffrin RM (1968) Human memory: a proposed system and its control processes. In KW Spence & JT Spence (eds), The Psychology of Learning and Motivation (Vol. 2). London, UK: Academic Press.

Baddeley AD (1986) Working Memory., Oxford, UK: Oxford University Press.

Baddeley AD, Hitch G (1974) Working memory. In GH Power (ed.), The psychology of learning and motivation (Vol. 8). London, UK: Academic Press.

Bartlett FC (1932) Remembering: a study in experimental and social psychology. New York: Cambridge University Press.

Brandon S, Boakes J, Glaser D, Green R (1998) Recovered memories of childhood sexual abuse: implications for clinical practice. British Journal of Psychiatry, 172, 296–307.

Brewin C (1996) Scientific status of recovered memories. British Journal of Psychiatry, 169, 131–134.

Brown J, McNeill D (1966) The 'tip of the tongue' phenomenon. Journal of Verbal Learning and Verbal Behaviour, 5, 325–337.

Brown R, Kulik J (1977) Flashbulb memories. Cognition, 5, 73–79.

Carney S, Geddes J (2003) Electroconvulsive therapy: recent recommendations are likely to improve standards and uniformity of use. British Medical Journal, 326, 1343–1344.

Cohen NJ, Squire LR (1980) Preserved learning and retention of pattern-analysing skill in amnesia: dissociation of knowing how and knowing that. Science, 210, 207–210.

Conway MA (1996) Autobiographical knowledge and autobiographical memories. In DC Rubin (ed.), Remembering our Past: studies in autobiographical memory. Cambridge, UK: Cambridge University Press.

Craik FJM, Lockhart RS (1972) Levels of processing: a framework for memory research. Journal of Verbal Learning and Verbal Behaviour, 11, 671–684.

Crook P, Bartus RT, Ferris SH, Whitehouse P, Cohen GD, Gershon S (1986) Age-associated memory impairment: proposed diagnostic criteria and measures of clinical change. Report of a National Institute of Mental Health workgroup. Developmental Neuropsychology, 2, 261–272.

Ebbinghaus H (1885) Uber das gedachtnis [On thinking]. Leipzig: Dunker. (Translation by H Ruyer & CE Bussenis (1913) Memory. New York : Teachers College Press, Colombia University Press.

Folstein MF, Folstein SE, McHugh PR (1975) Mini-mental state: a practical method for grading the cognitive states of patients for the clinician. Journal of Psychiatric Research, 12, 189–198.

Godden DR, Baddeley AD (1975) Context-dependent memory in two natural environments: on land and under water. British Journal of Psychology, 66, 325–331.

Goodwin DW, Powell B, Bremer D, Hoine H, Stern J (1969) Alcohol and recall: state-dependent effects on man, Science, 163, 1358.

Ikeda M, Mori M, Hirono N, Imamura T, Shimomura T, Ikejiri Y, Yamashita H (1998) Amnestic people with Alzheimer's disease who remembered the Kobe earthquake. British Journal of Psychiatry, 172, 425–428.

Kopelman MD (1995) The Korsakoff syndrome. British Journal of Psychiatry, 166, 154–173.

Kopelman MD, Stanhope N (1997) Rates of forgetting in organic amnesia following temporal lobe, diencephalic or frontal lobe lesions. Neuropsychology, 11, 343–356.

Kopelman MD, Wilson BA, Baddeley AD (1990) The Autobiographical Memory Interview. Bury St Edmunds, UK: Thames Valley Test Company.

Linton M (1986) Memory for real-world events. In DE Norman & DE Rumelhart (eds), Explorations in Cognition. San Francisco, CA: WH Freeman.

Lishman WA (1997) Organic Psychiatry: the psychological consequences of cerebral disorder. Oxford, UK: Blackwell Science.

Osterrieth P (1944) Le test de copie d'une figure complexe. Archives of Psychology, 30, 206.

Rose D, Wykes T, Leese M, Bindman J, Fleischmann P (2003) Patients' perspectives on electroconvulsive therapy: a systematic review. British Medical Journal, 326, 1363–1365.

Roth M, Tym E, Mountjoy CQ, Huppert FA, Hendrie H, Verma S, Goddard R (1986) CAMDEX: a standardised instrument for diagnosis of mental disorder in the elderly

with special reference to early detection of dementia. British Journal of Psychiatry, 149, 698–709.
Rubin DC, Wetzler SE, Nebes RD (1986) Autobiographical memory across the lifespan. In Rubin DC (ed) Autobiographical memory. Cambridge: Cambridge University Press.
Schacter DL (1999) The seven sins of memory: insights from psychology and cognitive neurosciences. American Psychologist, 54(3), 182–203.
Small GW (2002) What we need to know about age-associated memory loss. British Medical Journal, 324, 1502–1505.
Squire LR, Slater PC, Miller PL (1981) Retrograde amnesia and bilateral electroconvulsive therapy. Archives of General Psychiatry, 38, 89–95.
Tulving E (1972) Episodic and semantic memory. In E Tulving & W Donaldson (eds), Organisation of Memory. London, UK: Academic Press.
Victor M, Adams RD, Collins GH (1971) The Wernicke–Korsakoff syndrome. Philadelphia, PA: FA Davis.
Warren EW, Groome DH (1984) Memory test performance under three different wave forms of ECT for depression. British Journal of Psychiatry, 144, 370–375.
Wechsler D (1987) Wechsler Memory Scale – Revised Manual. San Antonio, TX: The Psychological Corporation.

FURTHER READING

Baddeley AD (1997) Human Memory: theory and practice. Hove, UK: Psychology Press.
- A comprehensive text on the psychology of memory.

Schacter DL (1999) The seven sins of memory: insights from psychology and cognitive neuroscience. American Psychologist, 54(3), 182–203.
- An interesting account of the malleability of memory.

Berrios GE, Hodges JR (2000) Memory Disorders in Psychiatric Practice. Cambridge, UK: Cambridge University Press.
- An excellent text on memory disorders.

Kopelman D (2002) Disorders of memory. Brain, 125, 2152–2190.
- An up-to-date review of the current status of our knowledge of the subject.

8

Psychological measurements: their uses and misuses

'Measure all that can be measured and render measurable all that defies measurement.'
Galileo Galilei

'Not everything that counts can be counted, and not everything that can be counted counts.'
Albert Einstein

The words 'test' and 'measurement', as used in psychology, are misleading because of the implied similarity to scientific measurements and medical tests. Conventional psychological testing is quite different from scientific measurements in natural sciences. What is accomplished by the application of psychological measurement is an estimation of a psychological construct. Psychological tests and measurements of personality, intelligence, attitude and motivation are fundamentally different from quantitative measurements in physical sciences such as height, weight and blood urea. Paul Kline, one of the foremost exponents of psychometric theory clarifies the issue as follows: 'There are no units of [psychological] measurement and no true zeros. Whatever psychological measurement is, it is not scientific measurement as defined in natural sciences ... If we consider what is meant by intelligence or extraversion, just for example, it is by no means clear what units of measurement might be used or what the true zero may mean. This problem applies to the majority of psychological concepts and variables' (Kline, 2000).

Besides, it is often mistakenly believed that psychological tests are 'objective', meaning that their findings and scores reflect an outside existence (as opposed to being subjective) and are real or at least approximate something close to it, as in laboratory tests, for example. The term objectivity has an entirely different meaning when applied to psychological tests or measurements. It refers to the standard ways in which they are administered, recorded and interpreted. This semantic difference has to be kept in mind when using the results of psychological tests. Psychological tests, then, are not tests of mental structures or entities as physical tests, neither are they objective in terms of physical or real existence – they are tests of psychological constructs and are useful to the extent that the underlying theoretical construct and the tests used to measure them are valid (Michell, 1997). It is important to keep these caveats in mind when reading the following account of psychological measurements.

Nevertheless, the term 'psychological measurement' appears to capture the findings of psychological tests better than any other. The terms measurement and test are used interchangeably in this book. Thorndike's often-quoted statement 'Whatever exists at all, exists in some amount' together with dictum, 'anything that exists in amount can be measured' may be said to form the basis of the science of measurement of mental or psychological factors, which is known as psychometry.

Despite the difficulties in quantification of psychological characteristics mentioned above, the field of psychometry is a thriving enterprise and, in fact, the ability to 'measure' human psychological attributes is considered to be one of the major advances in psychology.

What are psychological tests?

The definition of a psychological test provided by Anastasi (1982) cannot be bettered:

A psychological test is essentially an objective and standardised measure of a sample of behaviour.

Objectivity and standardisation in this context means that the administration, scoring and interpretation are carried out in a uniform and standard manner. For example, in the use of IQ tests the same test is administered in the same way to all subjects using the same material. It is scored and interpreted according to the strict rules set out in the manual so that the procedure is always consistent. The application of the test and its interpretation do not involve the examiner's subjective judgement. What is measured by tests ultimately is behaviour.

It is to be noted that behaviour, as described here, sometimes involves feelings, motives, interests and other aspects of mental functioning. The tests are designed to capture a representative sample of behaviour that is of interest. The test constructor is faced with the responsibility of devising an array of test items that adequately sample the universe of the domain that is under scrutiny. The information or data obtained by testing is converted to quantitative information or test scores.

Typically psychological tests have been used in three different areas: (1) in occupational settings tests are employed in personnel selection and vocational guidance; (2) in education they are useful for selection through examinations and identification of learning difficulties; and (3) in clinical work psychological tests are used as adjuncts to clinical decision making. This chapter is concerned with clinical applications and what follows is a summary of the various types of tests and their usefulness in clinical settings.

CRITERION-REFERENCED (KEYED) TESTS AND NORM-REFERENCED TESTS

Before discussing the characteristics of good psychological tests, it is important to distinguish between two types of tests: criterion-referenced tests and norm-referenced tests. The method of construction and statistical analysis of the two types are quite different. Tests that compare performance of an individual against agreed outside criteria are called *criterion-referenced tests*. The driving test is a good example. A properly conducted driving test allows a conclusion such as 'the applicant has demonstrated mastery of 75% of the driving skills necessary to be proficient at driving'. The skills that are considered necessary are selected with the explicit purpose of discriminating between two groups: those who are fit to drive on the road and those who are not. Thus criterion-referenced tests divide the subjects into two groups: those who meet the pre-set criteria and those who do not. These tests are most often used in educational, vocational and clinical settings where the purpose of testing is clear, such as passing an examination, selection for a job or categorisation into diagnostic groups. The contents of the test have no other meaning than their use. Psychiatric diagnostic systems using DSM-IV or ICD-10 (research criteria) are essentially criterion-referenced tests where it is made explicit that a specific number of symptoms and signs be present before making a diagnosis of a particular condition. Those meeting the criteria are deemed 'cases' and those who do not fulfil the criteria are deemed to be 'non-cases'. Thus, criterion-referenced tests, yield all-or-none responses indicating whether the subject has or has not attained the defined criteria. Criterion-referenced tests have been criticised by many for the lack of psychological meaning in their scales and items and the arbitrariness of their cut-off points.

Most tests used in clinical psychological practice are *norm-referenced*, i.e. the subject's test scores are judged against typical test scores from a representative group of individuals (norms). This involves the application of the test to an appropriate group of subjects and the construction of normative data. Such scores are assumed to be normally distributed and the subject's score is interpreted against group norms. Normative data are supplied by the test manufacturer and are available in the test manual. Thus, the conclusions from norm-referenced tests are comparative (there is no set criterion). In the example of the driving test, a norm-referenced test would conclude as follows: 'the examinee has performed better than 65% of all candidates who took the test'. The process of setting up normative data is called test standardisation.

Norms and standardisation

The numerical report of a person's performance on a norm-referenced test or scale ('raw scores'), is of little significance by itself. Interpretation of test scores are meaningful only when the scores are compared with those of a group of individuals of similar age, sex, social class and other important variables. Standardisation of a test involves testing a large sample population, for which the test is designed, in order to obtain a set of norms against which individual scores can be compared.

To be meaningful in interpreting test scores the standardisation procedure should take into consideration two important factors:

1. *Size of the standardisation sample.* The sample should be sufficiently large to reduce standard error of measurement. In studying individual variations such as personality and intelligence, one requires large samples – a factor that makes the procedure tedious and expensive.
2. *Representativeness of the sample.* Adequate comparisons can be made only if similarity exists between the group or individual being tested and the standardisation sample, which should therefore be representative of the

population for whom the test is intended. For example, if a test is designed for those aged 70 years, the normative or standardisation sample should consist of a sample of those aged 70 and above.

Thus, standardisation involves first defining the population for whom the test is designed, and drawing a sample from the population such that it is representative of that population. Inevitably it also involves stratification of the samples into homogeneous groups by such variables as age, sex, social class, level of literacy, and so on. Each subgroup needs a sufficient number of subjects, usually a minimum of 300, to make up an adequate sample. Thus, for a general population study of, say, intelligence, a very large number of subjects are required, in the order of several thousands. The standardisation sample for WAIS-III was 2450 people stratified according to age (thirteen age groups were created), sex, ethnicity, geographical region and educational level.

Expressing the results of norm-referenced tests

Raw scores obtained from tests are converted into standardised scores so that an individual's status with respect to his or her score can be compared with that of the normative group. There are two common methods of reporting performances on psychological tests: percentiles and standard scores. This serves two purposes: it makes scores comparable and, in the case of standard scores – but not in the case of percentiles – it permits the data to be statistically analysed.

Percentiles. Percentile scores provide an index of where one's score stands relative to all others on a scale of 1 to 100. Thus if an individual's IQ is reported to be on the 15th percentile, it means that only 15% of the standardisation sample received scores at or below the score the subject attained. Percentiles have the advantage of being easy to understand and easy to calculate. They are calculated by dividing the number of scores below the index score by the total sample size and then multiplying it by 100. Percentiles are on an ordinal scale (see below) and the difference between percentile units are not equivalent throughout. Hence they do not lend themselves to statistical analysis.

Standard scores. These show how far the individual's raw score deviates from the mean for the relevant normative sample. They are expressed in terms of the mean and the standard deviation of the raw scores for the normative group. The common standard score methods are:

- *T-scores* – a commonly used system with a mean of 50 and a standard deviation of 10.
- *IQ format scores* (also called deviation IQ) – this has a mean of 100 and a standard deviation of 15 (some tests use an *SD* of 16).
- Z-scores – these have a mean of zero and a standard deviation of three.
- *Stantine* (meaning standard as nine) – used less often, they have a mean of 5 and standard deviation of 2.

Standardised scores and their percentile equivalents are shown in Table 8.1. Box 8.1 provides brief definitions of the psychometric terms described so far.

Table 8.1 Percentiles and their equivalents in the standard score systems

Percentile score for normal population	*Z-score (Mean = 0) (SD = 1)*	*T-score (Mean = 50) (SD = 10)*	*Deviation IQ (Mean = 100) (SD = 15)*	*Stantine (Mean = 5) (SD = 2)*
–	*– 4 SD*	*10*	–	–
1	*– 3 SD*	*20*	*55*	–
2.5	*– 2 SD*	*30*	*70*	*1*
16	*– 1 SD*	*40*	*85*	*3*
50	***0***	***50***	***100***	***5***
84	*+ 1 SD*	*60*	*115*	*7*
97.5	*+ 2 SD*	*70*	*130*	*9*
99	*+ 3 SD*	*80*	*145*	–
–	*+ 4 SD*	*90*	–	–

CHARACTERISTICS OF GOOD PSYCHOLOGICAL TESTS

In order to be deemed good, a psychological test requires the following properties. It should:

- be reliable;
- be valid;
- possess good norms, i.e. be properly standardised (or fit similar models); and
- be appropriate for the person's age, cultural, linguistic and social background.

Box 8.1 Definitions of some of the common terms used in psychometrics

- *Factor analysis* – a statistical technique used to isolate underlying relationship between sets of variables
- *Normalised scores* – scores obtained by transforming raw scores in such a way that the transformed scores are normally distributed and have a mean of 0 and a standard deviation of 1 (or some linear function of these numbers)
- *Norms* – a list of scores and corresponding percentile ranks, standard scores, or other transformed scores of a group of examinees on whom a test was standardised
- *Standardisation* – administering of a carefully constructed test to a large, representative sample of people under standard conditions for the purpose of determining norms
- *Standard scores* – scores that express an individual's distance from the mean in terms of the standard deviation of the distribution, e.g. *T*-scores, deviation IQs, *Z*-scores and Stantines
- *Raw scores* – an examinee's unconverted score on a test, e.g. number of correct answers
- *Deviation IQ* – intelligence quotient (IQ) obtained by converting raw scores on an intelligence test to a score distribution having a mean of 100 and a known standard deviation, e.g. 15 for Wechsler tests

Scales of measurement

Psychological tests assign numbers to, and yield, numerical scores. But the resulting numbers may mean different things depending on the nature of the scale of measurement. There are four basic scales of measurement, of which only two are applicable to psychological tests:

1. *Nominal*. This classifies subjects on mutually exclusive categories as in male–female, consultants–trainers–administrators. Nominal scales are discrete.
2. *Ordinal*. This represents position in the group and is ranked according to first, second, third, and so on, which gives the order in which individuals are placed but does not tell us how far apart the people in various positions are, e.g. as in ranking by height or weight.
3. *Interval*. This measurement uses equal intervals such as minutes, degrees (temperature), number of words recalled in a memory test or percentage scored in an exam. Intervals on the scale are of equal size, so that 10 to 15 minutes is the same interval as 20 to 25 minutes. For interval scales there is no true zero.
4. *Ratio*. These are interval scales with a true zero point. Most measurements of physical qualities such as height, weight, time and distance are ratio scales.

Interval and ratio levels of measurement provide the greatest information when measuring a variable. For statistical analyses (parametric tests) one needs interval data or ratio data. Most psychological tests provide interval measurements, thus permitting transformation and comparison of scores.

Reliability

Reliability may be defined as the extent to which the outcome of a test remains unaffected by irrelevant variations and procedures of testing. It addresses the extent to which test scores obtained by a person are the same if the person is re-examined by the same test on different occasions. In other words, it is the accuracy with which the test measures a given psychological characteristic. In essence, reliability is the extent to which test scores are free from measurement error. Charles Spearman was the first to point out that all measurements are open to error and that an individual's score on a particular test can vary from time to time and from one situation to another. This theory of true scores, also called the classical theory, states that the observed test score X is the sum of the true score T and error component E. Thus:

$$X = T + E$$

The true score T is the ideal measurement that one strives for and is postulated to be a constant, while the error component E is assumed to be randomly distributed and cannot be eliminated completely. Such errors arise from various sources: degree of distraction, stress in the examinee, variations in the conditions of the test, and so on. But, the important assumption that E is randomly distributed permits the calculation of the reliability coefficient. A reliability coefficient of 0.7 means that 70% of the variability of test scores can be accounted for by true-score variance and 30% is accounted for by error-score variance. The basic procedure for establishing reliability is to obtain two sets of measurements and compare them, usually using a correlation coefficient. The minimum permissible figure for test reliability is thought to be 0.8. Below this level the test becomes less meaningful. Most psychometric tests in current use yield reliability coefficients of 0.9 or above.

There are several methods of estimating reliability (see Box 8.2):

Internal-consistency reliability

One part of the test needs to be consistent with other parts of the test. That is, different parts of the test should be measuring the same variable. The question that needs to be answered is: 'Is the test consistent with itself?' Thus, in personality test measuring introversion, the items that are designed to measure introversion must be tapping the same domain – introversion. The commonest method used to measure internal consistency reliability is the *split-half reliability*. Here the test is split into two halves so that a random allocation of half the test items or, more commonly, odd and even items, could be scored and compared with the other half and the correlation coefficient calculated. There are several methods of measuring consistency of a test's contents and homogeneity of items (e.g. split-half coefficient, Cronbach's (coefficient) α) and standard statistical software packages are routinely used to compute such measures. In *alternate-form reliability*, a somewhat different approach to the estimation of internal consistency is to use parallel-form reliability, also known as alternate-form reliability. In this approach each subject is given two versions of the same test and the correlation coefficient is calculated. The two tests need to be carefully constructed to resemble each other as much as possible. Many tests of cognitive ability and personality have alternate forms.

Test–retest reliability

The question here is: 'Does the test produce similar results when applied on different occasions?' In order to answer this question the test is administered at least twice to the same group of individuals after an interval, usually of

Box 8.2 Reliability and types of reliability of psychological measurements

The consistency with which a test measures what it is supposed to measure

- *Split-half reliability* – the scores on a randomly chosen half of the test items are correlated with scores on the other half
- *Test–retest reliability* – scores on the test administered to the same persons are correlated with those obtained on separate occasions
- *Alternate-form reliability* – two forms of the test are administered and the correlations calculated
- *Inter-rater reliability* – extent to which two independent raters scoring the test are correlated

about three months (to obviate the effect of memory for the test), and the correlation coefficient computed. Factors such as fatigue, anxiety, boredom, guessing, and poor test instructions are typical sources of measurement error. There may also be 'practice effects' such that more difficult items can be answered correctly on the second occasion. This is a particular problem for abilities tests.

Inter-rater reliability

Whenever the score of a test is dependent on the judgement of the person doing the scoring, it is important to establish the inter-scorer (rater) reliability of the test. Inter-rater reliability is established by comparing the scores of two independent examiners to determine the extent to which they agree in their observations. In examinations, essay questions are notorious for their poor inter-scorer reliability while scoring of multiple-choice questions (MCQs), particularly using computer programs, is accurate and highly reliable. Inter-rater reliability is improved by providing clear and structured guidelines, using test manuals, providing training and practice. Inter-rater reliability can be calculated for the whole scale or for each item. Of the several possible correlation coefficients that can be calculated from the observations of two or more examiners the kappa (κ) provides the best measure of reliability because it takes into consideration the fact that raters can agree by chance.

Validity

Validity refers to what the test purports to measure and how well it measures the characteristic in question. It must be shown that the test actually does measure what it claims to assess.

Validity is, therefore, the meaningfulness of the test. Strictly speaking, validity is not a property of a test but of the use of the test. It can be considered as a measure of the appropriateness and usefulness of the test. In constructing a test, two important issues that have to be taken into consideration are: (1) the construct to be tested (e.g. intelligence) must be theoretically described accurately; and (2) specific test questions should be developed to measure it adequately. Scientific research leading to accumulation of evidence to support the validity of the test is known as test validation. Test manuals are expected to provide the validity of their tests, including the purposes and populations it is valid for. Unlike reliability, there is no single measure of validity or validity coefficients.

For best results it is advisable to use as many different methods as is practically possible to assess the validity of the test. Four types of validity, which are discussed below, are summarised in Box 8.3:

Content validity. The question here is: 'Does the test adequately cover all the important aspects of the domain that is being measured?' For example, in measurement of empathy, construction of the test would have to take into account the cognitive, affective and behavioural dimensions of empathy and not limit the test to one or two of facets of it. It is also important to exclude

Box 8.3 Validity and types of validity of psychological measurements

The extent to which the test measures what it claims to measure

- *Content validity* – the extent to which the test probes the domain adequately
- *Construct validity* – the extent to which the test correlates with other tests measuring similar variables
  - —*Divergent validity* – the extent to which the test successfully discriminates between related constructs
  - —*Convergent validity* – the degree to which the test is positively correlated with other tests measuring the same variables
- *Criterion validity* – the degree of correlation between the test and an external criterion
  - —*Concurrent validity* – the test measure and the criterion are measured at the same time
  - —*Predictive validity* – the criterion is measured after the test
- *Face validity* – the degree to which the test appears to measure the variable

items from the test that could be attributable to other variables. In the case of empathy it may be important to exclude items measuring sympathy. Likewise, in a test of arithmetic ability measuring performance on multiplication only would be considered poor, while at the same time only tests of arithmetic should be included, not algebra. The test designer needs to define carefully and map out the elements in the domain under study including the boundaries of such domains – in short, he or she should be clear about both what goes in and what stays out of a test.

Construct validity. As mentioned at the beginning of this chapter, in psychology many domains that are studied and measured are hypothetical constructs such as honesty, self esteem, marital satisfaction, intelligence and so on. Often, measurements are based on observable behaviour (including self-reports of behaviour, thoughts, and feelings) and it is assumed that from such reports the underlying construct can be inferred. It is often derived by producing as many hypotheses about the construct as possible and testing them out in empirical studies. In constructing intelligence tests, for example, one sets out a series of hypotheses such as how it will correlate with other tests of intelligence, academic performance, occupational status and factor analytic studies, and so on. Inevitably, hypotheses may need revision. Construct validation is thus a gradual, and often protracted process, during which different workers using different methods assess the same construct. Eventually this leads to the accumulation of a considerable quantity of empirical data, which either supports or refutes the construct. Two types of construct validation deserve mention:

Divergent (discriminant) validity. This refers to the lack of correlation among measures that are thought to measure closely related but different constructs.

Donvergent validity. This refers to the agreement among the different measures that claim to measure the same variable.

For example, one would expect different scales measuring empathy to be highly correlated (convergent validity) while at the same time being poorly related to scores on scales that measure sympathy (divergent validity).

Criterion validity. This is the degree of agreement between the test score and a set of external criteria. Unlike other forms of validity it does not involve theoretical constructs or an explanation of the variables – it is the statistical relationship between measures of test (predictor) and the outside criteria. Generally speaking, the criteria need to be definable, acceptable and easily measurable. For example, in testing blood-alcohol levels for drink driving the results of the test are compared with criteria determined by the legal limit of blood-alcohol concentration (this is most often carried out by the breathalyser test), the assumption being that the alcohol levels in the expired air is a reliable index of blood alcohol levels. While the criterion here is somewhat simple and straight forward – the legal blood-alcohol level – in the case of psychological tests the criteria are often scores obtained by other psychological tests that are considered to be the 'gold standard' at the time of test construction. Any test of intelligence that one may want to devise at the present time would inevitably involve comparison with the WAIS, the industry standard in tests of intelligence

Two commonly used types of criterion validity are concurrent validity and predictive validity. The essential difference between these two forms of validity depends on whether test measure and criterion measure are carried out at the same time or not.

Concurrent validity. Here the test under construction and the test measuring the criterion are administered at the same time. For example, a putative test of intelligence and WAIS are administered at the same time, or close together, and the correlation between the two is computed. In many instances the criterion or 'gold standard' may not exist (if it does there is no need to construct a test in the first place!). In many cases one would expect to improve on already existing tests, refine them, make them shorter or use them for different purposes altogether. For example, one may want to devise a short clinical test of intelligence that could be used as a screening measure in day-to-day usage in a population with learning disabilities. In this case, concurrent validation against the WAIS or WISC would be reasonable and desirable. Difficulties arise when there are no such benchmark tests and one has to be satisfied with using closely related tests that provide moderate degrees of correlation.

Predictive validity. This refers to the effectiveness of the test in predicting an individual's performance on a future criterion measure – thus the criterion is measured later. The question for the test developer is: 'How successful is this test in predicting the criterion at a future date?' In the case of intelligence tests in children the selected criterion may be successful in academic tests. Unfortunately, for most psychological tests defining the criterion is beset with a great many problems. For some characteristics like extroversion it is almost impossible to set up criterion measures. The converse is true as well. One of the major challenges for test developers is to design tests for well-known outcome measures or criteria such as violence (towards person or property) or criminality. Lack of predictive power of most tests of personality to predict future offending behaviour, violence or criminality, is a major failing of all existing psychological tests. This arises partly because of the importance of situational and other factors that contribute to human behaviour and it would be naive to expect a test or a battery of tests to be able to predict such complex behaviours.

Table 8.2 Methods of data collection

Source of data	*Method of collection*	*Example*
Behaviour observation	Direct observation and coding	Strange situation procedure
Test procedures	Tested with test material	WAIS, matrix test
Questionnaires and inventories	Yes–no items	EPQ, MMPI
Rating scales	Likert scales	NEOP-R, attitude tests
Projective tests	Interpretation of pictures or other stimuli	TAT, Rorscha's

Face validity. Face validity is concerned with whether a test 'appears' to measure what it is supposed to measure. It is a subjective evaluation by both those taking the test and those using the test. There are no statistical measures to estimate face validity. But it is important for the people taking the test to have an understanding of what is being measured, to motivate them and to help them cooperate with the examiner. The disadvantage of high face validity is that examinees would be able to guess the purpose of the test and provide desirable answers or purposely distort their responses.

METHODS OF DATA COLLECTION

The information necessary for analysis is collected in various ways depending on the psychological construct under consideration. The most common methods of data collection used in psychological measurements are shown in Table 8.2.

Direct observation. A simple approach to measuring behaviour is, of course, to observe it directly. If, for example, it is decided to measure the wandering behaviour in an in-patient with Alzheimer's disease, close observation and 'event or time sampling' would provide a relatively accurate picture of the extent of the behaviour. Unfortunately, direct observation may not be appropriate or feasible for many psychological constructs.

Test procedures. Here the examiner requests the subject to carry out actions using standard methods and materials. In applying the WAIS the testee is presented with verbal and performance tasks and scored according to set rules.

Self-reports. These are statements about the subject's own account of his or her feelings, thoughts or behaviours. Items are selected on the basis of the theoretical construct under study (e.g. extroversion) using rational and empirical approaches and questionnaires are constructed to cover all aspects of the domain. Tests based on self-reports have been criticised for assuming that people show self-knowledge of the attribute they are questioned about. Another potential problem is that people may feel differently about themselves depending on the time and situations. The different methods of recording responses to the items are:

- *Forced-choice method.* Some questionnaires use a dichotomous True/False or Yes/No forced-choice method. The testee is asked to indicate whether he or she agrees with the statement or not.
- *Likert scale.* One of the most popular scales was developed by Likert in 1938. Subjects are presented with the statement of the item and asked to indicate on a five- or seven-point scale how strongly they agree or disagree. For example in the NEO five factor inventory an item on extraversion is, 'I like to be where the action is', and the examinee is asked to select one of the following responses: strongly disagree, disagree, neutral, agree or strongly agree. A numerical value is attached to each response.

Two other methods of marking items, used exclusively in tests of attitude (see Chapter 9), are:

1. *Thurstone scale.* The subject chooses from a large number of independent statements, each with a numerical value; the intervals between statements are approximately equal. For example, in developing a scale for measuring attitude towards abortion, about 21 statements judged on an eleven-point scale by a panel are selected for the scale and the subject is asked to indicate all the statements that they are in agreement with (Table 8.3). Their attitude is the average of these items.
2. Osgood's semantic differential scale. This entails ratings, on a seven-point scale, of an attitude towards an object, person, or idea on numerous bipolar adjectives scale. For instance, in a scale to measure attitude towards mental illnesses the following bipolar adjectives may be employed:

   Curable -- Incurable
   Predictable -- Unpredictable
   Innocuous -- Dangerous

Tests based on self-reports make several fundamental assumptions. First, people are thought to have self-knowledge of the attributes they are being questioned about and are thought to be reliable observers of their own behaviour. Second, individuals are considered to feel the same way about themselves most of the time, irrespective of situations. Third, it is assumed that the person is motivated to disclose his or her true feelings, behaviours and attitudes.

Table 8.3 Example of a Thurstone scale to measure attitude

How favourable	*Attitude towards abortion. Value on 11-point scale*	*Item*
Least	1.3	Abortion is a punishable offence
	3.6	Abortion is morally wrong
Neutral	5.4	Abortion has both advantages and disadvantages
	7.6	It is up to the individual to decide about abortion
	9.6	Abortion is the only solution to many problems
Most	10.3	Not only should abortion be allowed, but it should be enforced under certain conditions

When administering a psychological test one needs to be aware of the effect on the test of interaction between the examiner and the testee. Because tests are carried out mostly under artificial or contrived situation (in the laboratory or clinic) and not under natural conditions, they are open to distortions. One such problem, the response set, is specific to the use of questionnaires. Two others occur under any experimental condition.

1. Response bias or response set. One possible source of error in using self-rating questionnaires and scales is that of response bias, which is also called response set. This refers to the systematic patterns in which the testees respond, which falsify or distort the validity of the test. Several types of response sets have been identified:

1. Response bias of *acquiescence* is the tendency to agree with the items in the questionnaire regardless of their content. It is most likely to occur when items are couched in general terms rather than being specific. For example, the question 'Are you a friendly person?' is likely to produce more positive answers than asking 'Would those close to you consider you a friendly person?'
2. Response bias of *social desirability* occurs when the testee responds to items in the question in ways that are socially more acceptable. This may be a conscious effort to deceive or an unconscious attempt to create a favourable impression.
3. Response bias of *extreme responding* is the tendency to select responses that are extreme. For example, in a Likert scale the testee responds by marking all the items 0 or 7.
4. Response bias *to the middle* is the likelihood of providing safe or non-committal responses and avoiding extreme responses.

Most questionnaires attempt to overcome response bias by incorporating items that are designed to identify clients who are under-reporting or responding randomly. Addition of the lie items to the scale is one such method. The EPI for example, has several lie items like 'Once in a while do you lose your temper and get angry'? An honest answer to this would be 'yes'. Judicious combination of lie items help in identifying response bias but is almost impossible to eliminate biased reporting altogether.

2. Halo effect. Judgement on the general aspect of the test may colour the answers to most other items and skew the responses in one direction. The first few items of the questionnaire may convince the subject that the rest of the items are similar leading to the same response to all the items. (A similar situation arises in interviews and oral examinations when the examiner's response to a particular aspect of the candidate, for example, being articulate and being well spoken may favourably influence their judgement of the candidate on other abilities as well.) In a broad sense this refers to the tendency to assume that if a person is good at one thing they are also good at others as well.

3. Hawthorne effect. This refers to a positive interaction between the subject and the test procedure that may influence the responses. Initially described in industrial psychology where the very fact of the presence of observers at the industrial plant in Hawthorne increased the activity of the workers and hence production, this effect is often evident when subjects feel that they are being examined or scrutinised.

CLINICAL USES (AND ABUSES) OF PSYCHOLOGICAL TESTS

Psychological tests are useful *adjuncts* to clinical decision making, but they should not be used in place of sound clinical judgement. The main role of the clinician in conducting an assessment is to answer specific questions and make decisions about management. In order to accomplish these the clinician must integrate a wide variety of information from diverse sources such as history, examination, observation, and informants including psychometric data. Tests are only one method of gathering information. The clinician's main task is to situate the test results in a wider perspective to generate hypotheses and aid in decision making. For instance, elevated scores on Scale 6 (Hypomania) in the MMPI in a chief executive may reflect a driven, ambitious and dominant personality rather than hypomania. Thus, the best statement that could be made is that elevated or low scores on a test are *consistent* with a particular condition; they are not *diagnostic*.

Results of psychological tests are liable to be misused in some instances. This is especially so when psychometric testing tends to form the basis of social and educational policies. For example, in the past, there has been a tendency to place children to be classed as having 'special educational needs' solely on the premise of having scored low on IQ tests. The result was that children from low-social-class families and minority groups were placed in 'special schools' where the curriculum was less challenging. Thus, the children were doubly deprived, they were performing poorly and were deprived of a proper education thereby increasing their chances of failing academically. This goes against the basic principles of equality of access to education, equal opportunities and human rights. As a result of legal action taken by parents in some states of the USA the WISC is banned from use in educational settings.

A good knowledge of the tests that are available to measure the psychological variable in question is essential. Information about tests may be obtained from *The Mental Measurements Yearbook* (MMY), which provides an up to date authoritative review of most tests. Tests are revised regularly, usually every five years or so, and need to be regularly updated (the 15th edition of MMY, published in 2003, is available on the web at buros.unl.edu/buros/catalog.html). Information is also available from test publishers in the form of manuals that come with the test. These provide instructions on the use and application of the test together with reliability, validity and normative data. Most important of all is whether the test is appropriate and suitable for the specific clinic situation. Most standard tests such as Wechsler intelligence tests and MMPI require training before one can use them. The test results are treated as confidential information and there are strict regulations governing their disclosure to third parties. Informed consent is necessary before administration and both the British Psychological Society and the American Psychological Association have set professional standards and guidelines for test usage. Psychological test publishing is big business and copyrights are usually reserved.

There are several thousands of tests and measurements across the entire field of psychology. These range from measurement of marital satisfaction to

Box 8.4 Commonly used psychological tests

1A. Measures of general or global mental abilities
- *Wechsler scales (WAIS, WISC, WPPSI)*
- *Stanford–Binet intelligence scale*
- *Raven's progressive matrices*
- *British abilities test (BAS)*

1B. Measures of specific mental abilities
- *Wechsler memory scale (WMS)*

2. Measures of personality
- *Personality questionnaires*
  - *—Sixteen personality factor (16 PF)*
  - *—Eysenck personality questionnaire (EPQ–R)*
  - *—Neuroticism extraversion openness personality inventory (NEO–PI–R)*
  - *—Minnesota multiphasic personality inventory (MMPI–2)*
- *Projective tests*
  - *—Rorschach test*
  - *—Thematic apperception test (TAT)*

3. Neuropsychological tests
- *Wechsler memory scale–revised (WMS–R)*
- *Wisconsin card sorting test (WCST)*

ratings of clinical conditions such as anxiety and depression. Most commonly the psychological measurements that are useful in clinical practice are: (1) tests of cognitive abilities; (2) personality tests; and (3) neuropsychological tests (Box 8.4). Brief outlines of the tests are given below, more details on the tests are found in the appropriate chapters.

1. Tests of mental abilities

Often called intelligence tests, tests of general cognitive abilities are the most commonly used tests in clinical and educational psychology. These are based on the psychometric theory of intelligence and the concept of *g* or general intelligence and the factor structure of human abilities; the subscales may be used to measure specific abilities such as arithmetic or reading. The two most common scales used to measure general intelligence are the Wechsler scales and Stanford–Binet scale (see Chapter 2). Tests for specific mental abilities include tests such as Wechsler Memory Scale (WMS) (see Chapter 7).

2. Tests of personality

Personality tests may be broadly grouped into two: projective tests and personality questionnaires.

Projective tests

These are idiographic tests, which are said to test the unique aspect of one's personality. The tests are generally based on the psychoanalytic concept of projection that when individuals are presented with an ambiguous stimulus, which has no 'real' meaning, they project their own feelings, thoughts and fantasies into it. These tests use stimuli that are ambiguous and the subject is free to respond within certain parameters. The reliability and validity of projective tests are relatively low. The two best-known projective tests are the Rorschach's inkblot test and the thematic apperception test.

The Rorschach test. Perhaps the best known projective test, the Rorschach test (Rorschach, 1921) consists of ten bilaterally symmetrical inkblots (faithfully reprinted in all textbooks in psychology), which the subject is asked to interpret. A variety of interpretations are possible for each ink blot. The individuals' responses are scored according to three general categories: (1) the *location*, or the area of the inkblot on which they focus; (2) *determinants*, or specific properties of the inkblot that they use in making their responses (e.g. colour, shape); and (3) the *content*, or the general class of objects to which the response belongs (animals, humans, faces). Interpretation of the information obtained in this way is thought to be a way of obtaining access to the persons psychological make up. Although popular with psychoanalytically oriented workers and therapists, the major problem for those studying personality characteristics is its low reliability and validity. Hence the test has fallen out of favour.

However, a sophisticated scoring system developed by Exner (1974) has overcome some of these objections. It has revitalised the test by providing a more reliable scoring system. So much so, in fact, that some have argued that the test is now as good as the MMPI in predicting a variety of clinical phenomena.

Thematic Apperception Test. In this test (TAT; Murray, 1943) the subject is presented with a series of cards (about 10) with pictures on them. For example, Card 1 of TAT depicts a boy staring in contemplation at a violin and Card 2 shows a rural scene with a young girl in the foreground holding a book, a pregnant woman watching and a man labouring in a field in the background. The subject is told that it is a test of imagination (not intelligence) and is asked to make up a dramatic story for each of the cards. More specifically, he or she is asked to: (1) tell what has lead up to the events shown in the picture; (2) describe what is happening at the moment; (3) say what the characters are feeling and thinking at the moment; and (4) describe what will happen next. The stories are recorded verbatim, including pauses, questions and other remarks. The areas of interpretation are broken down into three categories: story content; story structure; and behaviour observation.

The assumption is that when presented with such ambiguous stimuli the subjects' stories reflect their personality and characteristic modes of interacting with the environment. Subjects are thought to create TAT stories based on a combination of at least three elements: the card stimulus, the testing environment and the personality or inner world of the individual. The term *apperception* was coined to reflect the fact that subjects do not just perceive, rather they construct stories about cards in accordance with their personality, characteristics and life experiences. Several scoring systems have been developed in attempts to standardise the interpretation of TAT material. The TAT has been used in research and psychotherapy. McClelland (1985) used TAT extensively in his studies on Need for achievement (see Chapter 5, p. 122). It has been used in prediction of overt aggression, identification of defence mechanisms and for mapping interpersonal relationships.

Personality questionnaires

These are the most popular personality tests. The commonly used questionnaires are based on the trait theory of personality and their contents are derived through factor analysis. They are easy to use, norms are easily available and are easy to interpret. However, validity of such tests is dependent on the theory and model of personality that underpins the test, the assumption being that personality dimensions are stable and that behaviour is consistent over a range of situations. One other problem is that the questions, and hence the answers, are to a degree crude and lack refinement. For instance, the following question is from the Eysenck personality inventory: 'Do you find it very hard to take no for an answer?' This is answered 'Yes/No' and is scored on the neuroticism scale if positive, which then raises a second question: 'Under what situation and with whom?'

Factor analysis. The principal psychometric technique used in most studies of personality traits is *factor analysis* and the key statistic involved is Pearson's correlation coefficient (r). Factor analysis is a method for investigating the dimensions or factors that underlie the correlation between more than two variables. It has been used extensively in the psychometric study of personality and intelligence. The purpose of factor analysis is to explore how the variables are interrelated and thereby examine the meaningful elements that they have in common and are responsible for their correlation.

A hypothetical example may illustrate the principles. Supposing we collected data on five scales using questionnaires that describe a sample of people on the following aspects: friendliness; helpfulness; empathy; dominance; and assertiveness. Next we work out the correlations among the five scales and arrange them in a correlation matrix as shown in Table 8.4.

As can be seen from the correlation matrix, the three measures, friendliness, helpfulness and empathy appear to show positive correlations between .70 and .80, whereas the correlation between the first three scales and the last two, dominance and assertiveness is very low (less than .25). But the last two measures, dominance and assertiveness, show high correlations (more than .65). From these observations we could reasonably conclude that a common construct underlies the first three traits while a different factor accounts for the similarities of the last two traits. All that is left for us to do is to name these two first-order factors.

Table 8.4 Correlation matrix for five scales (see text)

Scale	*Friendliness*	*Helpfulness*	*Empathy*	*Dominance*	*Assertiveness*
Friendliness		.75	.70	.15	.20
Helpfulness			.80	.20	.25
Empathy				.10	.20
Dominance					.75
Assertiveness					

Thus, it could be said that two factors have been 'extracted' from the items and, conversely, the respective items of the scales could be said to have been 'loaded' with the particular factors. They are said to be 'orthogonal factors' and can be represented graphically by two lines at right angles to each other. After the initial analysis, in some instances, the factors that emerge (the first-order factors) may be more or less correlated with each other. These can be subjected to further factor analysis and second-order factors obtained. Usually second-order factors are not correlated to one another and can be considered to be different, independent elements that constitute the universe of personality. Factor analysis is a complex area of statistics. An easy introduction to the method may be found in Kline (1994).

Common measures of personality

Despite the potential objections to the use of personality questionnaires to 'measure' personality traits, they are popular with psychologists, especially researchers in the field. The personality tests most often used by psychologists are mentioned below (see also Chapter 3).

16 Personality factor questionnaire. The 16 PF (Cattell, Eber & Tatsuoka, 1970) is a self-administered questionnaire consisting of 187 trichotomous items. It is thought to be a psychometrically sound instrument based on data from almost 25 000 people and has been used mainly in research. It is thought to provide a good instrument for measuring normal adult personality. The original 16 PF provides a profile of the subject's personality on all 16 factors (see Chapter 3). Cattell considered the 16 factors to be primary, meaning that all 16 were necessary for a comprehensive measure of personality. However, recent workers have extracted five second-order factors. The latest version of 16 PF, the 16 PF-5, is designed to be scored on the five factors: extraversion; neuroticism; tough poise; independence; and control.

Eysenck personality questionnaire–revised. The EPQ-R (Eysenck & Eysenck, 1991) is a well-known measure of the three Eysenck personality factors (see Chapter 3) and it has been used in hundreds of studies. It has 100 dichotomous 'yes/no' items. Along with scales measuring the three personality dimensions of extraversion, neuroticism and psychoticism, it also includes a lie scale. It has been normed on almost 5000 subjects, and has high reliability. Its factor analytic validity for the dimensions, especially extraversion/introversion, is good. However, the EPQ has been not popular with clinicians.

NEO personality inventory. The 'big five' dimensions of personality (see Chapter 3) form the basis of the NEO personality inventory (NEO-PI-R; Costa & McCrae, 1992). The NEO-PI-R is a self-administered questionnaire consisting of 240 items designed for use with adults. Each item is rated on a five-point Likert scale, from 'strongly agree' to 'strongly disagree'. Each facet (lower level trait) is assessed by eight statements, such as: 'I am not a worrier' (neuroticism, N) and 'I like to have a lot of people around me' (extraversion, E). A shorter version of the questionnaire comprised of sixty items is also available (NEO-FFI). The test is considered to be reliable and well validated. The main problem with the instrument is that the data derived from it is too general for clinical decision making. Nevertheless, theoretical research using the NEO-PI-R holds future promise for building bridges between (normal) personality psychology and psychiatry.

The Minnesota multiphasic personality inventory. This instrument (MMPI; Hathaway & McKiney, 1983) is one of the most extensively used and researched tests of personality assessment, especially in the USA. It is a 567-item pencil and paper test. Test items are of the true/false type grouped into validity, clinical and content scales (Box 8.5). Norms for the various scales have been developed on the basis of responses from the normal and clinical groups. It stands out from other personality tests in that it was developed using the criterion keying method rather than factor analysis. For example, patients who had received a diagnosis of depression (and no other) comprised the criterion group. Having made sure that they had an agreed diagnosis of depression, the responses of these patients to the item pool were compared with a group of normal controls. Items that discriminated significantly between the two groups were selected.

The MMPI was originally developed with the purpose of assisting in diagnosis of psychiatric conditions. Experience in using the MMPI has shown that patients usually show elevation in more than one scale. Thus, the MMPI provides a profile of the subject's scores and, over the years, a massive amount of data has accumulated that enables clinicians to identify patterns of *profiles*

Box 8.5 Scales in the Minnesota multiphasic personality inventory (MMPI–2)

1. Validity scales – seven scales
2. Clinical scales
   - *Hypochondriasis (Hs), Scale 1*
   - *Depression (D) Scale 2*
   - *Hysteria (Hy) Scale 3*
   - *Psychopathic deviance (Pd), Scale 4*
   - *Masculinity–femininity (Mf), Scale 5*
   - *Paranoia (Pa), Scale 6*
   - *Psychasthenia (Pt), Scale 7*
   - *Schizophrenia (Sc), Scale 8*
   - *Hypomania (Ma), Scale 9*
   - *Social introversion (Si), Scale 0*
3. Content scales
   - *Anxiety (ANX)*
   - *Fears (FRS)*
   - *Obsessiveness (OBS)*
   - *Depression (DPS)*
   - *Health concerns (HEA)*
   - *Bizarre mentation (BIZ)*
   - *Anger (ANG)*
   - *Cynicism (CYN)*
   - *Antisocial practices (ASP)*
   - *Type A (TPA)*
   - *Low self-esteem (LSE)*
   - *Social discomfort (SOD)*
   - *Family problems (FAM)*
   - *Work interference (WRK)*
   - *Negative treatment indicators (TRT)*

(profile analysis) that assist the clinician in treatment planning and predicting future functioning. The MMPI has been studied intensively and has more than 10 000 research articles to its credit. Computerised interpretive services are available. The scale was updated and revised to increase the utility of the instrument. The MMPI-2 published by Pearson Assessments in 1989 has surpassed its predecessor in its value to clinicians and is now one of the most popular personality tests used by psychologists. A common criticism of the MMPI is the usage of scale names such as depression, which may suggest that the subject shows features of the clinical syndrome. This is not true. Elevated scores on the depression scale reflect characteristics such as apathy, tendency to worry and self-depreciation. Thus the scales represent measures of personality traits rather than diagnostic categories.

3. Neuropsychological tests and assessments

These are tests designed to assess the psychological functioning of patients with cerebral damage. Often they are used to identify deficits in psychological variables such as memory, executive function or intelligence following brain damage or cerebral impairment. They are also used to localise brain lesions (see Chapter 7).

Clinical judgement

When assessing a patient or client the clinician attempts to gather information from a variety of sources (history, examination, past medical notes, accounts from informants and any psychological tests), synthesise and integrate these data and make an informed judgement on the diagnosis and make a sound aetiological formulation of the case. Each of the processes involved in clinical decision making affect their reliability and validity. Errors in clinical judgement are not uncommon. It is crucial to understand the process of decision making and be aware of relevant literature on clinical judgement if we are to improve the accuracy of it. Research has highlighted the following areas (Garb, 1998):

1. The accuracy of judgement is increased by semistructured approaches to interviewing rather than subjective methods based on theoretical knowledge or experience. This is particularly important where judgements on risk are involved. When diagnoses are made it is important to adhere to the specific criteria set out in ICD-10 or DSM-IV.
2. It has been shown that the more confident clinicians feel about their judgements, the less likely they are to be accurate. Interestingly, clinicians with greater knowledge and experience are less confident regarding their judgements and tend to keep an open mind.
3. Clinicians should be aware of the two possible biases to which they are liable when making clinical decisions. One results from the *primacy effect*, where the initial presentation (or referral information) influences information collected later. The implication is that clinicians need to pay sufficient attention to data collected at every stage of the assessment. Another source

of error arises from *confirmatory bias*. Here the clinicians selectively seek out information that confirms their initial judgements. Doctors are particularly prone to make 'instant' diagnoses and thereafter attempt to derive information to justify the decision. Since a diagnosis is nothing but an initial hypothesis, it is crucially important that clinicians carefully attempt to elicit information that may disconfirm their hypothesis as well as support it. Taking a meta-view of the consultation process, which includes the clinician and clinical situation, facilitates balanced decision making and avoids various forms of bias.

REFERENCES

Anastasi A (1982) Psychological Testing (5th ed.). New York: Macmillan.

Cattell RB, Eber HW, Tatsuoka MM (1970) Handbook for the Sixteen Personality Factor Questionnaire. Champaign, IL: Institute for Personality and Ability Testing.

Costa PT, McCrae R (1992) Revised NEO Personality Inventory (NEO-PI-R) (NEO-FFI) Professional Manual. Odessa, FL: Psychological Assessment Resources.

Exner JE Jr (1974) The Rorschach: a comprehensive system. New York: Wiley.

Eysenck HJ, Eysenck MW (1991) The Eysenck Personality Questionnaire – Revised. Sevenoaks, UK: Hodder & Stoughton.

Garb HN (1998) Studying the Clinician: judgement research and psychological assessment. Washington, DC: American Psychological Association.

Hathaway SR, McKiney JC (1983) The Minnesota Multiphasic Personality Inventory (Manual). New York: Psychological Corporation.

Kline P (1994) An Easy Guide to Factor Analysis. London, UK: Routledge.

Kline P (2000) The Handbook of Psychometric Testing (2nd ed.). London, UK: Routledge.

McClelland D (1985) Human Motivation. Glenview, IL: Scott, Foresman.

Michell J (1997) Quantitative science and the definition of measurement in psychology. British Journal of Psychology, 88, 355–383.

MMY (2003) The Mental Measurements Yearbook (15th ed.). [buros.unl.edu/buros/catalog.html]

Murray HA (1943) Manual to the Thematic Apperception Test. Boston, MA: Harvard University Press.

Rorschach H (1921) Psychodiagnostics. Berne: Hans Huben.

FURTHER READING

Anastasi A (1982) Psychological Testing (5th ed.). New York: Macmillan.

- A definitive text on the principles of psychological measurements.

Harding L, Beech JR (eds) (1996) Assessment in Neuropsychology. London, UK: Routledge.

- A good introduction to neuropsychology.

Kline P (1994) An Easy Guide to Factor Analysis. London, UK: Routledge.

- Factor analysis made simple.

Kline P (2000) The Handbook of Psychometric Testing (2nd ed.). London, UK: Routledge.

- A good introduction to the subject including summaries of common tests.

Social psychology

9

'Philosophers have interpreted the world in various ways; the point is to change it.'
Karl Marx

Man is a social animal. In order to function effectively and interact with his fellow human beings, man has had to develop a sense of other people's feelings, behaviours and intentions and his own behaviour. Social psychology is the scientific study of how people think, feel and behave in social situations. It attempts to understand and explain how the thoughts, feelings and behaviours of individuals are influenced by the presence of others. The underlying principle in social psychology is that people are active agents who influence and are influenced by the social world around them. Man is seen as being shaped by, as well as shaping, the social environment.

The field of social psychology is vast and forms interesting reading. Some of the most interesting and innovative experiments in psychology have been in the field of social psychology. This chapter focuses on four prevailing themes in the field: *social influence*, *attitude*, *attribution* and *group processes*. These are outlined below in order to give the reader a flavour of the subject. Readers interested in perusing the subject further are referred to the books recommended at the end of the chapter.

SOCIAL INFLUENCES

People tend to behave differently when others are present than they do when they are on their own. It is a common experience that the presence of another person changes one's behaviour. In experimental studies the interaction between the baby and the mother has been shown to change when the father enters the room. Since all human behaviour occurs in a social context, others exert a pervasive influence on our actions, thoughts and beliefs, although often we are not aware of these influences. Various experiments in social psychology have demonstrated a number of such social influences, the more important ones receive mention below.

Social facilitation and social loafing

One of the earliest experiments in social psychology was carried out by Ringelmann in the 1880s. He demonstrated that the more people there were in a tug-of-war team, the less hard each person in the team pulled. His findings have been replicated in subsequent experiments showing that, at least on some tasks, the presence of others reduces performance. This has been called *social loafing*. Other studies have shown that the presence of others sometimes increases task performance. Clapping or cheering by a crowd in a football match is an example of such *social facilitation*. Clearly both facilitation effects and inhibition effects are the result of the interaction between the individual, the group and many other factors. There do not seem to be any hard and fast rules as to when facilitation occurs and when social loafing occurs. However, the awareness of the effect of onlookers on task activity and productivity is important, especially in work situations.

Group polarisation

People in groups tend to make decisions that are more extreme than the positions held by individual members prior to the discussion. This phenomenon, known as *group polarisation*, refers to group discussions resulting in more extreme decisions than people would ever make alone. In experiments where subjects are asked to make group decisions on topics about which they had already indicated their individual preferences, it has been consistently found that the group decisions were more extreme in one direction or another than the members' individual choices. This has sometimes been called the *risky shift* because groups tended to take more risky decisions than individuals (Stoner, 1961). Subsequent work has shown that group decisions are not always more risky, rather that the shift is more extreme in the initially preferred direction (e.g. in a interview panel, the subject becomes more sure of the candidate already chosen by him).

The polarisation effect is particularly common where group members have not met each other before and where there is no group leader. It is less likely in situations where the group members know one another or where there is an influential leader. Group polarisation is of interest because groups that meet for the first time make many important decisions. For instance, jurors, examiners and interview panels make important decisions where polarisation effects have been observed to occur. A number of explanations have been proposed to explain polarisation effects. One reason may be that the exchange of information occurring during the group discussion influences the view of each individual in the group. It has also been suggested that each member wants to define their point of view more strongly in contrast to other members of the group and hence the need to be more extreme in expressing their opinions.

Conformity

Conformity is said to occur when people change their behaviours or beliefs towards that of a group's majority view as a result of real or imagined pressure from the group. When in a group people tend to agree with group judgements rather than stand out even when there is no explicit requirement to do so. Two experiments have become classics in studies on conformity.

The first is a study by Sherif (1936) in which participants were asked to observe a stationary light in a dark room and estimate its movement. The experiment made use of the *autokinetic effect*, an optical illusion that a stationary point of light in a completely dark room appears to move. This was carried out first on each individual and later in groups. Later when people were asked to shout out their answers, as a group, their estimates tended to converge towards a group norm. When the individuals were tested alone afterwards they continued to hold to the group norm.

The second experiment, carried out by Asch (1951), provides additional proof of the profound effects of conformity in groups. Asch asked participants in groups of 7 or 9 individuals to judge which of a set of three lines was the same length as the one that they were initially shown (Figure 9.1). All the participants, except the subject, were confederates. The 'stooges' were instructed to give the wrong answer. The experimental subject's turn always came last to ensure that they were always subjected to the group's majority view. It was found that, on average, one in three participants agreed with the incorrect response 37% of the time.

Asch's line judgement experiment differs from Sherif's procedure in one major aspect: the task set out by Asch is unambiguous and easy. Nevertheless, the erroneous answers given by the participants in these studies testify to the effect of group pressure. It should be noted that only around one third of the subjects conformed to the majority decision, whilst two thirds of his subjects consciously resisted conforming to peer pressure, indicating that there is wide individual variation in conformity.

Asch's experiments have been replicated in hundreds of studies using minor variations. The main findings from the various studies on conformity show that people tend to conform to social pressure under certain conditions:

1. When the situation is ambiguous or the task is unfamiliar. In Sherif's studies the autokinetic effect deliberately introduced an element of uncertainty. The low rates of conformity in Asch's experiments may be accounted for by the straightforwardness of the task. Several authors have attempted to explain why ambiguous situations lead to greater conformity. When reality is unclear or vague, people tend to use the group as a frame of reference. Festinger (1954) explained conformity on the basis of *social comparison*. In his words, 'When physical reality becomes uncertain, people rely more and more on "social reality"'.
2. When there is unanimity within the group. Groups' agreement enhances conformity. Disagreement within the group leads to a drastic reduction in conformity. Even if one person disagrees with the majority, conformity is

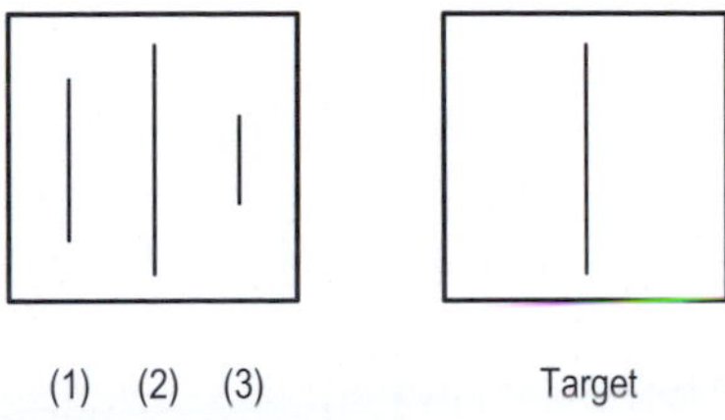

Fig. 9.1 Line judgement experiment (Asch, 1955)

dramatically reduced. In Asch's experiments it dropped to 10% if one confederate disagreed.

3. Small groups. The size of the group appears to be important. In Asch's experiments, conformity increased when the group size increased up to four, but further additions had little effect.
4. Group acceptance. Those who feel accepted by the group have been shown to find it easier to deviate from the group.

Several explanations have been put forward to account for conformity, such as social comparison, as mentioned above, avoidance of conflict and increased self-awareness, but it appears that different mechanisms may be operative in different situations.

Minority influence

While conformity to group norms is a universal phenomenon, the influence exerted by minorities in group decision making should not be underestimated. In contrast to the Asch experiments, Moscovici (1976) showed in a series of experiments that, over time, minorities in a group were effective in bringing about a change in the views of the majority provided that they were consistent in their responses. He designed a colour-judging task in which a minority were instructed consistently to describe a blue-green colour as green. The minority, confederates in this case, repeatedly and persistently gave the same answers in a series of trials. It was found that the views of the majority subjects changed over time to that of the minority. However, further research has shown the situation on minority influence to be more complex.

Obedience

Obedience refers to a change in behaviour that occurs in response to a command, order or demand from an authority figure. In conformity the behaviour change is the result of group pressure and there is no overt demand for behaviour change, whereas in obedience, the requests are firm, taking the form of instructions or orders. In all societies obedience to authority is culturally sanctioned to a lesser or greater degree. Indeed, all societies rely on internalised codes of reasonable conduct. From an early age children are socialised so as to follow parental authority, obey teachers and adhere to standards of moral behaviour. As adults we take orders from the police, firemen, the tax man or our superiors where appropriate.

After the Second World War a question that troubled social psychologists was how thousands of German soldiers could imprison, torture and kill millions of people, Jews, gypsies and communists, because 'authorities' decreed so. One hypothesis put forward soon after the war was that of the 'Germans' character'. Stanley Milgram put this theory to test and came up with results that were just the opposite: that most people, under certain conditions, would obey authority figures and punish others. Milgram (1963) conducted a number of experiments in which he attempted to get subjects to punish other participants by the use of electric shocks. Since his early work the Milgram experiments on obedience have become classics in the field of social psychology and have been replicated both by him and by others. Similar experiments have also been carried out in a number of other countries and have produced remarkably comparable and consistent results.

In his original experiment carried out at the prestigious Yale University in the USA, a white-coated 'professor' told volunteers from a cross section of society that they were taking part in an experiment to study the effects of punishment on tasks testing memory. Whenever the 'learner' made incorrect responses in a paired word-association test, the 'teacher' (subject) was to deliver shocks of increasing intensity. In reality the 'learner' was a stooge or confederate who responded to simulated shocks in a standardised way. Shocks were 'delivered' by a machine that looked authentic and shocks ranged from 15 to 450 volts. The intensity of the 'shock' was clearly marked from slight shock to extremely intense shock to danger and, ultimately, XXX. The 'learner' was instructed to moan as the shocks got higher and at more than 200 volts to protest verbally, demanding to be released. At 300 volts he was asked to yell and pound at the walls and beyond this to become silent and unresponsive, mimicking a collapsed state. In the initial experiment the 'learner' was placed in an adjacent room, so that the 'teacher' could not see him. The experimenter (the white-coated 'professor') urged the 'teacher' to continue, in standard ways by saying, 'Please continue' and, 'You are requested to continue'. (Remember that the subjects under study were the 'teachers' who administered the shocks.)

The findings came as a surprise to all: 65% of all participants continued to give shocks up to the maximum intensity of 450 volts. Prior to the experiment Milgram had asked a panel of students, middle class adults and psychiatrists to guess beforehand how many would continue with the shocks. All three groups predicted that subjects would not exceed the 'intense shock' level. As can be seen from Table 9.1, almost 90% of the subjects went beyond this limit.

Although the Milgram experiments have been the subject of criticism on ethical and methodological grounds, they demonstrate the extraordinary

Table 9.1 Shock levels and percentage of subjects administering the shocks (Milgram, 1963)

Shock levels as marked on the instrument	*Current levels (volts)*	*Participants continuing with the experiment (%)*
Slight	15–60	100
Moderate	75–120	100
Strong	135–180	100
Very strong	195–240	100
Intense	255–300	87.5
Extremely intense	315–360	76.5
Danger, severe	375–420	65.0
XXX	425–450	65.0

power of authority figures on people's behaviour. Milgram has carried out variations of the experiment and subsequent work has clarified several situational and social variables that influence people's willingness to obey instructions from an authority figure:

- *Legitimacy.* The first experiment was carried out at the prestigious Yale University and in conditions of an experimental laboratory. When the experiment was repeated at a run-down office building, the level of obedience fell to 48%, i.e. only 48% administered the maximum shock. When orders were given not by a white-coated 'professor' but by an 'ordinary person' the obedience levels went down to 20%.
- *Proximity of learner.* In the original experiment the 'learner' and the 'teacher' were in separate rooms. When the conditions of the experiment were altered such that the 'learner' and the 'teacher' were in the same room, only 40% administered shocks at the maximum level. When the 'teacher' had to take the hands of the 'learner' and put it on the switch to deliver the shock because the subject was reluctant to administer the shock, obedience levels went down to 30%.
- *Proximity of authority figure.* If the experimenter left the room or gave instructions over the phone, obedience was reduced to 20%, including attempts to cheat by pretending to flick switches.
- *Disagreement between authority figures.* Conflict in commands given by two authority figures brought about a dramatic reduction in obedience, with none giving maximum shocks.
- *Defiance by peers.* The variable that most reduced obedience was the presence of an example of defiance. When a fellow volunteer refused to deliver the shocks at strong shock levels (150 volts), 20% defied the authority and gave up. If a second confederate rebelled at 240 volts there was a remarkable increase in the level of defiance, which escalated now to 60% or more refusing to follow instructions. However, it is important to note that 10% of the subjects continued to give shocks up to maximum levels in the presence of non-obedient peers, indicating that peer rebellion has little effect on some obedient souls! (It should perhaps be noted that the participants were tested before the experiment, to make sure that they were psychologically well-adjusted people.)
- *Gender.* Contrary to popular belief, females were equally likely to deliver shocks up to the maximum level.

To what extent are the results of Milgram's experiments applicable to 'real-life' situations? One example of a naturalistic study is that conducted by Hofling and colleagues on nurses and doctors (Hofling et al., 1966). In this study, each nurse was telephoned by a doctor and asked to administer 20 mg of a drug called Astropen to a patient on the ward. This violated accepted rules in several ways. Doctors were not supposed to order medication on the phone, the medication was not on the authorised ward list of drugs, the doctor's name was not familiar to the nurses and the drug container said that 10 mg was the limit and that higher doses could be fatal. In spite of such warnings and deterrence, 21 of the 22 nurses in the experiment were about to administer the drug and were stopped by one of the researchers. This study, carried out under real-life conditions was a compelling demonstration of the detrimental effects of obedience to authority.

These disturbing findings from experiments by Milgram and others on obedience to authority are difficult to explain. Several explanations have been offered and some are outlined below:

- Milgram introduced the concept of *agentic state* to explain the shift that occurs in people's thinking when obeying others. According to Milgram there are two states of consciousness: the autonomous state and the agentic state. In the former, individuals see themselves as independent agents who can exercise choice, make decisions on the basis of moral judgements and take responsibility for their actions. In the agentic state, people consider themselves to be acting as agents of others in the hierarchy and do not feel as much individual responsibility. A subject is thought to shift between these two states, depending on situational factors. The Nazi party members who committed vicious crimes were 'ordinary men' who were parents, husbands and employees, but as members of the establishment they became agentic and obeyed orders from their superiors.
- *De-individuation*. This refers to a process in which individual's control over their own behaviour is weakened as a result of being part of collective action, thereby becoming less concerned about moral standards and consequences of one's own behaviour. Zimbardo's prison experiments, which demonstrated the phenomenon of de-individuation most powerfully, are discussed below.
- *Binding forces*. A group of workers, who studied crimes committed by those at subordinate levels, have proposed that in certain situations the individual appears to be psychologically tied to the authorities' definition of the situation (Kelman & Hamilton, 1989). This is commonly seen in massacres carried out by armed forces that follow the command of one or more superior officers. In such situations the followers' behaviour is thought to be *rule and role orientated*.

Social role

All human interactions involve social roles. The term social role refers to the part people play in society. Roles such as parents, friends, manager, boss, doctor, helper, are socially constructed patterns of behaviour involving certain duties, obligations and rights. Social roles are also associated with role expectations concerning how a person is supposed to behave in particular situations. For example, a child is expected to be compliant and obedient, a parent caring and protecting.

Whereas in obedience situations social influence is exercised by persons in positions of authority, in some situations roles exert social pressure and influence over individuals as much as authority figures. A classic study on social roles is the famous Stanford Prison experiment carried out by Zimbardo and colleagues (Haney, Banks & Zimbardo, 1973; Zimbardo et al., 1973). Twenty-one male volunteers were selected for the study, nine of them were assigned to the role of 'prisoners' and the rest were to act as 'guards'. The experiment was made as realistic as possible with the 'prisoners' being arrested by the police and brought to prison. The prison was situated in the basement at Stanford University. It had cells similar to real prisons, together with an observation room for guards. The 'guards' wore uniforms and sunglasses, and were equipped with batons and whistles. The 'prisoners' were strip searched, deloused and given prison clothes and numbers. The 'guards' were to run the prison the way they pleased. The experiment was planned to last for two weeks but it had to be abandoned after just five days. The 'guards' started humiliating the 'prisoners' and became increasingly hostile and brutal. For example, they made it a 'privilege' to go to the toilet, they used foul language, brandished their batons at the 'prisoners' and were overtly cruel. The 'prisoners' showed some initial protest but soon became docile and withdrawn, some showed hysterical crying and screaming. Five 'prisoners' were taken out of the experiment because they were showing acute symptoms of depression and anxiety.

The Stanford Prison experiment demonstrated forcefully the expression of role expectations. Those individuals who acted as 'guards' had acted very much in keeping with their beliefs about the role of a prison guard and so did the 'prisoners' who acted helplessly. Zimbardo explained these findings on the basis that the 'guards' were experiencing *de-individuation*. De-individuation involves the loss of one's sense of personal individuality and identity. It also involves the merger of such identity with those of another person or group. Zimbardo (1971) expressed the conclusion of the experiment most eloquently: 'In less than a week the experience of imprisonment undid a lifetime of learning; human values were suspended, self concepts were challenged and the ugliest and the most base pathological side of human nature surfaced'. (The recent reports of abuse of Iraqi prisoners should come as no surprise to those familiar with the Stanford experiment.)

Helping behaviours

Both clinical psychology and psychiatry have shown a tendency to study and describe antisocial behaviour, rather than the sorts of behaviours in which people interact in ways that benefit one another. In contrast, prosocial behaviour, that is behaviour that is of help to someone else, has received less attention. Research into various forms of positive behaviours between individuals has focused on four themes: simple helping behaviour; altruistic behaviour; bystander intervention; and cooperative behaviour.

Simple helping

This refers to behaviour that provides assistance to others in need. Simple helping is not sacrificial and may involve expectation of some form of reward. People frequently weigh up the cost/benefits in a given situation and offer help when rewards exceed costs. Often the reward is emotional or avoidance of a negative state, like embarrassment or punishment.

Altruism

In social psychology altruism refers to behaviour that is undertaken with the intention of benefiting another without the expectation of any personal benefit. In short, it is voluntary self-sacrificing behaviour. Social history has recorded numerous instances of unselfish behaviours in which individuals had taken extraordinary trouble to help other people. Altruistic behaviour has been observed in animals (see Chapter 11). What motivates people to help others without any expectation of personal reward? Several views have been put forward:

1. *Empathy*. Several studies have addressed the question of empathy-based altruism. Empathy is the ability to understand someone else's point of view and to share the emotional state of the other. Empathy develops early in childhood; infants as young as 18 to 30 months have been shown to exhibit obvious concern when they saw other children in distress.
2. *Sociobiological view*. An evolutionary perspective of altruistic behaviour views altruism as a trait that has evolved as a result of the human struggle for survival. Human beings have to cooperate and help one another in order to survive and over the years helping behaviour is thought to have become hard wired into the human genetic code. According to this theory it is social organization that interferes with the innate altruistic tendency and causes people to behave otherwise.

Bystander intervention

A particularly appalling state of affairs in our times is that when someone is attacked violently in public and no one comes forward to help the victim. A frequently cited case is that of Kitty Genovese, a 28-year-old woman who was stabbed to death in New York as she returned from work early in the morning in March 1964. Thirty-eight people witnessed the murder from their apartments but none intervened in spite of the fact that she screamed for help and the incident took more than half an hour. The Kitty Genovese case shocked social psychologists and set in motion a series of investigations into bystander intervention and the factors that make people help (or not help) others in distress.

A study by Pillavin and colleagues (1969) in a New York underground railway station serves to illustrate the main factors that contribute to intervention by onlookers. In this experiment people witnessed a confederate stagger and collapse under one of two conditions: in one he carried a black case and appeared ill; and in the other he carried a bottle of alcohol and smelled of alcohol. It was found that: (1) onlookers were more likely to help when the individual appeared to be ill (95%) than when he appeared to be drunk (50%); and (2) the longer the emergency continued without help forthcoming, the more likely it became that individuals would leave the area or start discussing the situation without helping. In mixed-race groups, there was a tendency for same-race helping.

A number of studies carried out under various conditions have revealed that bystander intervention is influenced by a number of personal and situational factors:

1. Situational characteristics.
   - If the situation appears to be a real emergency (e.g. a heart attack), onlookers are more likely to provide assistance.
   - If it is perceived that the victim and the perpetrator know each other, bystanders are reluctant to be involved. In the case of Kitty Genovese many people may have assumed that the attacker and she had a close relationship.
   - Presence of other bystanders has been shown to inhibit going to the aid of another person in distress. The more people there are to witness an emergency, such as witnessing smoke coming into a waiting room, the less likely that any of them will take action (Latane & Darley, 1968).
2. Victim characteristics.
   - Bystanders are less likely to help if they feel that the condition is self-imposed as in the case of the 'drunk' in the New York underground study.
3. Bystander characteristics.
   - Men are more likely than women to intervene when there is a danger to a person. Those with relevant skills and expertise (e.g. resuscitation) come forward to help more than others.

Two different explanations have been put forward to explain the reluctance of people to help another in distress: (1) *diffusion of responsibility* – each individual member in a group feels less responsible to intervene when in a group than when alone; and (2) *pluralistic ignorance* –a belief that the other bystanders interpret the situation as harmless.

LEADERSHIP

Leadership is generally regarded as one of the crucial factors in the success or failure of any social activity from governance of nations to management of organizations. The core ideas of leadership are the same be it politics, social reform or war. Leadership is important because the human and financial cost of failure of leadership is very high indeed. Battles have been lost because of incompetent leadership, millions of people suffer because of poor leadership and incompetent management of organisations costs millions in lost revenue. Several studies that examined organisations such as large hospitals, large aerospace companies and corporations have reported the base rate for incompetent management to be around 60% (Hogan, Curphy & Hogan, 1994). Deficient political leadership has been held responsible for the failure to prevent wars and other deadly inter-ethnic conflicts, which have resulted in thousands of lost lives.

One definition of leadership is that it is 'the process whereby the individual influences a group of individuals to achieve a common goal' (Northouse, 2001). Leadership only occurs when others voluntarily adopt, for a period of time, the goals of the group as their own. Thus, leadership involves building cohesive and task-orientated teams, persuading and motivating the team to work willingly towards the achievement of the group's goals in a given situation. The role of leaders is two fold: first, to develop a vision of the future; and, second, to motivate the members of the group to achieve them. Leadership and motivation are inextricably linked and successful leaders bring out the best in people. Leadership, therefore, embodies three main elements: power, persuasion and vision.

1. Power. Power is the ability to influence others and, in the context of leadership, it refers to the ability of the leader to get others to adopt common goals. The leader is vested with power that other members of the group do not possess. The leader may be:

- Appointed by the organisation and given the authority over the group (position power).
- Elected by the group.
- 'Emergent' – informally acknowledged by the group.

Six types of *social power* have been described (Collins & Raven, 1969):

1. Reward power – the power to provide rewards.
2. Coercive power – the power to punish.
3. Referent power – power through identification with the leader.
4. Expert power – power resulting from having greater knowledge or skills.
5. Legitimate power – power bestowed by virtue of social position.
6. Informational power – power arising from possession of valued information that is unknown to others.

2. Persuasion. Persuasion is the ability to motivate and enthuse the group to pursue the goal. It differs from coercion where power is used to enforce change through rewards and punishment. Modern leadership, as defined above, is the very antithesis of coercion because it involves some degree of consensus rather than just blind obedience; it is more concerned with gaining commitment than compliance.

3. Vision. Leadership implies having a vision, being ahead of the team. Formulation of an idealized vision and providing a means to achieve it is, by far, the main task of the leader. It is this unique ability that distinguishes a good leader from a manager of affairs.

Studies on leadership have focused on four key variables: the leader, the task, the group (team) and the situation or context.

Theories of leadership

The oldest theory of leadership is the *great man theory*, which attributes a set of distinct, unique characteristics to leaders as compared to non-leaders. But it has proved impossible to identify the particular traits that distinguish leaders from others. Of the hundreds of traits that have been studied two characteristics that show some weak correlation are intelligence and talkativeness (Handy, 1993).

A second approach to studying and understanding leadership is to examine the patterns of *behaviour* rather than characteristics of personality. Three *styles of leadership* based on the behavioural patterns of leaders have been described:

1. *Autocratic* leadership refers to when the leader is aloof, dominant, makes all the decisions and is very task centred.
2. *Laissez-faire* leadership style is where the leader's input is minimal, limited to supplying material and information.
3. *Democratic* leadership style involves decision by group discussion aided by the leader.

The above taxonomy of leadership behaviour was originally described by Lewin and colleagues in their classic 1930s' study (Lewin, Lippett & White, 1939) in which three groups of school boys were exposed to the three styles of leadership by confederates in a task involving carving models from soap bars. Ever since, the democratic style of leadership has been upheld as the effective and desirable one. However, in some instances other types of leadership may be more appropriate. Some situations may call for urgent action, and in such situations an autocratic style of leadership may be the best. In the case of a team that has developed to be confident, motivated and capable, a laissez-faire leader may be effective by handing over ownership and empowering the members of the team to achieve the goal.

Leadership style – task orientation versus relationship orientation

Studies in the 1950s analysed a number of variables concerned with leadership behaviour in high- and low-productivity groups. Three seminal pieces of work, the well-known Michigan studies (Likent, 1961), the Ohio Studies (Vroom, 1983) and the Harvard studies (Bales, 1951) have described two important dimensions of leadership: task orientation (TO) and relationship orientation (RO). Although these studies conceptualise the two dimensions slightly differently and use different names to describe them, many subsequent studies have produced similar descriptions and some of the new models of leadership incorporate the two dimensions.

- *Task-orientated leadership*. This reflects how much a leader is concerned with the actual task in hand. TO leaders are more directive, and more concerned with task needs than the needs of the team. They are, therefore, more focused on the organisation of the work process, such as the allocation of tasks.
- *Relationship- or people-orientated leadership*. This reflects how much the leader is concerned for the members of the team, providing support and encouragement. RO leaders are considerate to subordinates, pay more attention to relationships at work, exercise less direct supervision and encourage team member's participation in decision making.

In general, high productivity has been shown to be associated with RO leadership style but relationship between style and outcome is more complex and is dependant on contextual factors (see below). Moreover, task-centred leadership is more effective when the circumstances are either highly favourable or highly unfavourable than it is in situations with the average range of appropriateness (Bass, 1990). To an extent, therefore, leadership is dependent on situational factors and the relationship between style and outcome is more complex.

Leadership – Contingency theories

Contingency theories hold that group performance is dependant (contingent) upon a number of factors apart from leadership style. The best-known contingency theory is that of Fielder. Fielder (1965) argued that group performance depends on two factors: leadership style and situational favourableness. In his view, effectiveness of leadership is contingent upon the leader adopting an appropriate style of leadership in the light of the relative favourableness of the situation. He enumerated three important variables that determine situational favourableness:

1. *Leader–member relations* – the degree to which the leader is accepted and supported by the group members.
2. *Task structure* – the extent to which the task is clear and defined, with explicit goals.
3. *Leader's position power* – the extent to which the leader has the power to enforce compliance and control group members through reward and punishment.

The most favourable contingency is when: (1) the leader–member relationship is good; (2) the leader is invested with substantial legitimate power; and (3) the task is highly structured and the goals and methods are clear. At the other extremes of these conditions the situation is said to be least favourable. There is substantial evidence, based on studies of leadership style, that goes to show that when situational favourability is moderate or in the mid-range, the RO leaders are more successful, while in the two extreme conditions of favourability the TO leaders are more effective (Figure 9.2). Several measures are now available for assessing managers on the two dimensions of task orientation and person orientation. Fielder's work also suggests that it may be easier for leaders to change the situation to achieve effectiveness, rather than change their leadership style. Fielder's theory has resulted in a great deal of research and discussion and the results have been mixed.

Leadership and management

Often leadership is confused with management. A good manager may be a poor leader. A leader may have no organisational skills but his vision unites people behind him. It has been said that 'managers do things right and leaders do the right thing'. Leaders think radically, managers think incrementally. Leaders question assumption, they seek out the essence of the situation, they are innovative and let vision guide their action. A leader is someone who people follow naturally through their own choice, whereas a manager must be obeyed.

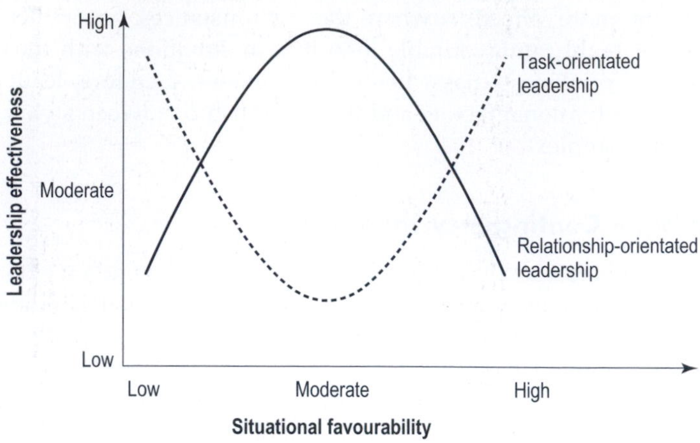

Fig. 9.2 Contingency theory of leadership: leadership style and situational favourability (Fielder, 1965)

Leaders are strategic formulators of a vision, whereas managers are implementers of strategy. Leadership is what counts in any organisation that really wants to move forward. It is an exercise in imagination and inspiration. The leader inspires others to share his vision, motivates them to set aside, even if it be temporarily, their selfish aims and take part in sharing his/her vision voluntarily for the greater good. Diverse historical figures such as Alexander the Great, Napoleon and Lenin have proved their leadership precisely by their ability to combine their strategic vision (which we may or may not share) with a remarkable capacity to persuade others to follow their foresight and dream. It is this unique quality of leadership that has made men to lay down their lives in the process of attaining the aims articulated by their leader.

Management is a process that enables organisations or teams to set and achieve their goals by planning, organising and controlling their resources including motivation of their employees or team members. The definition of management provided by Henri Fayol in 1916 is held to be a classic statement:

> *To manage is to forecast and plan, to organise, to command, to coordinate and to control.* (Fayol, 1949)

Later writers have substituted the term motivation for command. The main aim of the manager is to maximise the output of the organisation or deliver the expected outcomes through administrative implementation. In order to achieve the results the managers involve themselves in a variety of activities. These, known by the acronym POMC, may be summarised as follows:

- Planning – deciding on the objectives or goals and deciding how to achieve them.
- Organising – putting the plans into operation by allocating tasks, coordinating activities and providing the resources.

Table 9.2 Leadership and management

Leaders	*Managers*
Think radically	Think incrementally
Formulate a vision and a strategy	Implement the strategy
Inspire others to share and join (follow) their vision	Organise, try to motivate and control followers
'Followers' unite voluntarily	Impose their will
Power: referent	Power: legitimate, reward and coercive

- Motivating – obtaining the commitment of the employees/team members in fulfilling the goals.
- Controlling – Establishing standards of performance, measuring progress and taking corrective action.

Although leadership and management are qualitatively distinct, we expect our managers to be leaders to some degree. Managing and leading are two different ways of organising people. The manager enables the organisation or team to set and achieve their objectives whilst the leader is visionary and effectively persuades others to share his/her vision through inspiration and appeal to emotions (Table 9.2)

In conclusion, although studies on leadership over the last 50 years have not produced a great many 'facts', they have provided fertile ground for new thinking, not least in the area of management training. The most effective leaders are those who can develop a range of leadership styles and who also know when to apply each. These styles are easily recognisable but it is less easy to be consciously aware of the need to use a particular approach at a given time. Leadership study is an ever-expanding subject and there has been a proliferation of theories of leadership. For a detailed account of the various theories see Northouse (2001).

ATTRIBUTION

Whether one is aware of it or not we, as human beings, have a strong tendency to explain and understand what is going on in the world around us. Whenever we observe a piece of behaviour or action, such as witnessing a traffic accident or seeing a patient who had taken an overdose, it is in our nature to try to ask the question *why* such things happened. This is true not only when we observe other people's actions but also applies to our own actions and experiences. For example, if one experiences pain in some part of the body, one looks immediately for causal explanations. It is important to remember that people make different types of attributions to other people's (and their own) actions, such as intent, motivation and responsibility, but in social psychology the term 'attribution' is used only when they imply *causality* or offer explanatory judgements. Thus to make an *attribution* is to determine a cause for something.

Attribution theory is an influential body of knowledge in social psychology concerned with how people explain the *causes* of their own and other people's behaviour. Heider (1958), the pioneer in this field, suggested that people systematically seek to explain causes of behaviour in a commonsense search to understand why things happen. He described attribution as the process of making 'causal inferences'. In making causal attributions, the sequence of events is:

Behaviour (or experience) → search and collection of information → construction of an implicit theory that explains behaviour

Heider suggested that human beings act as 'naïve psychologists' proposing hypotheses for actions of their own and others.

People attribute causes to almost all behaviours. Although we may seek out information, causal inferences are made on the basis of minimal information and seem to happen almost automatically and often spontaneously. Making such causal attributions seems to help us to understand other people's (and our own) behaviour and predict what could happen in the future. The implications of attribution theory for everyday social interaction are that people may, and indeed do, make different attributions for the same behaviour.

Heider (1958) distinguished between two types of attributions.

1. *Internal (dispositional) attributions*. These assume that other people's actions are caused by internal characteristics or dispositions of those people.
2. *External (situational) attributions*. Here someone's behaviour is attributed to external causes or the current situation.

For example, when we witness an accident, an internal or dispositional attribution would be that the driver made a mistake, was careless or was drunk, while an external or situational attribution would be that the road was slippery or that the brakes of the vehicle were faulty.

Attribution is a subjective process because attributions are how people *perceive* behaviour to be caused, rather than how it is *really* caused. Not surprisingly, attributions are open to errors. Some erroneous attributions are systematic distortions of perceptions of causes of behaviour that have been observed to occur in various situations. Three common attributional biases are:

1. *Fundamental attribution error*. This is the tendency to make internal attributions for other people's behaviour and ignore situational factors or causes. As naïve psychologists we constantly assess how much an action is due to the person as opposed to situational causes and our inclination is to overestimate the degree to which actions and behaviours reflect the dispositions of individuals and underestimate the importance of situational determinants. In short, we have an inherent tendency to make internal or dispositional attributions rather than external attributions. Numerous experiments and studies have confirmed this inherent flaw in human thinking and judgement.
2. *Actor/observer difference*. It has been shown that people show systematic bias in attribution when it comes to their own (actor) behaviour as compared with other people's (observer) behaviours. People are inclined to attribute other people's behaviour to internal or dispositional causes, while at the

same time attributing their own behaviour to external factors. This is particularly evident when assessing unexpected or unusual or negative events. For example, failing an exam is often attributed by the candidate to difficulties in the test or a fault of the examiners (external attribution) while when another person fails the examination it is often ascribed to his/her lack of suitability, or lack of preparation, and so on. This self/other difference is a robust finding that had been repeatedly demonstrated in a number of studies.

3. *Self-serving bias*. People show a strong bias towards attributing their success to internal causes, while attributing failures to situational causes. Thus if you pass an examination it is because of your cleverness and hard work; if you fail it is because it was an unfair paper! There is strong evidence for self-serving bias. It has been argued that self-serving bias helps maintain self-esteem.

Dimensions of attribution

Attribution theory has been developed and modified over the years. Research into the nature of attribution has established several important dimensions of attribution (Seligman et al., 1979).

1. *Locus*. Internal versus external – internal attributions locate the cause in the person, such as ability, effort, personality trait, mood, and so on, while external attribution refers to causes outside the person, such as situational factors, actions of others, difficulty of the task, etc. (as described by Heider).
2. *Stability*. Stable versus unstable (permanent versus temporary) – stable causes are relatively permanent, unchanging and lasting, while unstable attributions are temporary and fluctuating.
3. *Generality*. Global versus specific – global causes are perceived as applicable to most, if not all, actions of the person, whereas specific attributions pertain to those that are restricted to certain domains or situations.
4. *Controllability*. Controllability versus uncontrollability – attributions that are controllable are perceived as beyond one's effort, autonomous and independent, whereas controllable causations are seen as manageable and prone to containment or mastery.

These insights into attributional processes have been usefully applied to clinical situations, especially to depression. The best-known and most studied attributional phenomenon is that of learned helplessness (see Chapter 1).

Misattributions

It is only to be expected that some of the causal and explanatory attributions would be inaccurate, incorrect or wrong. In day-to-day social interactions it is common for the initial attributions to be wrong and such misattributions may be amended or changed after reflection or when new evidence comes to light. While some misattributions may be revised or corrected, others tend to be enduring, resulting in a pattern of recurring misattributions that may not be apparent to the subject. Some examples of the misattribution of bodily symptoms are as follows:

- Misattribution of bodily sensations is commonly encountered in general practice when patients experiencing a physical symptom, such as chest pain, attribute it to angina or heart attack while, in fact, it may be due to a relatively innocuous cause like muscle pain.
- Primary hypochondriasis is a condition in which somatic symptoms, often minor pain or discomfort, are believed by the subject to be due to serious physical illnesses in spite of reassurance by several medical professionals. The central feature of primary hypochondriasis is the enduring tendency to misattribute innocuous bodily symptoms to physical illness. The subject ignores alternative interpretations of symptoms and persists in misattributing the meaning of the symptom so much so that it becomes ingrained as a false belief or overvalued idea.
- Ideas of reference is a term used in phenomenology to describe misattribution of other people's actions to aspects of self. For example, the subject interprets casual conversations between two people as something associated with self. Such self-conscious behaviour is common in most people at some time or other but is usually transient and context related. It is more common in adolescents when identity, egocentricity and self-image are important. Persistent and pervasive ideas of reference are a feature of paranoid states.

Attributions in clinical encounters

In clinical encounters clients and patients discuss their concerns or complaints, which are most often seen as symptoms or 'presenting complaints'. Invariably, behind such complaints are causal attributions such as their belief about what the symptoms are due to and what may be producing them. According to attribution theory, patients would have their own theories about the origin of their symptoms and being naïve scientists they may well have made efforts to think about and even collect information regarding their symptoms in an attempt to make sense of their difficulties. Often these attributions remain unspoken. It is incumbent on the clinician to elicit the unvoiced attributions that patients have made and to be able to bring forth such attributions and discuss them in the open.

Causal attributions that patients and family members make about their symptoms or illnesses are an important component of what Kleinman has called *explanatory models* – the notion that people have about the causes of an episode of their problems. These beliefs profoundly influence care-seeking behaviour and adherence to recommended interventions. Understanding the sufferer and carer's explanatory model is an essential element in all forms of clinical practice (Kleinman, 1980).

ATTITUDE

Attitude refers to our tendency to think, act or feel consistently in a favourable or unfavourable manner towards entities in our environment. For example, one might have an attitude towards capital punishment, abortion, immigration or mental illness. The entity towards which people hold an attitude (e.g. capital punishment) is called the attitude object or the psychological object. Such objects include abstract entities, one's own behaviour (e.g. drinking), ideologies, ideas or concrete objects. Attitude is distinguished from other related concepts by three distinct features:

1. *Attitudes are learned.* People are not born with a specific attitude towards certain objects or ideas. Attitudes are acquired from parents, family, friends and society and to an extent reflect cultural predispositions.
2. *Attitudes are evaluative.* Attitudes involve subjective judgements such as being sympathetic–unsympathetic, liking–disliking, good–bad and beneficial–harmful. Human beings appear to have an inherent tendency to appraise, judge and evaluate psychological objects. Individuals register an instantaneous and automatic judgement of good/bad, towards psychological objects that they come across. Research has demonstrated that attitudes can be activated automatically. No doubt this involves preconscious automatic processing. There is also evidence to show that evaluative judgements (e.g. categorisation of the food items into good and bad) involve large parts of the right hemisphere of the brain whereas in non-evaluative judgements (e.g. categorisation of food items into vegetables and non-vegetables) the left hemisphere is implicated (Crites & Cacioppo, 1996). People also show individual variations in their need to evaluate.
3. *Attitudes tend to be relatively persistent.* Attitudes remain remarkably consistent over time and several studies have shown that, although attitudes do change and can be changed, by and large, attitudes are relatively stable. Bringing about changes in attitudes of groups of people is central to discourses such as psychotherapy, political propaganda, and advertising and marketing.

Attitudes have three main components (called ABC of attitude): the affective component involves feelings and evaluations; the behavioural constituent consists of ways of acting towards the psychological object; and the cognitive element concerns one's beliefs. Attitudes are usually measured using self-report questionnaires (see Chapter 8).

Do attitudes predict behaviour? The relationship between attitude and behaviour is complex and is influenced by numerous social factors. Behaviour usually, but not always, reflects attitudes. This is particularly true when aggregates of behaviours, i.e. behaviours in general, are taken into account rather than a single behavioural act. However, as everyone knows, attitudes can be concealed or suppressed and not revealed in behaviour. A number of factors beyond attitudes influence behaviour including desirability of the behaviour and situational factors. It is not unusual for individuals to hold positive and negative attitude towards an attitude object, a mental state known as *ambivalence*. Holding ambivalent attitudes produces an uneasy feeling in people and has been shown to affect judgement and behaviour in profound ways.

The issue of the attitude/behaviour relationship is an important one because it affects a wide range of issues from conduct towards minority groups to changing voting preferences. Health promotion is aimed at changing people's attitude towards exercising and risk factors such as smoking and drinking. Can attitudes be changed? The answer is a qualified 'yes'. Two important areas pertaining to attitude change are *cognitive dissonance* and *persuasive communication*. The theory of cognitive dissonance credibly argues that people adopt various strategies to maintain their attitudes whereas persuasion is about convincing people to change their attitudes. These are discussed below.

Cognitive dissonance

Individuals prefer, and therefore seek, to hold beliefs and cognitions that are consistent with each other and their behaviour. People seek to maintain a degree of cognitive consistency and avoid inconsistencies in their beliefs and ideas. Holding two contradictory attitudes simultaneously is unpleasant and individuals try their best to reduce the conflict in their mind by various means. The state of psychological tension that occurs when an individual holds two cognitions that are psychologically inconsistent is known as *cognitive dissonance*.

Leon Festinger's (1957) theory of cognitive dissonance has been one of the most influential theories in social psychology. He used the example of a heavy smoker to illustrate his theory. The smoker's cognition, 'Smoking is dangerous to my health' is dissonant with the cognition, 'I smoke'. The two cognitions are inconsistent or dissonant with each other and the conflict leads to an unpleasant state of arousal. Festinger asserted that, faced with such a state of dissonance, people are motivated to try to reduce it by whatever methods are possible. Logically speaking, the simplest way to reduce dissonance in this case is, of course, to stop smoking. But a person who has been unable to stop smoking may try a number of dissonance reduction methods. There are three main ways of reducing dissonance (Figure 9.3):

- *Removing the dissonant cognitions*. Dismissing the dissonant cognition is a common way of dealing with cognitive dissonance. The smoker may tell him/herself, 'I will consider it when the time comes', 'There is no evidence that smoking is harmful' or, 'I refuse to think of it'.
- *Reducing the importance of the dissonant cognition*. Trivialising, minimising or disqualifying the dissonant cognition is another way of dealing with the unease generated by dissonance. Thus, the smoker may compare the risk of smoking with the risks of road traffic accidents and conclude that the risks from smoking are minimal, or he/she may modify the cognition so as to minimise its significance by believing, 'I do not smoke that much'. He/she may even discredit the source of information, 'There is no real evidence that smoking is harmful' or he/she may be selective about noticing information that supports the cognition such as not counting the number of cigarettes smoked in a day or saying, 'So and so smokes more than me but is well and healthy'.
- *Adding new consonant cognitions*. Adding a third cognition to neutralise the dissonant cognition is a well-known method of reducing dissonance. For example, the smoker may consider that smoking reduces tension or keeps

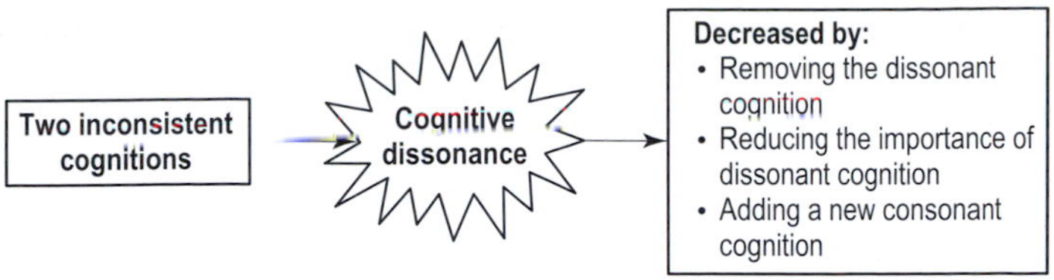

Fig. 9.3 Cognitive dissonance and methods of reduction (Festinger, 1957)

his/her weight down. He/she may tell him/herself, 'I have a strong personality and I will not get addicted'.

It is evident that cognitive dissonance theory is based on the assumption that people rationalise in order to maintain their attitude. Cognitive dissonance research has produced a number of findings and paradigms since its enunciation by Festinger in 1957. Several types of cognitive dissonance have been identified:

Post-decisional dissonance. This occurs when a commitment or decision has been made to a course of action, for example buying a car. Often it is reduced by emphasising the positive aspects of the chosen alternative. Thus, people who have bought new cars read more advertisements about the cars they have purchased than about the cars they had considered buying; house buyers are more likely to rate their houses better *after* having bought them; governments try to justify their blatantly wrong actions (such as going to war) to reduce dissonance among the people. An extreme form of post-event dissonance-reducing strategy is *justification of cruelty*. Several experiments have shown that those who cause suffering and hurt to others often justify their cruelty by belittling or demonising their victims ('They deserved it /Asked for it'). It is interesting to note that they are less likely to derogate their victims if they believe that the victims are able to retaliate.

Forced (induced) compliance dissonance. This occurs when people are made to carry out acts that conflict with their prior beliefs or attitudes. In such situations changing the belief or attitude to correspond with the (induced) behaviour reduces dissonance. For example, in one experiment, subjects (army recruits) made to eat fried cockroaches justified their behaviour by saying, 'After all it was not too bad' or, 'There must be a good reason for getting us to do this' (Zimbardo et al., 1965). It has been shown that when individuals are made to repeatedly say or do something that is counter-attitudinal (the opposite to their own attitude) such as writing an essay that is against their beliefs, it is likely to leads to an actual change in attitude or belief.

Belief-disconfirmation dissonance. This arises when people are exposed to information that is inconsistent with their prior beliefs. In a study of a religious group that believed in a prophecy that a flood would destroy the world on a given day, it was found that when the doomsday did not occur, members of the group maintained their belief by adding a new cognition that the flood did not materialise because of the group's prayers (Festinger, Riecken & Schacter, 1956)!

Effort-justification dissonance. This occurs whenever people expend energy and effort on an unpleasant activity in order to attain a desirable outcome that in the event turns out to be a poor one. People are more likely to persuade themselves that the goal is more attractive and worthwhile than it actually is. Initiation rights to join societies and clubs make the membership of such organisations more valuable to the individual.

Although the concept of cognitive dissonance appears simple and straightforward its importance lies in the fact that it reveals a basic tendency in man – the strong desire of individuals to maintain their attitudes and their employment of a number of different strategies, including self-deception, in their efforts to justify and rationalise both those attitudes and their consequent actions. Festinger's cognitive dissonance theory has generated a great deal of research and been applied to a wide variety of psychological topics involving motivation, cognition and emotion. As a theory of attitude maintenance it has provided valuable insights into the resistance encountered when attempts are made to change attitudes either in clinical encounters or social situations. Research has shown that dissonance is not inevitable and that certain conditions have to be met for dissonance to occur (Cooper & Fazio, 1984). For dissonance to occur the individual must:

- be aware of the inconsistency;
- take responsibility for the behaviour, belief or attitude;
- experience a certain amount of arousal as a result of dissonance; and
- attribute the unease felt to the inconsistency in his cognitions.

These findings have significant implications for psychotherapeutic interventions for psychological and psychiatric problems. Motivational interviewing is one such technique that is used to induce dissonance in bringing about change in the treatment of clients with alcohol-misuse problems (see Chapter 5).

Persuasion and persuasive communication

A second way of changing attitudes is through persuasion. In everyday relationships, in the workplace, in politics and in the market place, persuasion plays an important role in trying to change people's attitudes. Because of the importance of persuasion for society as a whole, there has been extensive research on persuasion and methods of persuasion. A selective account of persuasions and persuasive communication is given here. Each of the statements mentioned here has had support from many studies, too numerous to be cited. The reader is referred to a textbook on persuasion and communication for further information (Stiff & Mongeau, 2002, see further reading).

Persuasion is the conscious attempt to change attitudes through communication of some message. The communication model developed by the Yale Group (Hovland, Janis & Kelly, 1953) and subsequent work by others focuses on the four main variables in persuasive communication: the source (the communicator); the message (the characteristics of the message); the audience or recipients (the target at whom the message is directed); and the channel or medium through which the message is delivered.

Source variables

A number of source variables influence the effectiveness of the messages. The most important characteristics of the communicator that influence effective persuasion are:

Credibility of the communicator. By far the most important factor that influences attitude change in the audience is the reliability of the person delivering the message. When the communicator is of high status (e.g. a judge) people listening to the message are more likely to be persuaded than they would be by those delivered by low-status communicators.

Expertise. Those who are perceived to have expertise in the field have more influence on people's attitudes than those presumed to have less expertise. This is the case even when the recipients of the message do not know the actual level of expertise of the communicator.

Attractiveness. In general, good-looking communicators are better at persuading people than their unattractive counterparts, a concept exploited by the advertising industry.

Likeability. A related factor is the likeability of the communicator as judged by the audience. The verbal and non-verbal cues, mannerisms, gestures and style of the presentation and delivery of the message, exert a positive influence on the audience.

Similarity of the communicator. The more similar the communicator is to the audience in terms of age, gender and ethnic background, the greater is the appeal. Many studies have shown that the background and values held by the communicator have a better effect on the audience if the audience is able to identify with them. This factor is made use of in advertising. For example, when selling cosmetics, the models are young and the appeal is for people of the younger age group, whereas when selling pensions, the models tend to be older.

Message variables

Message variables are concerned with the content of the information provided in the communication and the way it is delivered.

Confident delivery. Messages delivered with confidence are more persuasive. Using phrases such as 'obviously', 'beyond doubt', etc., is more convincing than using tentative expressions like 'it appears that', 'I need to check this', 'I am unsure of this', and so on.

Fear appeals. The emotional impact of a message is an important factor in changing people's attitudes. One of the most studied factors is fear. Advertising campaigns that produce a certain amount of fear and anxiety in the audience, such as cancer warnings in smoking advertisements, are to a certain degree effective and produce the desired outcome. Inducing too much fear, however, is less effective, presumably because extreme emotions interfere with information processing and the audience tends to ignore the message. Thus, fear-arousing messages appear to follow Yerkes–Dodson's law (see Chapter 4).

Two-sided messages. The audience responds to the one-sidedness and two-sidedness of the message in different ways. One-sided messages are most effective with subjects who have had little education in situations where the communicator presents his arguments convincingly. On the other hand, two-sided messages are more effective in persuading: (1) those who initially disagree; (2) people who are well informed on the subject; and (3) an audience that is going to hear counter-arguments in the future. Presenting a strong argument together with a weak version of arguments counter to your position is called *inoculation*.

Order of presentation. The order in which the messages are presented has a moderate degree of effect on their persuasiveness. Messages to audiences show both primacy and recency effects (see Chapter 7). When the message is of personal relevance, the primacy effect seems to be stronger.

Humour. Humour and light-hearted discussions have a positive effect in convincing the audience as long as they are relevant to the key message

Repetition and conclusions. Messages that are repeated are more effective than messages delivered once only. A firm summarising statement about the message is also useful.

Audience variables (the target)

There are individual differences in the susceptibility to persuasion. The personality of the receiver of the message may affect attitude change. Intelligence, self-esteem and anxiety all influence how well the message is understood and processed. People who already hold views closer to the position propounded by the communicator tend to absorb the message better than those holding more extreme or different views. This process has been described as *assimilation*. Thus, starting from a position not so far removed from that of the audience produces a better persuasive effect than simply stating one's strongly held beliefs.

Channel variables (transmission of message)

The method of delivery and the style of presentation have a significant effect on persuasion. Fast-talking speakers give the impression of credibility. However, fast-talking also interferes with systematic message processing and so it would be more effective with audiences who are initially in opposition to the view held by the communicator. Similarly, a speech delivered with enthusiasm and conviction is felt to be powerful. Powerful speeches include good eye contact, the appearance of deep-felt conviction and a flexible stance. Speeches that include hesitations, qualifiers and disclaimers are considered weak and are less effective in persuading people.

Measuring attitudes

This topic is covered in Chapter 8 (see p. 192).

Prejudice and discrimination

Prejudice is defined as an attitude (usually negative) towards members of some group, based solely on their membership in that group. It is important to distinguish between prejudice and discrimination. Prejudice is a negative *attitude* directed towards people simply because they are members of a specific social group. Discrimination is a negative *action* towards members of a specific social group. Thus, if someone dislikes a minority group, such as homosexuals, but the dislike does not affect their behaviour towards members of that group, then that person shows prejudice but not discrimination. Discrimination, on the other hand, involves negative actions such as aggression, segregation or exclusion, directed at the members of the minority group.

Prejudice has been considered as an attitude that predisposes a person to think, feel and perceive in favourable or unfavourable ways about a group or its individual members. Like any other attitude, it is composed of cognitive, affective and behavioural components. The affective content is expressed by prejudice, the behavioural component by discrimination and the cognitive component by stereotyping.

Historically, prejudice has had disastrous consequences, the most notorious being ethnic cleansing and genocide. Allport (1954) proposed five stages of ethnic discrimination:

1. *Antilocution*. Hostile talk, verbal attack and denigration directed against some other group.
2. *Avoidance*. Systematic avoidance of the other group. Segregation is an extreme example of avoidance.
3. *Discrimination*. Exclusion in terms of civil rights, jobs and educational opportunities.
4. *Physical attack*. Violence against people and property of the other group, including racial riots.
5. *Extermination*. Deliberate killing and murder of members of the other group.

Children acquire prejudices early in life, even before coming into contact with those against whom the prejudices are held. Most often they are transferred prejudices from parents and other family members. Unfortunately, prejudices are stable over time. Most often, they only loosen when social and cultural norms change. Higher social class, education and intelligence are associated with lower levels of prejudice. Some manifestations of prejudice are racism, sexism and homophobia. Prejudice is most likely to develop under certain social conditions:

1. Intergroup competition. Prejudice and discrimination are more likely when there are group conflicts, especially over scarce resources.
2. Prejudice may develop as a way of justifying oppression. Unequal power distribution within society is a common contributor to discrimination and prejudice. The majority often develops negative attitudes towards the victimised minority as a means of self-justification.
3. The desire to enhance social identity is a factor that promotes prejudice in certain circumstances. In order to maintain high levels of self-esteem, the majority group tends to maintain a favourable opinion of their own group and to derogate the outgroup.
4. Authoritarian personality trait is associated with hostility and prejudice towards other groups.

5. Religious beliefs and prejudice have been shown to be associated. Religious people have been shown to be more prejudiced than others under certain circumstances. Human history abounds with wars fought in the name of religion.

Stereotypes

Stereotyping is the attribution to a person of a number of characteristics or traits, which are assumed to be typical of the group to which the individual belongs. Thus, the presumed characteristics of the group are generalised and applied to all individuals of the group. Stereotyping is a normal part of the thinking process – it helps us simplify information, categorise it and use it with ease. Compartmentalisation is an easy shorthand way of dealing with complex information. Stereotypes are social schemas – simplified representations similar to those governing perception of objects – about groups of people that influence the perception, beliefs and expectations. Stereotyping has been called the 'dark side' of heuristics.

Some typical stereotypes are: Blacks are inferior to Whites; Jews are money grabbers; women are weak/inferior to men; and homosexuals are sick people. Often stereotypes are based on minimal information derived from second- and third-hand information (e.g. TV, radio and newspapers) and the prejudiced person has little direct experience of the outgroup. They are based on evaluative judgements predicted in advance on the basis of some arbitrary characteristics presumed to be possessed by the target group. Stereotyping is, therefore, defined as the tendency to place a person in categories according to some easily and quickly identifiable characteristics such as age, sex, ethnic membership, nationality or occupation and then to attribute to him/her qualities believed to be typical of members of that category (Box 9.1).

Another feature of stereotyping is that when people are presented with information that does not fit the global stereotype, they often create subtypes or subcategories to explain the difference. Stereotypes are resistant to change and persist in spite of evidence to the contrary.

Methods of reducing prejudice

Reducing prejudice and discrimination is of vital importance for the harmonious functioning of civil societies. The danger of ignoring nascent prejudice and discrimination, as outlined by Allport (see above), is that failure to

Box 9.1 Characteristics of stereotypes

1. Categorised on the basis of the most noticeable features, e.g. colour, race, and sex
2. All members of the social group are considered to possess the same characteristics
3. Any individual belonging to the group is attributed with possessing the stereotypic characteristics
4. Based on minimal, second-hand, or outdated information

address the important issues associated with prejudice could rapidly lead to disastrous outcomes for the entire society. One way of reducing prejudice and its adverse consequences is to bring about frequent contact between the two groups. The *intergroup contact hypothesis*, as it is known, holds that frequent social contact and interaction between the two groups disconfirms the assumption that everyone in a group is similar. Allport (1954), the originator of the contact theory, was quick to point out that contact by itself ('mere contact') was not sufficient to bring about reduction in prejudice. He held that the positive effects of intergroup contact occur only in situations marked by four key conditions:

1. *Equal status within the situation*. Ingroup bias increases with status differential. It is important that both groups expect and perceive equal status in the situation. Equal status also implies that both groups feel that power distribution is relatively equal.
2. *Common goals*. Prejudice reduction through contact requires that the two groups actively strive to achieve common goals (superordinate goals). Mixed race sporting teams provide prime examples of this principle.
3. *Intergroup cooperation*. Achieving common goals must involve interdependent effort without intergroup competition. In Sherif's summer camp experiment (see later) the two groups were shown to overcome previously held prejudices when they had to strive together to attain common goals. Cooperative action by the groups must achieve positive results, otherwise it leads to blame and recrimination.
4. *Support of authorities, law and/or custom*. Explicit social sanction and authority support is essential to produce positive results. Research in military, religious and business institutions shows that when authority support is readily available, contact is effective in bringing about positive results. On the other hand, individual or minority-group efforts that do not enjoy the support of 'authorities' lead to failure in reducing prejudice.

Allport's predictions have received overwhelming support from numerous field studies across a variety of situations, groups and societies. It has proved to be one of the most robust predictions in social psychology. Recent research (Pettigrew, 1998) has added a fifth condition:

5. *Friendship potential*. The contact situation must provide the participants with an opportunity to become friends. Optimal intergroup contact requires time for cross-group friendships to develop. It also implies that contact and interaction should occur not just in one situation, such as work or school, but in a variety of situations for the effects to generalise.

However, it is a mistake to overestimate the influence of individual and group factors in the formation and maintenance of prejudice. In the ultimate analysis, the structure and organisation of society and economic factors are the major factors that are able to neutralise our predisposition towards prejudice. Moreover, effective leadership is a critical factor in preventing the escalation of conflicts between groups and nations that may lead to 'deadly conflicts' and war (Hamburg, George & Ballentine, 1999).

Stigma

The word stigma is derived from the Greek word 'στιγμα', a mark placed on slaves so as to identify them. Thus, stigma and the process of stigmatisation consist of two fundamental elements: (1) recognition of the differentiating 'mark'; and (2) subsequent devaluation of the person or persons bearing the 'mark'. The idea of stigma was first developed by the American sociologist Erving Goffman. He defined stigma as any physical or social attribute or sign that devalues a person's identity such as to disqualify him or her from full 'social acceptance' (Goffman, 1968). He described three types of stigma: physical defects; social stigma (e.g. membership of an ethnic minority); and personal blemishes (e.g. a police or prison record). The most striking aspect of stigma is its universality. Throughout history and in almost every culture groups of persons have been stigmatised. People with mental illness, disabled people, certain minorities, homosexuals, criminals, and drug addicts have all been singled out by society for stigmatisation. Goffman emphasised that it was society at large that, by its definition of normality, constructed an ideology about those stigmatised in order to justify its own fear, rejection and discrimination. The following account focuses on the stigma of mental illness but the principles apply to most other forms of stigmatisation (Box 9.2).

Stigmatisation is an extreme form of discrimination arising from negative stereotyping, which, in turn, is the result of prejudicial attitudes.

$$\text{Prejudice} \rightarrow \text{Stereotyping} \rightarrow \text{Stigma}$$

In the case of mental illness, the majority of the general public harbour negative evaluations ('Mentally ill people are violent') and negative emotional reactions ('They scare me'). This view of mentally ill people is applied to *all* people considered to have a mental illness. Thus, all people with mental illness are stigmatised and the impact of such stigmatisation has been shown to result in three different responses (Corrigan & Watson, 2002):

1. *Fear and exclusion*. People with mental illness are perceived to be unpredictable and dangerous. They are, therefore, kept out of mainstream society.
2. *Authoritarianism*. People with mental illnesses are perceived as lacking 'insight' or as being irresponsible. Hence, society needs to make decisions for them, including compulsory institutionalisation.
3. *Benevolence*. Those with severe mental illnesses are seen as helpless and to be in need of care. Benevolence may result in patronising attitudes and a lack of respect for the individual's rights.

Unlike the case of physical disabilities, mentally ill patients are perceived by the public to be, in some way, responsible for their plight and it is therefore felt that

Box 9.2 Stigmatising beliefs about mental illness

- People with mental illnesses are dangerous to others (e.g. 'homicidal maniacs')
- Mental illness is imaginary or feigned
- Mentally ill people are weak
- Mental illness is self-inflicted

they ought to be in control of their disabilities. Often the illnesses are attributed to weakness of character or are believed to be self-induced. The public reaction to such perceptions is usually one of anger and a belief that help is not deserved.

The behavioural component of stigma is discrimination and it takes many forms:

- *Social avoidance*. Persons with mental illnesses are excluded from social interaction. Obtaining good jobs and housing, living in ordinary neighbourhoods and socialising with others turn out to be problematic. An extreme form of social avoidance is the refusal of someone to marry a person from a family in which another individual suffers from a mental illness. This is a particularly common stigmatising attitude in collectivist societies (e.g. Southeast Asian countries).
- *Withholding help*. People with mental illness are perceived to be less in need of help than, for example, those with physical illness. The lack of will to help those with mental illnesses operates at many levels. General medical wards are keen to get them discharged, patients taking overdoses are treated with contempt and the resourcing of mental-health services is far lower than other parts of the health service.
- *Coercive treatment*. Some sections of the public believe that people with mental illnesses should be treated against their will or detained (and punished) for the 'protection' of others!
- *Segregation in institutions*. Studies have repeatedly shown that the public endorses segregation of the mentally ill in institutions.

According to Goffman's original formulation, the stigma of mental illness can be either discrediting (when it is obvious to others) or discreditable (when it is not obvious to others). The latter, *self-stigma*, has been a neglected area of study until recently. Whereas *public stigma* is the reaction of the members of the public to people with mental illness, self-stigma refers to the prejudice which people with mental illness hold against themselves (Corrigan & Watson, 2002). Self-stigma results from internalisation of the negative attitudes held by society at large – the mentally ill person comes to agree with the negative evaluation of him or her by others and feels disempowered. Low self-esteem and lack of confidence in oneself arising from self-stigmatisation lead to limited attempts to pursue employment, housing and other opportunities. Perceived stigma prevents people from disclosing their difficulties, accepting the diagnosis and adhering to treatment.

Strategies for changing public stigma

Three different approaches have been adopted to change public stigma (Corrigan & Penn, 1999):

1. *Protest*. Recently there has been an outcry by various professional and voluntary groups (including the Royal College of Psychiatrists in the UK) against the hostile portrayal of mental illness in the media. The protest movement has been effective, to some extent, in getting stigmatising images withdrawn.
2. *Education*. Changing the public's erroneous perceptions of mental illness has been the aim of education campaigns (e.g. 'The Changing Minds' campaign organised by the Royal College of Psychiatrists).

3. *Contact*. Interpersonal contact with persons with mental illness is one of the most effective ways of changing public perception of mental illness and reducing stigma, especially when members of the general public meet with persons with mental illness who are well functioning and of equal status.

GROUP PROCESSES

Insanity in individuals is something rare – but in groups, parties, nations and epochs, it is the rule.

Friedrich Nietzsche

It was noted at the beginning of the chapter that behaviour of two people towards each other is different when a third person is present. How people think and act when in small groups (two is a dyad, three is a group) is even more different and the behaviour of groups towards one another is yet more dissimilar. It has been demonstrated in various studies and across different situations and cultures that people's actions, perceptions and behaviours differ depending on whether they are acting as individuals alone, in the presence of others or collectively as groups. Thus, there are at least three social contexts in which human behaviour may be studied (Figure 9.4):

1. *Interpersonal behaviour*. The actions of an individual with a unique set of personality characteristics towards similar individuals (e.g. John is friendly, amiable and helpful to others).
2. *Intragroup (within-group) behaviour*. Behaviour of members of a group towards one another (e.g. miners are united, helpful to one another).
3. *Intergroup (between-group) behaviour*. Individuals acting as group members towards other groups (e.g. Protestants toward Catholics).

Groups and group processes

Some of the earliest writings about groups were by Sigmund Freud. Group psychology, according to Freud, is concerned with the individual man as a

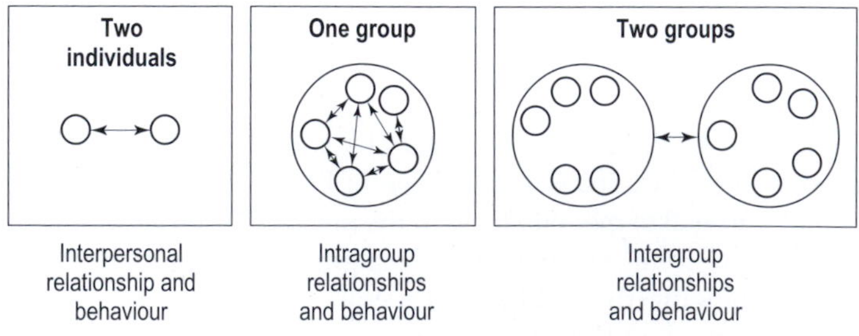

Fig. 9.4 Diagrammatic representation of interpersonal, intergroup and intragroup relationships

member of a race, caste, profession or nation who have been organised for a definite purpose. He wrote: 'An individual belonging or forming part of a group differs from the isolated individual' (Freud, 1921). This emphasises a basic fact – that the thinking, feeling and behaviour of individuals in a group are fundamentally different from those of the individual person.

But a mere collection of people is not the same as a group. For example, the audience in a meeting, a football crowd or a collection of people in a waiting room do not constitute a group. Groups are distinguished from crowds and other gatherings by the following criteria:

1. *Interaction over time*. Members of a group interact over a period of time, not momentarily. In short, they have continuity of existence over time or history of having been together and have some lasting relationship. Small groups are thought to go through a process of development that involves various stages: forming (being accepted); storming (resolving conflicts); norming (attaining consensus); performing (achieving goals); and adjourning (disbanding) (Tuckman & Jensen, 1977).
2. *Group identity*. Over time persons perceive themselves as members of the group and adopt an identity with the group.
3. *Emotional ties*. Group members come to know one another and form emotional bonds.
4. *Shared goals*. The individuals develop a sense of purpose and shared goals.
5. *Group norms*. Groups develop common views about standards of conduct (norms). Often the rules are implicit, unspoken and taken for granted. Such rules specify what one ought to do and members become aware of them only when rules are broken. In addition, some groups may make the rules formal and explicit. Groups form their own traditions, customs, habits and rituals (e.g. family dinners, team meetings). Group norms are remarkably resistant to change.

The structure of the group varies depending upon its type. Common, naturally occurring groups include: (1) families; (2) friendship groups; and (3) work groups. Multidisciplinary teams, staff groups in wards, teams on production lines and aircrews are examples of work groups with specified tasks. Functional differentiation and specialisation within teams are common. Communication networks form within the group. Rules and roles and emotional bonds develop resulting in cohesion within the group. Cohesion is essential to keep the group together. Group members develop a sense of loyalty and realise that the benefits accruing from group membership are worth sacrificing their individuality for. The underlying features and dynamics of larger groups like religious and ethnic groups, races, communities and nations are similar to those of small groups but may take more specific forms.

A striking feature of group behaviour is the difference that has been consistently observed between how groups behave towards their own members, known as the ingroup (intragroup behaviour), and how they behave towards those defined as belonging to another group, known as the outgroup (intergroup behaviour). Observations in natural settings and findings from numerous experiments in social settings have repeatedly demonstrated that intergroup behaviour tends to be remarkably different from intragroup behaviour in several aspects. This difference was most convincingly demonstrated by two outstanding experiments in social psychology, the summer camp experiment and the 'minimal group paradigm' study.

The summer camp experiment

Two groups of 11-year-old boys with no previous record of psychological problems were taken to a summer camp in the Robber's Cave State Park near Oklahoma City. The experiment took place in three phases. In the first stage the boys took part in games and group activities in their respective groups. But they were unaware of each other's existence. They were given names, the Eagles and the Rattlers, and each group was designated a flag. In the second phase of the experiment they were told that there was another group nearby and the staff arranged for competitive sports, including baseball, a tug-of-war, treasure hunt and other events. Both groups practised hard and cheered their team mates but they also started booing and insulting the other group. Soon the hostilities escalated and extended well beyond the playing field. For example, after being defeated in a game, one group burned the banner left by the other group. This was followed by raids on the other camp site and fist-fights. By the end of the two weeks the experiment had transformed 22 well-adjusted boys into two gangs who behaved aggressively towards each other and were bent on extracting revenge.

The two groups were next brought together under conditions that involved no objective competition. This included common events like movies, dinners and socialising events. Instead of reducing conflict, these events simply served as an opportunity for mutual recrimination. Having demonstrated that contact alone was not helping in the reduction of intergroup hostilities, in the third stage of the study, the researchers introduced a series of goals called 'superordinate goals', which could be achieved only through cooperation between the two groups. The experimenters contrived to create 'problems' that could only be solved if the two teams worked together. For example, they staged a break down of the water supply and the boys worked together to trace the pipeline to its origins. A breakdown of the camp truck was also arranged and the two groups had to get together to restart the truck by pulling the vehicle. On another occasion they were told that a movie that both groups liked was too expensive to rent and both groups ended up contributing money in order to rent it. Although superordinate goals did not improve intergroup relationships immediately, after a week of cooperation the name calling and other hostilities had greatly decreased. On the last day they opted to travel home together on the same bus and, in fact, took their seats on the bus next to members of the other group. Some even exchanged telephone numbers and shared refreshments bought with the money that they had won in the competitions.

This summer camp experiment by Sherif et al. (1961) has become a landmark in the study of intergroup cooperation and conflict. Numerous experiments carried out along similar lines have come to the same conclusions, which may be summarised as follows:

- Groups form quickly, especially when they are involved in common activities. Such activities promote group cohesion and group identity.
- Under conditions of competition, group hostilities develop rapidly and the conflict escalates to the point of attacks on each other. Competition in one situation, for example on the playing field, extends to other settings.
- Common goals, shared by members of both groups, that can only be met by mutual cooperation (superordinate goals) reduce conflict and promote cooperation and understanding.

'Minimal group' experiment

Another social psychological experiment that is recognised as a seminal piece of research on intergroup relations is the one carried out by Henry Tajfel and his colleagues (1971). In this experiment, boys aged between 14 and 15 years from the same school were brought together to a room to participate in a study of visual judgement consisting of clusters of dots flashing on a screen in a series of 40 slides. In the next phase of the experiment the boys were told about their performance in the initial task of dot estimation. Half the group were told that they were overestimators and the other half were classified as underestimators. In fact these assignments were made randomly. Thus the dot-estimation task was used to divide participants into two categories on an arbitrary basis. After being assigned to a group, in the next phase of the experiment, each boy was given the opportunity to distribute rewards worth a small amount of money to two other individuals. For example, he might be asked to divide, in any way he wanted, 15 points between two other boys, who were identified only as, for example, member number '10' of the 'W' group or member number '17' of the 'X' group. That is, each participant knew the group to which the other boy belonged only on the basis of over-estimators and under-estimators and there was no face-to-face contact. It was found that when making allocations only for individuals who belong to their own category, participants tended to choose the most equal point allocations. However, when the participants belonged to both groups they consistently allocated more points to members of their own group and fewer points to members of the opposite group.

Tajfel interpreted the findings of the experiments in terms of intergroup discrimination. More importantly, he pointed out that participants, with no previous history of group interaction, classified arbitrarily into groups decisively discriminated in favour of members of their own group and against members of the other. Thus *mere categorisation* into two separate groups appears to be *sufficient* to produce intergroup discrimination. This paradigm has been called 'the minimal intergroup membership'.

As evidenced from the studies cited above, group behaviour is characterised by a number of distinctive features, which may be summarised as follows:

1. *Intergroup bias*. Groups show a systematic tendency to evaluate their own group (the ingroup) and its members more favourably than the outgroup and its members. More specifically, the group-serving tendency takes the

form of favouring the ingroup (ingroup favouritism) and/or derogating the outgroup (outgroup derogation). In a study of school children categorised only on the basis of identification badges (green or blue), where each child was asked to rate another child's performance in a simple task such as providing an account of him/herself, both groups showed moderate but significant ingroup favouritism (Rabbie & Horowitz, 1969), thus confirming Tajfel's observations in minimal group experiments. This bias towards 'us' appears to be a general tendency whatever the group – class, religion, ethnic group or nation.

2. *Outgroup homogeneity effect*. A key feature leading to own-group favouritism is the tendency of groups to minimise differences between members of the outgroup and perceive them as homogeneous and undifferentiated. The belief that the outgroup is homogeneous and similar is an important factor in generating stereotypes and group prejudice. One explanation for the outgroup homogeneity effect is the cognitive process of categorisation. As indicated earlier, in order to make sense of the myriad of events, objects, people, ideas and concepts that impinge on our thinking processes, human perception and cognition rely on the process of grouping them into categories. Two types of categorisation have been described – natural categories or classification of objects (e.g. birds, furniture) and social categories such as ethnic groups, races, and teams. According to Allport (1954) categorisation plays an important role in producing prejudice. He outlined the features of categorisation as follows:
   - It helps form large classes and guides daily adjustment.
   - It helps gather together as much of the group as possible.
   - It enables us quickly to identify related members.
   - The category saturates all its contents (and leads to stereotyping).
   - Categories are formed on what appears to be rational differences.
3. *Accentuation effect*. Groups have a propensity to overestimate their differences. Amplification of group differences has been demonstrated among various ethnic groups. Most studies show that intragroup (within group) variations are greater than those between groups on various dimensions such as beliefs, preferences and behaviours. Despite these objective findings group members exhibit a strong tendency to accentuate the differences between them and the outgroup.
4. *Intergroup competitiveness*. Groups are more competitive than individuals. In the summer camp experiment carried out by Sherif, intergroup competitiveness emerged very quickly with devastating effect. Group competitiveness does have its positive effects, for example when teams compete to increase production or performance, but conflict is usually not too far away.

Why do these group differences and intergroup attitudes arise? This apparent universal tendency of human beings to differentiate their group from 'others' and behave differentially towards the outgroup involves more than intellectual categorisation. Often it has a strong emotional component encompassing feelings of loyalty, attachment, belonging and social identity. Several theories have been advanced to explain these intergroup processes:

1. *Social identity theory*. As proposed by Tajfel (1978), one-way of explaining the ingroup favouritism and outgroup negative bias is to consider people as making *social comparison* between their group and the outgroup. Just as we strive to view ourselves positively and in a self-centred way (egocentrism), we tend to make social comparisons because we need to provide ourselves with a positive social identity (ethnocentrism). Social identity refers to conceptualisation of the self that derives from membership in emotionally significant social categories or groups. This is different from personal identities, which are identifications that define the individual in relation to or in comparison with other individuals. As much as we strive to view our individual selves positively, we also want to view our social identities in positive terms. The group thus becomes an extension of self.
2. *Realistic conflict theory*. The summer camp experiment provides ample proof that conflict is almost inevitable when competition arises between groups for scarce but valued material resources. Several research studies have confirmed that competition for resources leads to deterioration of intergroup relations and results in conflict. As the 'Rattlers and Eagles' demonstrated, group competition can escalate rapidly from hostility to verbal aggression to violent attack. In real life, competition for resources is a fact of life that causes friction between classes, groups and nations.

Perhaps the last word on intergroup relations should go to Freud who, long before the birth of social psychology as a discipline, pronounced with remarkable insight:

> *It is always possible to bind together a considerable number of people in love, so long as there are other people left to receive the manifestations of their aggressiveness.*
>
> Freud (1929)

REFERENCES

Allport GW (1954) The Nature of Prejudice. Reading, MA: Addison-Wesley.
Asch SE (1951) Effects of group pressure on the modification and distortion of judgements. In H Gretzkow (ed.), Groups, Leadership and Men. Pittsburg, PA: Carnegie Press.
Bales RF (1951) Interaction Process Analysis. Reading, MA: Addison-Wesley.
Bass BM (1990) Bass and Stogdill's Handbook of Leadership: theory, research and managerial application (3rd ed.). New York: Free Press.
Collins BE, Raven BH (1969) Group structure: attraction, coalition, communication and power. In G Lindzey & E Aronson (eds), The Handbook of Social Psychology (2nd ed.). Reading, MA: Addison-Wesley.
Cooper J, Fazio RH (1984) A new look at dissonance theory. In L Berkowitz (ed.), Advances in Experimental Social Psychology (Vol. 17, pp. 229–264). Orlando, FL: Academic Press.
Corrigan PW, Penn DL (1999) Lessons from social psychology on discrediting psychiatric stigma. American Psychologist, 54, 765–776.
Corrigan PW, Watson AC (2002) Understanding the impact of stigma on people with mental illness. World Psychiatry, 1, 16–20.
Crites SL Jr, Cacioppo JT (1996) Electrocortical differentiation of evaluative and non-evaluative categorisations. Psychological Science, 7, 318–321.
Fayol H (1949) General and Industrial Management. London, UK: Pitman.
Festinger L (1954) A theory of social comparison processes. Human Relations, 7, 117–140.

Festinger L (1957) A Theory of Cognitive Dissonance. Stanford, CA: Stanford University Press.

Festinger L, Riecken HW, Schachter S (1956) When Prophecy Fails. Minneapolis, MN: University of Minnesota Press.

Fielder FE (1965) A contingency model of leadership effectiveness. In L Berkowitz (ed.) Advances in Experimental Social Psychology, vol 1, PP 59–112. New York: Academic Press.

Freud S (1921) Group psychology and the analysis of the Ego. In Civilisation, Society and Religion (Vol. 12, p. 96). London, UK: Penguin Books.

Freud S (1929) Civilisation and its discontents. In Civilisation, Society and Religion (Vol. 12, p. 305). London, UK: Penguin Books.

Goffman E (1968) Stigma. Harmondsworth, UK: Penguin Books.

Hamburg DA, George A, Ballentine K (1999) Preventing deadly conflict: the critical role of leadership. Archives of General Psychiatry, 56, 971–976.

Handy C (1993) Understanding Organisations (3rd ed.). London, UK: Penguin Books.

Haney C, Banks WC, Zimbardo PG (1973) Interpersonal dynamics in a simulated prison. International Journal of Criminology and Penology, 1, 69–79.

Heider F (1958) The Psychology of Interpersonal Relations. New York: Wiley.

Hofling CK, Brotman E, Dalrymple S, Graves N, Pierce CM (1966) An experimental study in nurse–physician relationships. Journal of Nervous and Mental Diseases, 143, 171–180.

Hogan R, Curphy GJ, Hogan J (1994) What we know about leadership: effectiveness and personality. American Psychologist, 49(6), 493–504.

Hovland CI, Janis IL, Kelly HH (1953) Communication and Persuasion. Newhaven, CT: Yale University Press.

Kelman HC, Hamilton VL (1989) Crimes of Obedience: towards a social psychology of authority and responsibility. New Haven, CT: Yale University Press.

Kleinman A (1980) Patients and Healers in the Context of Culture. Berkley, CA: University of California Press.

Latane B, Darley JM (1968) Group inhibition of bystander intervention in emergencies. Journal of Personality and Social Psychology, 10, 215–221.

Lewin K, Lippett R, White PK (1939) Patterns of aggressive behaviour in socially created 'climates'. Journal of Social Psychology, 10, 271–299.

Likent R (1961) New patterns of management. New York: McGraw-Hill.

Milgram S (1963) Behavioural study of obedience. Journal of Abnormal and Social Psychology, 67, 371–378.

Moscovici S (1976) Social Influence and Social Change. London, UK: Academic Press.

Northouse PG (2001) Leadership: theory and practice (2nd ed.). Thousand Oaks, CA: Sage.

Pettigrew TF (1998) Intergroup contact theory. Annual Review of Psychology, 49, 65–85.

Pillavin IM, Rodin J, Pillavin JA (1969) Good Samaritanism: an underground phenomenon? Journal of Personality and Social Psychology, 13, 289–299.

Rabbie JM, Horowitz M (1969) Arousal of ingroup–outgroup by chance win or loss. Journal of Personality and Social Psychology, 13, 269–277.

Seligman MEP, Abramson LY, Semmel A, von Baeyer C (1979) Depressive attributional style. Journal of Abnormal Psychology, 88, 242–247.

Sherif M (1936) The Psychology of Social Norms. New York: Harper & Row.

Sherif M, Harvey OJ, White BJ, Hood WR, Sherif CW (1961) Intergroup Conflict and Cooperation: the Robber's Cave experiment. Norman, OK: University of Oklahoma.

Personality and Social Psychology (Vol. 9). Newbury Park, CA: Sage.

Stoner JAF (1961) A Comparison of Individual and Group Decisions Involving Risk. Cambridge MA: Massachusetts Institute of Technology.

Tajfel H (1978) Differentiation Between Social Groups: studies in the social psychology of intergroup relations. New York: Academic Press.

Tajfel H, Bellig M, Bundy R, Flament C (1971) Social categorisations in intergroup behaviour. European Journal of Social Psychology, 1, 149–178.

Tuckman BW, Jensen MAC (1977) Stages of small group development. Group and Organisational Studies, 2, 419–427.
Vroom V (1983) Leadership. In M Dunette (ed.), Handbook of Industrial and Organisational Psychology. New York: Wiley.
Zimbardo PG (1971) Psychological power and pathology of imprisonment. Statement prepared for United States House of Representatives Committee on the Judiciary: Subcommittee Number 3: Hearing on Prison Reform, 25 October. San Francisco, CA.
Zimbardo PG, Banks WC, Craig H, Jaffe D (1973) A Pirandellian prison, the mind is a formidable jailer. New York: Times Magazine, April 8, 38–60.
Zimbardo PG, Weisberg M, Firestone I, Levy B (1965) Communication effectiveness in producing public conformity and private attitudes. Journal of Personality, 33, 233–256.

FURTHER READING

Allport GW (1954) The Nature of Prejudice. Reading, MA: Addison-Wesley.
- The classic and groundbreaking work on prejudice. One can only wish that the world would take notice of this 50-year-old piece of wisdom.

Harmon-Jones E, Mills J (eds) (1999) Cognitive Dissonance: progress on a pivotal theory in social psychology. Washington, DC: American Psychological Association.
- A formidable volume, the latest on the subject.

Northouse PG (2001) Leadership: theory and practice (2nd ed.). Thousand Oaks, CA: Sage.
- A well-written, brief introduction to the various theories of leadership complete with case examples.

Pennington DC, Gillen K, Hill P (2002) Social Psychology. London, UK: Arnold.
- A very readable and slim book, a good introduction to the subject.

Stiff JB, Mongeau PA (eds) (2002) Persuasive Communication (2nd ed.). New York: Guilford Press.
- A definitive textbook, worth dipping into.

Aggression

10

'Political history is largely an account of mass violence and expenditure of vast resources to cope with mythical fears and hopes.'
Murray Edelman, *Politics as Symbolic Action*

Aggression and aggressive behaviour are hugely important not only for clinical practice but also for civil society as a whole. For the clinician, assessment and management of risk of violence in patients in a variety of settings is a challenging task. Aggressive behaviour is a central feature in conduct disorder in children and various forms of personality disorders. It is also of interest to social psychologists because violent crimes, road rage, sports violence, domestic violence, sexual aggression and bullying are behavioural manifestations of aggression that need to be studied and, if possible, diminished. Ethnically and politically motivated violence is the most malignant form of human aggression, which both costs society dear and questions the very core values of civilisation.

According to the most widely accepted definition, aggression is any form of behaviour directed towards the goal of harming or injuring another living being who is motivated to avoid such treatment (Baron & Richardson, 1994). In short, aggression is the *intent to harm*. It should be noted that it is the person's *motivation* to harm that defines an act as 'aggression' and not the consequences of the act. The key word is intent. Since others make the attribution of intent, the judgement of the behaviour is dependent on the perspective of the observer(s), societal and cultural values and norms. The measures used in studies of human aggression have attempted to capture its different components: the intention to harm another individual; the behavioural manifestation of this intention (e.g. violent behaviour, criminality, murder); the accompanying emotion (ranging from irritation to rage); and aggressive personality traits (e.g. hostility). It is important to keep in mind the dependent variable being measured when reading the literature on aggression.

Aggression needs to be distinguished from assertiveness. Assertiveness is: (1) standing up for your rights in such a way that you do not violate another person's rights; and (2) expressing your needs, wants, opinion, feelings and beliefs in direct, honest and appropriate ways. Aggression inevitably involves violating or ignoring other people's rights in order to get your own way or dominate a situation. In interpersonal situations aggressive behaviour causes two counterproductive reactions in others, fight or flight. In other words, either aggression breeds aggression or people retreat in frustration and irritation. Inducing this sort of behaviour hardly achieves one's aims.

Aggressive acts can be grouped along various dimensions:

- *Instrumental vs. hostile aggression*. Premeditated means of obtaining some goal other than harming the victim (e.g. robbery) is referred to as instrumental aggression. Hostile aggression is unplanned, driven by anger and is intended to harm the other person.
- *Proactive vs. reactive aggression*. Proactive aggression refers to unprovoked aggression while reactive aggression is retaliatory in response to instigation.
- *Verbal vs. physical aggression*.
- *Physical vs. psychological aggression*.

Violence is harmful behaviour inflicted upon another person or property involving the use of force. Aggression may or may not result in violence but all violence is aggression. Violence is defined as the *act* that leads to physical harm or destruction. Physical assault, murder and rape are the result of personal violence whereas violence to property involves acts such as arson and damage to cars.

Developmental course of aggression

Aggressive behaviour outbursts are common in two to three year olds (the 'terrible twos'). These usually arise from habit training or behaviour control by parents and manifest as temper tantrums. After the age of four years, there is a marked drop in aggressive behaviour although there is some increase in instrumental aggression particularly during cooperative play. Aggression during primary school years has been studied in several populations and the main conclusion from these studies is that moderate to severe aggression at this age heralds future problems, such as behaviour difficulties. There is also considerable evidence for stability in aggression from pre-school period to adolescence. In one review of studies the magnitude of correlation was shown to be 0.60 over an interval of 10 years (Oliveus, 1979). Whether this is due to some underlying constitutional influence is unknown; available evidence indicates that it is multifactorial in origin.

ISSUES IN AGGRESSION

Why do people engage in aggressive behaviour? Numerous theories have been proposed none of which, unfortunately, comprehensively account for all instances of aggressive behaviour. As would be expected in a subject as complex and complicated as aggression there is no overreaching grand theory that satisfactorily explains all aspects of aggression.

Early ethologists maintained that aggressive behaviour was inborn, innate and genetically determined (see Chapter 11). Konrad Lorenz, in his book *On Aggression* (1966), defined aggression as 'the fighting instinct in beast and man which is directed against members of the same species'. His hydraulic model of aggression, now considered to be outdated, does carry an intuitive appeal to many laymen. The concept of aggression as an 'innate' condition that is part of human nature has its origin in the theories of Freud.

Psychoanalytic theories view aggression as the overt behavioural manifestation of an aggressive drive. The aggressive drive is thought to be one of the two primary instinctual drives (the other being the libido). It is considered to be innately hostile and destructive towards the object at which it is directed. Aggressive drives undergo modification and change under the neutralising influence of the ego, thereby limiting its destructive manifestations. Freud later reformulated aggression as a part of an innate self-destructive death instinct, 'thanatos' (see Chapter 13).

Contemporary theories of aggression are unanimous in acknowledging the importance of genetic, biological, social, cultural and psychological factors that contribute to aggressive behaviour. These are considered below.

Biological factors

Sex difference

A finding that stands out in all studies examining aggressive behaviour is that it is predominantly a male activity. Physical violence, rough and tumble play, violent crime and reactive aggression are more prevalent in males than females. Sex differences in aggressive behaviour are apparent in early childhood and are maintained through adolescence and adulthood. Male predominance in violent behaviour has lead to a lot of theorising but there has been little hard evidence as to its cause. Two obvious candidates that may account for the sex difference in aggression are the Y sex chromosomes and male sex hormones (androgens).

The Y chromosome

It has been tempting to speculate that aggressive behaviour arises from an extra Y or a large Y chromosome. The findings in the 1970s that XYY individuals were found in disproportionate numbers in secure hospitals and prisons lead to a number of studies that investigated the relationship between the presence of XYY genotype and criminality (not aggression specifically). The main conclusion from these studies was that there was little evidence for the role of the Y chromosome in determining aggressive behaviour.

Androgens

The role of testosterone has been the subject of many investigations (Archer, 1991). The best work in this area has been based on animal models. Generally speaking, in a variety of vertebrates there is clear evidence that testosterone increases aggressive behaviour (although there are clear exceptions) as measured by direct observation, i.e. by measuring the amount of fighting and threatening. In rodents, administration of testosterone increases aggression and castration decreases it. But there is also evidence that previous experience in aggressive encounters can override the influence of testosterone. For example, in the house mouse, castration carried out after maturity has little effect on aggression for some time afterwards, whereas castration before puberty (i.e. before experience of adult fights) results in a reduction of aggressive behaviours.

It has been well established that in animals the levels of circulating testosterone during foetal development may have important and lasting effects on aggressive behaviour. In the rhesus monkey, for example, it has been shown that *prenatal exposure* to testosterone typically causes higher levels of aggression in male infants. In one experiment (Chamove, Harlow & Mitchell, 1967), a group of rhesus monkeys separated from their mothers at birth, were raised in isolation for the first three years of life (thus effectively eliminating rearing variables, such as differential treatment of the sexes by mothers and peers). The isolates were then paired with randomly sexed infant monkeys. All the *male* isolates directed significantly more hitting at their companions than did the females (who, in fact, showed more nurturing behaviour).

It is generally accepted that, in animals, the hypothalamus plays a key role in the regulation of aggressive behaviour. It has been shown that there are structural differences between the brains of males and females, and that these differences lie in the hypothalamus. At birth the brain is undifferentiated between the sexes, but circulating levels of the male gonadal hormone testosterone, *immediately after birth*, stimulates the development of the male pattern in the hypothalamus of the male infant. If a male is castrated immediately after birth, he retains the female pattern. If a female is treated with injections of testosterone at a comparable age, she develops the male pattern. Thus, androgens play a vital role in the *initial differentiation* of male and female aggressiveness and this difference persists throughout the juvenile stage despite the absence of gonadal hormones. There is clear evidence, therefore, that androgens provide 'organisational' influence on aggressive behaviour in non-human mammals.

But what is the relationship between aggressive behaviour and male sex hormones in the adult? In a variety of studies on male rhesus monkeys it has been clearly established that those individuals with the highest levels of plasma testosterone tend also to be the most aggressive individuals. However, the relationship between testosterone and aggression is relatively weak and the association between the two are not straightforward. When testosterone levels are artificially raised there is no corresponding increase in aggression in rhesus monkeys or chimpanzees. When castrated rhesus monkeys are returned to their natural habitat they continue to show aggressive behaviour and are even able to fight and defeat larger males.

There are two reasons for exercising caution in interpreting the correlation. First, there is considerable evidence that aggressive behaviour may *lead* to elevated testosterone levels in both humans and primates. In rhesus monkeys, winning a fight is associated with increased levels of the testosterone, whereas defeat is followed by a fall in levels (Rose, Bernstein & Gordon, 1975). Similar findings have been reported in human subjects. For example, winners of a competition, such as a wresting match, show an increase in testosterone levels compared to losers (Elias, 1981). Thus, there appears to be a bidirectional relationship between androgens and aggression in primates and the level of plasma testosterone may *reflect* rather than *determine* the level of aggressiveness (Rose, Gordon & Bernstein, 1972).

Second, hormonal influence on aggression is relatively small. Social contexts have a powerful and immediate impact on the expression of aggressive behaviour. Alternatively, high testosterone levels may be related to personality characteristics such as sensation seeking, dominance and assertiveness. In humans, gender differences in aggression stem, in part at least, from contrasting gender roles, modelling and socialisation. In most cultures, males are socialised into, and are expected to display, more aggressive behaviour than females in a wide range of situations.

Another area of interest has been the effect of testosterone administration on achieving dominance status (see Chapter 11) in non-human primates. The underlying assumption here is that testosterone-induced aggression facilitates the establishment and maintenance of a dominant position within the hierarchy. But this does not seem to be the case. Numerous studies carried out on non-human primates such as rhesus monkeys and baboons have failed to show a correlation between measures of long-term dominance and levels of testosterone or its artificial administration. Learned patterns of behaviour during past aggressive encounters appear to override any potential influence of testosterone.

In summary, animal research has established that, although in some animals like rodents there appears to be a direct and positive relationship between testosterone and aggression, in primates, (including man) high levels or artificial administration of testosterone show no correlation with measures of aggression. There is no evidence to show that dominance status in non-human primates is related to testosterone levels. Moreover, raised levels of the hormone may be the consequence of aggressive behaviour rather than its cause.

Unlike in rodents, available evidence for the prenatal influence of androgens on aggression indicates that there is no effect in humans. Numerous studies carried out to investigate the possible link between androgens and aggression in humans have also revealed that there is little correlation between the two. As mentioned before, there appears to be a transient rise in androgen levels in male subjects who have won at competitive sports. This finding has been interpreted in various ways. Apart from a direct cause (win)–effect (increased testosterone) relationship, it is likely that the elevated mood leads to a rise in the hormone level, or the rise in status following his success results in both the elevated mood and higher testosterone levels. The obvious conclusion from all these studies is that the interrelationship between androgenic hormones and measures of aggressive behaviour in man is neutral (Archer, 1991).

Genetic factors

Compared to hormonal influences, the evidence for hereditary influence on aggression in humans and animals is strong. Mice that have been selectively interbred for aggression show excessive and extreme aggression. By twenty-five generations 'killer mice' were produced that immediately attacked any mouse placed in their cage. On the other hand, inbreeding of the least aggressive members of the group resulted in animals that were non-aggressive and refused to be provoked even when attacked (Lagerspetz & Lagerspetz, 1983). Studies of monozygotic (MZ) and dizygotic (DZ) twins in humans suggest a weak genetic component to aggression. For example, one study showed a correlation for MZ to be .40 and .30 for DZ based on questionnaire measures (McGue, Brown & Lykken, 1992). In general, studies on heritability of aggression have examined different variables related to aggression (e.g. delinquency, offending and violence) and produced mixed results. Overall, the contribution of genetic factors to aggressive behaviour per se appears to be small.

Psychosocial factors

Frustration–aggression theory

That frustration sometimes leads to aggression in man and animals is a common observation. Scientific study of frustration began with Dollard et al.'s (1939) attempts to study aggressive behaviour in human volunteers. They defined frustration as any interference with goal-directed activity. Their theory, known as the frustration–aggression theory, is based on the premise that aggression is a motivational drive similar to hunger and thirst, but instead of being internally determined the aggressive drive is instigated by external events that cause frustration. The main assertions of the theory are that: (1) frustration always leads to some form of aggression; (2) aggression always arises as a consequence of frustration; and (3) the discharge of the pent-up energy through aggressive acts produces a reduction in aggressive drive (catharsis).

Thus, according to the theory, frustration is both a necessary and sufficient condition for aggressive behaviour. The theory also holds that aggression can be inhibited by fear of punishment, in which case it is displaced onto other targets (Figure 10.1).

Although the hypothesis has a popular appeal, research has shown that none of the assertions made by the theory is true. Numerous studies have shown that: (1) frustration does not always lead to aggression, although at times it may have a role; (2) aggression can arise from many factors other than frustration; and (3) there is little or no support for the concept of catharsis; indeed, it has been shown that the very opposite may be true – aggression leads to indulgence in further aggression and can be self-perpetuating. Moreover, social factors, almost entirely disregarded by the theory, play a crucial role.

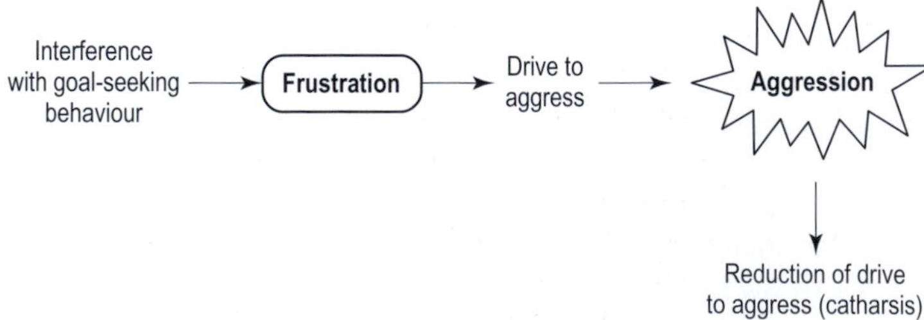

Fig. 10.1 The frustration–aggression theory (Dollard et al., 1939)

Since its formulation, the frustration–aggression theory has undergone a number of modifications, partly as a result of the finding that frustration alone is insufficient to induce aggression. A number of other factors have been identified that, in some measure, contribute to aggressive behaviour:

- *Provocation*. By far the most important single cause of human aggression is perhaps provocation by others. Provocations include insults, verbal aggression, personal physical attacks and perceived injustices.
- *Environmental cues*. Aversive stimuli are thought induce aggression but only in the presence of environmental cues. Heat, noise and overcrowding are said to promote aggression. Aggressive cues can be people or objects that acquire an aggressive cue value by conditioning, prior reinforcement or mere association. An intriguing finding is that the presence of a weapon promotes aggressive behaviour. In a well-known experiment subjects were asked to give shocks to a confederate in conditions where either a weapon or neutral objects (badminton racquets and shuttlecocks) were present. Half of the subjects were angered by the confederate prior to the experiment by having a negative evaluation of their performance. The angered subjects administered more shocks when in the presence of the weapon compared to those in the no-weapon condition. The *weapon effect* is considered to be an important but controversial finding (Berkowitz & Le Page, 1996).
- *Arousal*. Instead of focusing on drive as the prime cause of aggression, others have attempted to study arousal, which, unlike drive, is directly measurable through recording of sympathetic activity (heart rate, sweating, blood pressure). It has been observed that arousal dissipates slowly. Arousal arising from one event may be misattributed to a second event, especially if the two events are separated by a short interval. Arousal resulting from such activity as exercise, sexual excitement and noise have been shown to facilitate aggression provided the arousal state is attributed to the second, anger-provoking, stimulus. This has been called the 'excitation transfer theory of aggression' (Zillmann, 1971). Thus, arousal elicited by irrelevant sources can be mislabelled as anger in situations involving provocation, thus producing anger-motivated aggression.

Berkowitz, a well-known authority in the field, has attempted to incorporate these and other recent findings into the frustration–aggression theory to produce a coherent and more holistic model of aggression. According to this *cognitive neo-association theory* (Berkowitz, 1989, 1990), an aversive or unpleasant event such as frustration, provocation, loud noise or an uncomfortable temperature produces negative affect. The negative affect produced by unpleasant experiences automatically stimulates various thoughts and memories and physiological responses associated with fight or flight. The fight associations give rise to rudimentary feelings of anger, whereas the flight associations give rise to rudimentary feelings of fear. In addition, the cues present during an aversive event become associated with the event and the cognitive and emotional responses triggered by the event.

According to Berkowitz, aggressive thoughts, emotions and behavioural tendencies are linked together in memory. Concepts with similar meanings

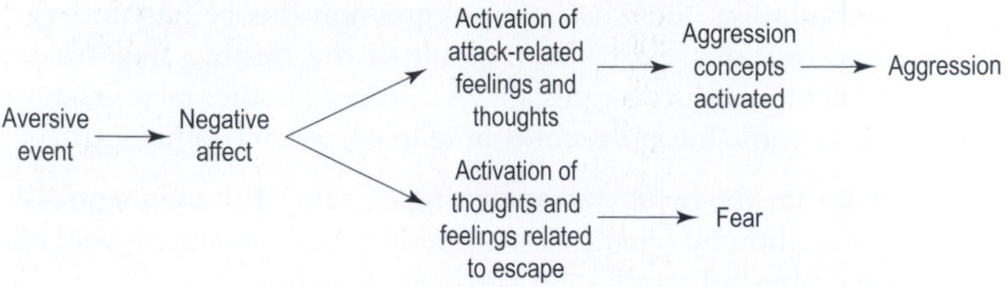

Fig. 10.2 Berkowitz's associative model of aggression

(e.g. harm, attack) and concepts that are frequently activated simultaneously (e.g. gun, shoot) develop strong associations. When a concept is activated, or primed, the activation spreads to related concepts and brings about their activation (Figure 10.2). The theory has provided a broad framework for the study of aggression and has generated a large amount of research.

Aggression as socially learned behaviour (social learning theory)

Aggression is primarily a form of social behaviour that is embedded in social relationships. Contextual factors play a major role in inducing, enhancing, regulating and eliminating such behaviour. Most psychologists have, therefore, come to the view that the causes of aggressive behaviour are neither in the person alone nor are they entirely due to environmental factors, but lie in the interaction between the two. The theory that best represents this view is the social learning theory (SLT) put forward by Bandura (1973, 1989). SLT elegantly combines both biological characteristics – genetic, hormonal and other individual factors – with situational, social and cultural factors in a coherent way that provides the best explanation so far for various empirical observations. Because of its sound theoretical underpinnings and support from research studies, SLT has found applications in institutions, secure units and forensic settings where management of aggressive behaviour is of paramount importance.

According to SLT, aggression is no different from other forms of social behaviour. SLT is firmly based on the premise that aggression is a set of acquired behaviours. It, therefore, emphasises the role of learning in the acquisition, instigation and maintenance of overt aggressive behaviour. The basic principles of SLT are outlined in Chapter 1. Its applications to aggressive behaviour are considered here.

SLT acknowledges the role of genetic, hormonal and other biological characteristics of the individual in the potential to aggress, but it holds that the probability of specific sorts of aggression is, in the main, learned. According to SLT the processes responsible for aggression are best understood in terms of: (1) acquisition or original learning of aggressive behaviour; (2) instigation of overt aggression at a given time; and (3) maintenance of aggression (Figure 10.3).

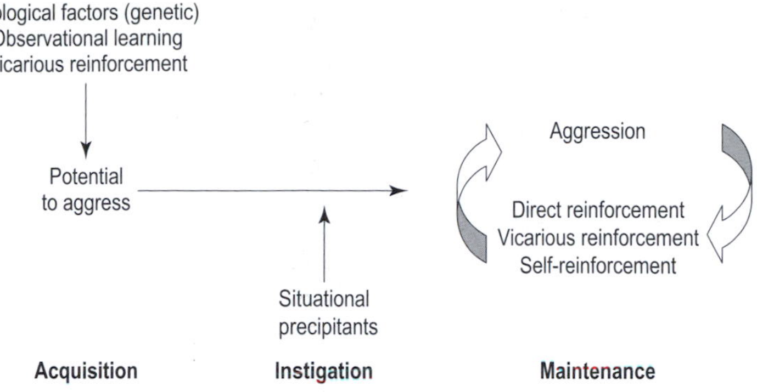

Fig. 10.3 Social learning theory of aggression (Bandura, 1989)

Acquisition of aggression

- *Biological factors.* Although the greatest emphasis for acquisition of aggression is placed upon learning processes, SLT acknowledges that genetic, hormonal and other biological characteristics influence individuals' capacity or potential to aggress.
- *Observational learning (vicarious learning).* Both children and adults acquire new and novel methods of aggression previously not in their repertoire of behaviour by observing similar behaviour in other people. This theory was originally demonstrated by the well-known Bobo doll experiment (see Chapter 1) and been replicated in numerous experiments subsequently. Also called vicarious learning or modelling, observational learning by exposure to aggressive behaviour by others occurs in three different contexts. Familial modelling has a powerful influence on the way children learn to behave. Witnessing and experiencing violence in the family is, by far, the most potent influence on acquisition of violent behaviours by children. Subcultural modelling is typified by learning the observation of peer aggression. Many researchers have documented symbolic modelling on media, desensitisation to violence and disinhibition caused by violent images as important sources of aggression. Newson (1994), in her review of available evidence on the link between TV violence and violence in children, concluded that the correlation was positive and substantial. But others have argued that most of the studies are flawed and that TV violence is one of the many factors that are associated with aggressive behaviour (Cumberbach, 1994).
- *Vicarious reinforcement.* When observers witness aggressive models – peers, parents or television characters – receiving positive reinforcement for behaving aggressively, they tend to adopt these actions themselves.

Maintenance of aggression

Whether aggressive behaviour is maintained, strengthened or extinguished is largely dependent on reinforcement contingencies in accordance with operant conditioning principles (S–R learning). Thus, rewards and punishments regulate aggressive behaviour. Bandura identified three groups of reinforcement contingencies.

- *Direct external reinforcements*. These extrinsic rewards may be tangible (e.g. money), social (e.g. status and privilege) or a reduction of aversive treatment (e.g. children rewarded for aggressive outbursts by being allowed to have their own way).
- *Vicarious reinforcement*. Already mentioned above.
- *Self-reinforcement*. Aggressive behaviours are often maintained by the individual's self-produced rewards and punishments. How one feels about ones' aggressive behaviour often influences the likelihood of a repetition of the act. Individuals who derive a heightened sense of self-esteem through aggressive acts are more likely to continue to aggress.

Instigation of aggression

Once an individual has learned to aggress, a number of different factors determine whether he/she actually behaves in an aggressive way or not. Aggression always occurs in interpersonal situations, as the actions, intentions and responses of others may instigate it. Provocations, frustration, environmental cues, and many other factors precipitate aggressive behaviour. A powerful predictor of aggression is opportunity. Presence of law enforcement authorities and witnesses act as constraints, whereas the presence of aggressive cues, aggression-prone individuals and relative anonymity promote aggression.

Disinhibition. This is a common precipitant of aggression. Normally, people are inhibited from expressing their aggressive potential by internal and external controls. Self-regulation is partly due to the fact that most people hold moral standards that they find difficult to disregard. Disinhibition resulting from alcohol and illicit drugs is well documented. Two other situations in which normal self-regulation may be overridden are in instances of victim dehumanisation and moral justification. Demonising, derogating and blaming the victim ('they deserve it' or 'asked for it') are typical ways of escaping from normal moral standards. War propaganda is an obvious example, but the process also operates in cases of rape, child abuse and genocide. Moral justification ('it is for their own good') is a particularly powerful form of self-justification because it is claimed to be carried out through benevolence and good will but can result in disastrous consequences.

REFERENCES

Archer J (1991) The influence of testosterone in human aggression. British Journal of Psychology, 82, 1–28.

Bandura A (1973) Aggression: a social learning analysis. Englewood Cliffs, NJ: Prentice Hall.

Bandura A (1989) Social Learning Theory. Englewood Cliffs, NJ: Prentice Hall.

Baron RA, Richardson DR (1994) Human Aggression (2nd ed., p.7). New York: Plenum Press.
Berkowitz L (1989) Frustration–aggression hypothesis: examination and reformulation. Psychological Bulletin, 106, 59–73.
Berkowitz L (1990) On the formation and the regulation of anger: a cognitive neoassociationist analysis. American Psychologist, 45, 294–503.
Berkowitz L, Le Page A (1996) Weapon as aggression-stimulating stimuli. Journal of Personality and Social Psychology, 7, 202–207.
Chamove AS, Harlow H, Mitchell G (1967) Sex differences in the infant-directed behaviour of preadolescent rhesus monkeys. Child Development, 38, 329–335.
Cumberbach G (1994) Media violence: science and common sense. Psychology Review, 3, 2–7.
Dollard J, Doob LW, Miller NE, Mowrer OH, Sears RR (1939) Frustration and Aggression. New Haven, CT: Yale University Press.
Elias M (1981) Serum cortisol, testosterone and testosterone-binding globulin responsiveness to competitive fighting in human males. Aggressive Behaviour, 7, 215–224.
Lagerspetz KMJ, Lagerspetz KYH (1983) Genes and aggression. In EC Simmel, Hatine M & JK Walters (eds.), Aggressive Behaviour. Hillsdale, NJ: Lawrence Erlbaum Associates.
Lorenz K (1966) On Aggression. London, UK: Methuen.
McGue M, Brown S, Lykken DT (1992) Personality stability and change in early adulthood: a behavioural genetic study. Developmental Psychology, 29, 36–109.
Newson E (1994) Video violence and the protection of children. Psychology Review, 1, 5–7.
Oliveus D (1979) Stability of aggressive reaction pattern in males: a review. Psychological Bulletin, 86, 852–857.
Rose RM, Bernstein IS, Gordon TP (1975) Consequences of social conflict on plasma testosterone levels in rhesus monkeys. Psychosomatic Medicine, 37, 50–62.
Rose RM, Gordon TP, Bernstein IS (1972) Plasma testosterone levels in the male rhesus: influence of sexual and social stimuli. Science, 178, 643–645.
Zillmann D (1971) Excitation transfer in communication mediated aggressive behaviour. Journal of Experimental Social Psychology, 7, 419–434.

FURTHER READING

Baron RC, Richardson DR (1994) Human Aggression (2nd ed.). New York: Plenum Press.

- A comprehensive textbook on the subject.

Ethology

'If you look into the eyes of a chimpanzee, you know you're looking into the eyes of a thinking, feeling being.'
Jane Goodall

Historically in psychology the study of animal behaviour has followed two trends. The North American tradition has been to study animals in the laboratory and was focused on the effects of the environment on behaviour. In contrast, most European research involved studying animals in their natural environment. The former has been loosely called *comparative psychology* defined as the scientific study of psychological processes in animals and their comparison with psychological functioning in humans. The latter, known as *ethology*, is the study of patterns of behaviour of animals in their natural environments.

Ethology emphasises the analysis of adaptation and evolution of animal behaviour patterns. When ethologists consider any class of behaviour they are mainly concerned with four issues (Hinde, 1982):

1. The immediate or proximal causes of the behaviour.
2. The development of the behaviour over the animal's life cycle (ontology).
3. The evolution of the behaviour within the species (phylogeny).
4. The useful consequences of the behaviour (function).

Ethologists rely on naturalistic observations as the main tool for their studies but they also modify the environment to investigate the role of particular environmental stimuli.

The pioneering work of European zoologists, Karl Von Frischer, Niko Tinbergen and Konrad Lorenz in the 1930s established ethology as a distinct discipline. In 1973 the Nobel Prize in medicine/physiology was awarded to the three of them for their contributions to the understanding of animal behaviour. Von Frischer is widely known for his analysis of the behaviour of bees, especially the bee dance, which communicates the source of flowers to others in the colony; Tinbergen and Lorenz are famous for their studies on innate animal behaviour and imprinting. In the following pages we discuss some ethological concepts that may be relevant to human behaviour and psychiatry.

Species-typical behaviour

In psychology the term *instinct* has been used in two fundamentally different ways. First, certain actions performed by animals in response to specific stimuli occur without previous learning, i.e. they occur 'naturally', and these have been referred to as instinctive behaviours. Biologists (introduced and) used the term instinct to explain behaviours that were thought to be 'natural' to the species that were determined primarily by heredity (e.g. nesting instinct, the instinct for seasonal migration, maternal instinct). Second, the word instinct has also been used to describe an internal drive or motivational force that impels animals, including humans, to achieve certain goals (similar to the Freudian concept of drive). The following discussion centres on the former application of the concept of instinct.

The classical view of instinct or instinctive behaviour was that detailed instructions for the performance of the behaviour and the recognition of the stimuli that elicit the behaviour were encoded in the genes. Thus, the environment was thought to play little part in the system, apart from providing a context for genetic expression. Instinctive behaviour was, therefore, thought to be characteristic of the species and believed to be made up of action patterns that were released by certain specific stimuli.

The concept of instinct has changed over the years with the growing realisation that all behaviour is the result of genetic and environmental influences and that the dichotomy between instinct and acquired behaviour is quite meaningless. Hence the term *innate* has come to be used for activities that are characteristic of the species. The term innate behaviour is a better alternative to instinct because it refers to the actual behaviour rather than the hypothesised cause of the behaviour. In order to refine the instinct/innate concept and overcome the nature/nurture debate as to the causation of the behaviour, psychologists have adopted terms like *species-specific* and *species-typical behaviours*.

Species-typical or species-specific behaviours are those behaviours that occur in a similar fashion in nearly all members of the species, although within the species the behaviour may not be identical but always bears a strong resemblance. In contrast to innate species-typical behaviour are the learned behaviours, such as chimpanzees' use of sticks as a tool (in termite feeding, for example, see later). Ethologists have used four criteria to define innate, species-typical behaviour (Cairns, 1979):

1. The behaviour is stereotyped (always appearing in the same sequence of actions) across individuals of the same species.
2. It is present without relevant previous learning that could have allowed it to be learned.
3. It is universal for the species (i.e. found in all members of the species).
4. Once established it remains relatively unchanged as a result of experience and learning.

Examples of species-typical behaviour are nest building (in birds), the honey bee 'dance', warning calls, bird song, and so on. All these behaviours have been called innate or species-typical.

Recent work has clearly demonstrated that species-typical behaviour is heavily influenced by environmental conditions and is not entirely innate as was once thought. *Birdsong* is a case in point. It has long been believed that birds inherit their calls and songs. While this is true of some species, in the case of the more common birds such as crows, hummingbirds and parrots the songs that the birds sing depend partly on learning.

Experiments by Thorpe (1961) on the development of chaffinch (*Fringilla coelebs*, a small song bird common in western Europe) illustrate some of the key issues. In natural conditions adult male chaffinches have a repertoire of a few typical songs. Birds that are reared in isolation from birth (so that they never had the chance to hear another bird of the same species) do develop a song, but the song is simple and lacks the richness and musical qualities of the normal adult song. If young birds are reared together with other birds of the same age but still in auditory isolation from other adult chaffinches, they produce a song that is a little more elaborate than the isolate pattern. If the birds are isolated after exposure to adult birds but before they start to sing, their song develops more or less normally. Isolated birds exposed to tape recordings of chaffinch song reproduce the song to which they have been exposed.

Thus, learning appears to play an important part in development of the song in the chaffinch. However, they do not learn songs of other birds. For example if such birds are exposed to tape recordings of songs of a differed species, they fail to reproduce the 'foreign' song; they learn only songs with a note quality similar to that of the chaffinch song. Moreover, there appears to be a 'sensitive period' when the learning of the song is most likely to occur. Modern ethologists have rejected the distinction between innate and learned behaviours – they now believe that both hereditary and environment contribute to most, if not all, innate or species-typical behaviour.

A specific form of innate behaviour is called *fixed action patterns* (FAP). This refers to a complex behavioural sequence that typically occurs in a fixed, stereotypic fashion. Examples of FAP are squirrels burying nuts, birds performing courtship dances, spiders spinning webs and sticklebacks (a type of fish) fighting to protect territory. In some species FAPs are quite elaborate. For example, the male bowerbird takes hours to build and decorate its love nest with flowers, shells, twigs and colourful beetles to attract a mate. FAPs usually serve an adaptive function such as defending, mating or eating.

FAP is considered to be triggered by a *sign stimulus* – a particular stimulus whose presence is thought to automatically release the FAP. Tinbergen is credited with discovering the role of sign stimuli in his studies on sticklebacks. He made the observation that the red belly of a male stickleback fish that intrudes into the territory of another provokes aggressive behaviour. He is said to have accidentally found that the sticklebacks in his tank became aggressive when a bright red post-office van passed by. In subsequent work, he was able to demonstrate that a model that only vaguely resembled the stickleback in shape but that was red in the lower half elicited the aggressive response, whereas an accurate decoy without the red area did not (Tinbergen, 1951).

On the basis of these and other findings, Tinbergen proposed that an innate behaviour is released by an *innate releasing mechanism* (IRM) when the appropriate external signal is present. A classic study by Lorenz and Tinbergen (Tinbergen, 1951) illustrates the concept well. Using a paper model that resembled a hawk when moving in one direction and a waterfowl when moved in the opposite direction, they showed that newly hatched ducks and geese showed fear when the model of the hawk was moved over their heads. When the model was moving in the opposite direction it looked like a harmless, long-necked waterfowl and produced no fear reaction. According to the researchers the short neck of the hawk model acted as an innate sign stimulus for the innate fear response.

Recent research has shown that FAPs are not as fixed as originally proposed by Tinbergen. They are more variable and are modifiable by environmental influences. They are now called *model action patterns* because of the variability of behaviour around average or modal forms (Barlow, 1977).

Are there comparable FAPs in humans? Many facial expressions such as smiling and crying are found in all cultures and can be regarded as species-typical FAPs comparable to those of non-human species. There is no doubt that the cry and the smile of the baby can be regarded as sign stimuli or social releasers. Caring responses elicited in parents by the facial features of infants may be considered to be another example of an FAP. For instance, Lorenz (1971) suggested that the infant's babyish appearance elicits care-taking behaviour in parents. Infants of many species, particularly mammals, have large heads in comparison to the body, a forehead that is large in relation to the face, large eyes and prominent cheeks, i.e. they appear cute (Figure 11.1). The suggestion that such cuteness of babies provokes innate care-giving behaviour in adults, especially parents, has received some experimental support (Sternglanz, Gray, & Murakami, 1971).

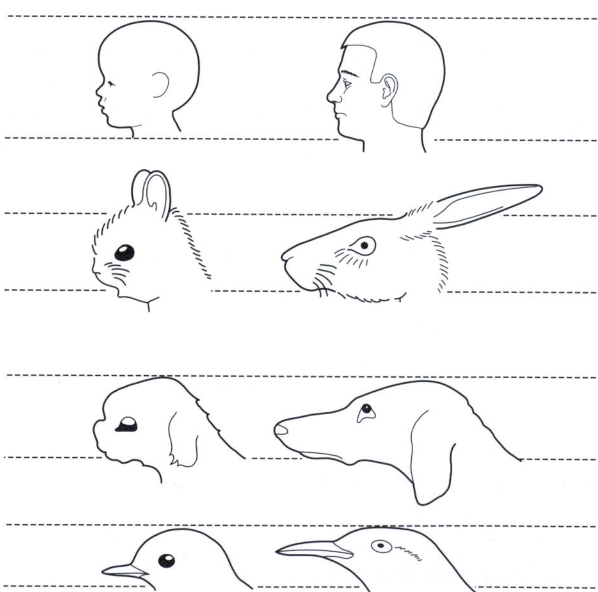

Fig. 11.1 Releasers of parental reactions in man. The sign-stimuli on the left release parental behaviour and are compared with the corresponding adult characteristics that do not release this behaviour. (Reproduced by permission of K Lorenz & N Tinbergen. From Mowbray RM, Rodger TF, & Mellore CS (1979) Psychology in Relation to Medicine (5th ed.). Edinburgh: Churchill Livingstone)

Imprinting

The young of birds and mammals that are relatively independent and are ambulant soon after birth (called precocial species), such as ducks, hens, sheep and deer, show a strong tendency to follow their mothers around. Lorenz studied the 'following responses' of ducklings and suggested the term *imprinting* to describe this distinctive process by which young newly hatched birds learn the characteristics of their mother and, therefore, their species. He went on to demonstrate that such newly hatched birds would follow any moving object that they saw within the first few hours or days but avoid or take flight at the sight of other objects. In short, imprinting occurred in a specific time period to specific sets of stimuli. Lorenz discovered that imprinting was somewhat indiscriminate, that young birds could become imprinted to electric trains, a set of yellow gloves, moving milk bottles and to human beings. Lorenz was able to get some ducklings to imprint on to him, so that they followed him everywhere.

Each species has particular preferences for imprinting on to certain stimuli. For example, domestic chickens most readily imprint onto blue or orange objects while ducklings prefer orange-green objects. The following response is enhanced if the object moves and emits appropriate sounds. Later studies have shown that barriers placed in the path of the young increases the following response. In natural conditions, imprinting occurs to the mother, since she is the one that the young encounter during the initial period after birth. The more an animal follows and becomes familiar with an object, the less it is attracted to others and, in fact, often shows the opposite response, fear, to other model objects.

According to Lorenz, the young animal becomes imprinted upon whatever moving object it encounters during a particular phase of development and that it subsequently directs its filial (offspring's), sexual and social behaviour towards this object. Lorenz's classical definition identifies five characteristics that distinguish imprinting from other conventional forms of learning (Salzen, 1998):

1. Imprinting is formed during a definite and brief period of development.
2. Once formed, imprinting is stable, long lasting and, even, irreversible.
3. It has long-term consequences for later social development, particularly sexual responses and preferences.
4. It helps the young to learn about specific characteristics of the same species and is species-specific.
5. Imprinting is fundamentally different from associative learning; neither reward nor reinforcement play any part in its development.

Ever since Lorenz's groundbreaking studies, imprinting has been investigated extensively, discussed and debated. It has also led to the general acceptance of Lorenz's main postulates about imprinting, albeit with certain revisions and modifications. Current understanding of the features of imprinting may be summarised as follows:

Critical/sensitive period. Lorenz believed that imprinting was entirely due to biological factors and that imprinting took place during a restricted period of time. He introduced the term 'critical period' to describe the brief time interval during which imprinting occurs. Subsequent research has established that the period during which imprinting takes place is not rigidly fixed as Lorenz had implied. We now know that the period during which imprinting occurs is affected considerably by experience. Many studies have shown that it is possible to significantly lengthen the critical period under certain conditions. For example, young ducklings kept in isolation developed imprinting well past the end of the normal critical period. (In previous experiments the birds had been kept together and therefore had imprinted on one another.) Conversely, exposure to an intensified sensory environment or early exposure to suitable imprinting stimuli could shorten the critical period. It is possible to produce imprinting even after the critical period has ended if the animal is exposed to the appropriate stimulus intensively for a long enough period of time.

Therefore, it is clear that the critical period is much more complex than was originally thought and it has now been termed the *sensitive period*. But Lorenz was right when he pointed out that imprinting occurred during a particular developmental period in that this was the time when the animal was optimally responsive to a specific kind of stimulation. But, as recent research shows, sensitive periods are not fixed and unmodifiable as was once thought. Thus, biology prepares the bird to learn from certain experiences and this predisposition to learn is optimal at certain periods in development. Sensitive periods have also been identified for behaviours such as learning bird songs, learning to distinguish males and females of the species and, in humans, forming attachment relationships.

Current evidence suggests that there are at least two types of sensitive periods – one for filial imprinting and another one for sexual imprinting. In experiments it has been found that when, after hatching, chicks are exposed to a moving model for various intervals (e.g. 0–15 days, 16–30 days and 31–45 days), those exposed for 1–30 days show strong filial imprinting whereas the sensitive period for strongest sexual imprinting was 31–45 days. It is worth noting that the latter coincides with the time when birds begin to take on an adult-like appearance and develop plumage.

Sexual imprinting occurs most readily to conspecifics (those of the same species) and less readily to inanimate objects or human beings. In the absence of any alternative, however, reliable sexual imprinting to other objects may occur and be long lasting. For example, birds that are hand reared become sexually imprinted on to the gloves used by the handler. In short, contact with the parent during the sensitive period has a long-lasting influence.

Irreversibility/reversibility. Initial studies on imprinting emphasised the long-term stability of the behaviour. For example, Lorenz showed that jackdaws raised by humans will join a flock of jackdaws but return to the human during the reproductive season and show courting behaviour towards him. Birds that are hand reared become sexually imprinted on people. Sexual preferences based upon imprinting often persist for a number of years. But, as a number of studies have shown, imprinting behaviour can be altered, or even reversed, by subsequent prolonged experience. Thus, it is possible to alter a previously established inappropriate sexual preference in an adolescent bird and get it to 're-imprint' on birds of its own species. This appears to be true for both filial and sexual imprinting.

In summary, there is evidence for a 'soft' form of imprinting rather than the 'hard' form enunciated by Lorenz in the 1930s. Imprinting is now thought to be a unique and special form of learning. It involves pre-programmed learning or certain learning predispositions (Hess, 1973). Concurrent and subsequent experience of behavioural interactions with members of the same species can enhance and modify imprinted preferences. Imprinting serves several adaptive functions for the animal: it serves the function of helping to recognise and follow members of one's own species and, from an evolutionary point of view, ensures that mating occurs with the same species.

Bowlby (1969) believed that the basic features of attachment are similar to imprinting. Attachment involves considerably more developmental complexity and reciprocity than classical motions of imprinting. Bowlby acknowledged that the findings of ethologists on the imprinting behaviour of animals made a significant contribution to his thinking on attachment (see Chapter 12).

Dominance hierarchies

One issue that has interested ethologists for a considerable period of time is the way that animal groups are organised. A central theme in social organisation is the idea of *dominance*. In 1922, Schjeldrup-Ebbe made the important observation that if hens were fed in such a way that only one of them could feed at a time, a 'pecking order' developed, such that the same hen would always feed first, the second would feed next, and so on. This behaviour would spread to non-feeding times and a dominance hierarchy was soon evident.

Most, but not all, group-living animals, especially primates, tend to form dominance hierarchies. It involves the distribution of power, especially access to resources such as food or mates, among group members by setting implicit 'rules' as to who can control whom. Animals higher in the hierarchy tend to displace lower ranking individuals from resources (food, mates, space). The hierarchy is not fixed and depends on a number of changing factors (age, sex, aggression) and may also depend on the support of others. The hierarchy is initiated and sustained by hostile behaviours, albeit sometimes of a subtle and indirect nature. The concept of dominance has been studied more intensely in primates presumably because of their close genetic relatedness to humans.

On the phylogenetic scale chimpanzees are our closest ancestors, sharing almost 99% of our chromosomes. It should come as no surprise, then, that chimpanzee society is one of the most intensely studied animal groups in the wild. The most comprehensive and impressive field study of chimpanzees was carried out by the primatologist Jane Goodall in the Gombe National Park, Tanzania (Goodall, 1990). The Gombe study focused on approximately 160 chimpanzees (*Pan troglodytes*) and recorded their behaviour patterns and social relationships in minute detail in order to piece together the overall patterns of chimpanzee life. The 'main characters' were given names and their activities followed over several hours each day together. The study lasted altogether 30 years, during which time Goodall and her colleagues meticulously collected and collated the data. This study provides the best insight so far into chimpanzees' life in their natural habitat.

Chimpanzees live in social groups called communities or unit groups. Among chimpanzees the males were observed to be the dominant sex. In the chimpanzee society in Gombe there was a clear-cut hierarchy among males, organised according to social rank. Within the community a male hierarchy was evident, ordered in a linear fashion with one clear alpha male, followed by a few, usually three, high-ranking males, about six middle-ranking males and five or so low-ranking males. The alpha is the highest-ranking male in the colony and he showed an intense motivation to dominate his fellows and was often feared by the others. All adult males dominate all females. Females have their own hierarchy.

The hierarchies of the adult males are relatively stable for years, but some low-ranking males can occasionally challenge them. The alpha male maintains his position by charging displays, threats and occasional fights. Once a male has established his position as the alpha male, the degree of aggression shows a dramatic fall, as the young males submit themselves to him. The middle-ranking males are often submissive to the alpha male, even when he begins to age and become infirm, showing that learned behaviour, in part, maintains the hierarchy.

Eventually the alpha male comes to be challenged by some young adult, low-ranking male and a reversal of dominance between the two takes place over a period of time, during which the lower-ranking male starts winning more and more fights. Often males enlist the support of others during conflicts. Goodall recounts how a 20-year-old chimpanzee called Figan came to dominate a 22-year-old alpha male named Evered. Figan formed an alliance with Faben, his older brother with a paralysed arm, and was supported by him in his aggressive encounters with Evered. Such coalitions are a crucial factor in attaining and maintaining rank. Loss of rank results in a fall within the hierarchy for the alpha male who is thereafter never able to regain his former position.

In the Gombe study, females did not show a clear-cut dominance hierarchy. However, there were females who were high ranking, one of whom often emerged as the alpha female, the remainder fell into middle-ranking and low-ranking classes. One factor that determined the rank of the females was the nature of her family. Coalitions between mothers and members of their immediate families was of overwhelming significance in attaining and maintaining high status.

Studies on dominance hierarchy among other animals have produced rather different pictures. Studies on baboons have produced quite surprising and confusing results. Contrary to the findings of previous studies, a remarkable study by Rowell (1972) demonstrated the importance of considering the type of environment in the social organisation of primates. Rowell studied three colonies of baboons living in three different environments, the 'monkey island' in the London zoo, the African savannah and the African forest. Rowel documented a rigid hierarchy in the baboons at the London zoo with a well-identified alpha male and a clear-cut pecking order; those living in the savannah showed a more flexible hierarchical structure; and those in the African forest exhibited no hierarchy at all. This variation in social hierarchy among baboons has been interpreted as a result of the competition for resources.

Baboons are biologically more distant from humans than chimpanzees, but their life-style and ecological setting have made the baboon model central to the reconstruction of the earliest stage in human evolution. Shirley Strum (1987) studied a troop of olive baboons (*Papio anubis*) in Kenya for 15 years. Olive baboons are savannah dwellers and, in comparison to chimpanzees, they were observed to have a different social system. For example, males leave the group in baboon society (among chimpanzees it is the adolescent females who leave the group). The males were not dominant or domineering. Males won attractive females by finesse rather than by force. Females and their kin were the stable core of the group, males came and went. Baboon kin groups are headed by an older female, and include her offspring and their offspring. These female-based units formed the core of the troop, and it was the females and their families, not the adult males, who could be ranked linearly into a stable dominance hierarchy. In this study, every member of the family of the alpha female (named Peggy) outranked every other member of every other matriline. Every family could be placed within the hierarchy in an orderly fashion. When the matriarch died her daughter took over.

It is clear from these and other studies that dominance hierarchies are not as common in the animal kingdom as was once assumed, that dominance varies from species to species and that the environment in which they live exerts considerable influence on their social organisation.

Attempts have been made to apply ethological methods of observational research to human groups. In one such study (Strayer & Strayer, 1976), videotapes of free play in a group of pre-school children were used to study dominance. Three groups of behaviours were used as indices of dominance behaviour: physical attacks; threat gestures; and struggles for position (e.g. be the first) or objects (e.g. toys). The children who used different strategies to win these encounters were considered to be more dominant. Analysis of the videotapes showed that among the pre-school children there was a relatively stable dominance hierarchy.

Territoriality

Group-living animals share an area of land within which they forage, sleep, raise their young and go about their other daily activities. An area occupied by one species of animals is described as a *home range*. Any part of this overall range that is *defended* against other conspecifics is a *territory* (Noble, 1939). Two key elements of territoriality are:

1. *Defence*. The territory owner, having established his boundaries, discourages others from using the area, often by fighting and proclaiming his presence by means of vocal and visual displays.
2. *Space*. After the initial aggressive demarcation of boundaries, neighbouring territory owners typically respect one another's property and further overt aggression is rare.

Territorial behaviour is widespread in the animal kingdom. Chimpanzees are intensely territorial. When conspecifics from neighbouring social groups intrude they are actively repelled. Members of the troop frequently visit boundaries in pairs or groups and monitor them. Ritualised aggressive displays are exchanged by neighbouring communities followed by retreat without conflict. Boundaries are usually respected for a number of years until communities split and make up new territories. In common with other aspects of animal behaviour, there is wide variation among species as to the level of territorial behaviour. While some animals, such as certain birds, fishes and chimpanzees, are intensely territorial others, like tigers and lions, do not guard their territories.

Displacement activity

A unique form of behaviour seen in some animal groups is *displacement activity*. This consists of behavioural acts that occur in conditions of high frustration or indecision. For example, domestic cocks engaged in an aggressive encounter would suddenly break off the fight and start feeding; the three-spined stickleback has been seen to engage in sand digging during territorial disputes; and displacement preening is common during courtship in mallards.

Displacement activities are characterised by the following features:

- The activity is similar to motor patterns that are normal for the species.
- The movements displayed appear to be irrelevant, and entirely out of context with the behaviour immediately preceding or following them.
- They occur in conflict situations when the discharge of surplus motivation through normal paths is somehow prevented.

The mechanism underlying displacement activity is unclear but it is thought to reflect arousal due to anxiety and social tension. Some have argued that obsessional behaviour in humans is similar to displacement activities and serves to reduce anxiety.

Peacemaking and reconciliation

Much has been written about aggression in animals (see Chapter 10) but more recently it has been found that reconciliation and peacemaking are common in the animal kingdom, especially in non-human primates. Reconciliation, defined as friendly reunion between two former opponents soon after an aggressive confrontation, is a conspicuous part of social life among non-human primates.

Observational studies in captive and wild populations of chimpanzees have revealed that former opponents frequently engage in friendly interactions not long after fights or angry confrontations. Numerous studies have shown that the number of friendly contacts between two animals that have just engaged in spontaneous fights is significantly greater than those in the same individual in the absence of previous aggression. Chimpanzees typically embrace, kiss on the mouth, groom or hold hands after confrontations (de Waal, 2000). The degree of sophistication shown by some species is astounding. For instance, some reconciliations have been shown to involve third parties! Such reconciliatory behaviour plays an important pacifying function and helps to maintain social relationships. Thus, through cycles of conflict and reconciliation, over time, relationships are negotiated within the groups without permanently disrupting them. The fact that primate societies are characterised by cooperation, reconciliation and conflict resolution has come as a surprise finding to many ethologists and psychologists who have been steeped in the tradition of instinctual aggression propounded by Lorenz.

Helping and altruism

Altruism is behaviour that benefits another individual without any consideration of personal gain. The most dramatic examples of altruism come from studies of captive chimpanzee colonies. In a chimpanzee island in Oklahoma, a three-year-old female fell into the moat and was found struggling in the water. An unrelated nine-year-old female chimpanzee was observed to jump into the water to rescue her. This is a remarkable example of altruism, because chimpanzees cannot swim and the 'helper' was taking a calculated risk. In a similar incident, an eight-year-old gorilla at the Chicago zoo was seen to save a three-year-old boy who had fallen six metres into the primate's enclosure. She was observed to rush and catch the boy then sit down on a log and cradled him in her lap, gently patting his back (de Waal, 2001). There are several examples of helping behaviour in animal societies. Adult chimpanzees of either sex have been observed to go to the aid of their infants or mothers, and family members have been seen regularly helping one another or those related by kinship.

Theory of mind in chimpanzees

There is now clear evidence that chimpanzees have a 'theory of mind' (see Chapter 12, p. 303) and are able to know what others in the group think. In an ingenious experiment carried out at the Max Plank Institute, two male chimpanzees, one dominant and one submissive, were placed in cages opposite so that they had visual access to each other. The experimenter hid a banana in a box in between the cages. When this was done so that both the animals could see the banana, the dominant animal quickly snatched it. The subordinate chimpanzee did not even attempt to come out of the cage. Next the experimenter hid the banana in such a way that the subordinate chimpanzee could see it but the dominant one could not. The question was: 'Did the subordinate ape know that the dominant one could not see the banana?' The subordinate animal was observed to quickly snatch the banana demonstrating that the subordinate chimp understood that the dominant one could not know that there was a banana there. Thus, chimpanzees appear to have an understanding of what another animal knows, i.e. they have a theory of mind. Most primatologists now believe that chimpanzees understand the needs and emotions of other chimpanzees and respond correctly.

Culture in non-human primates

One of the most remarkable findings by Goodall was that chimpanzees were able to create and use tools. She made the landmark observation that the chimpanzees of Gombe used twigs and branches to fish for termites. Until then it was assumed that making and using tools was an activity exclusive to humans. In fact, it was considered to be one of the important characteristics that distinguished man from animals. Over the years Goodall documented many examples of tool use in chimpanzees, including the use of stones for cracking nuts and using leaves as sponges to soak up water. Soon the scientific community realised that other workers in different parts of the world had already made similar observations. For example, Japanese workers had documented sweet-potato washing in Japanese macaques (*Macaca fuscata*) in Koshima, Japan. As early as 1953, Mito, a Japanese primatologist, had recorded her observations of an 18-month-old juvenile carrying a sweet potato to a stream and cleaning it in the water before eating it. Over the next few days the monkey refined the technique by going deeper into the water and rubbing off the mud and then washing the potato before eating it. The practice quickly spread to her peers and within five years more than three quarters of juveniles and young adults were engaged in regular potato washing (Kawai, 1965).

Now there is not only accumulating evidence of many learned behaviour patterns within communities of primates but also evidence that different populations of the same species engage in different forms of learned activities. Thus, different populations of chimpanzees use different tools and often the same tool is used in different ways by other colonies. These behaviours are transmitted intergenerationally so that it becomes a distinctive feature of a particular group.

Many primatologists contend that these behaviour patterns in non-human primates meet the minimal criteria for culture (Whitten et al., 1999). In biology, cultural behaviour is defined as behaviour patterns that are transmitted repeatedly across generations through social or observational learning to become a population-based characteristic. A close examination of various socially acquired behaviour patterns in chimpanzee colonies documented over the years shows that there are numerous behaviour patterns, including grooming, tool usage and courtship behaviours, that are customary and habitual in some communities but absent in others. These behaviour patterns are highly distinctive – so much so that they qualify to be called culture, thus far a phenomenon considered to a characteristic of humans only.

Aggression

Aggression and violence are regarded as 'animal characteristics'. For example, big fish feed on small fish, animals hunt other animals and animals that kill their own species are common. Lorenz regarded aggression as a basic drive common to most animals and man (Lorenz, 1966). It was described as an accumulating force that needed to be discharged, usually in response to specific stimuli (the hydraulic model). By definition aggression in humans is a motivational act impelled by the intent to harm (see Chapter 10). But in the case of animals, activities motivated by other factors such as protection of the young and feeding have been characterised as aggression. For example, Moyer (1968) described eight types of aggressive behaviour: (1) predatory (directed towards the prey); (2) inter-male (resulting from closeness to an unfamiliar male); (3) fear-induced; (4) irritable (as a response to frustration and deprivation); (5) territorial defence; (6) maternal (defence of offspring); (7) sex-related (related to sexual competition); and (8) instrumental (to gain a reward). The motivation for each of these instances is different indeed.

The aggression witnessed in chimpanzees may be more relevant to that seen in humans than the forms seen in the rest of the animal kingdom. One of the disquieting findings in the Gombe study was the degree of violence and aggression observed among the chimpanzees. During her period of study the group of chimpanzees split into two fractions. The rivalry between the two soon turned into a bloody civil war as they mounted vicious attacks on members of the other group. One group eventually killed most of the males and some of the females of the other group. It had been observed previously that the chimpanzees ate meat and killed other animals like baboons and ate them, but the brutality of their attacks on their own kind shocked the researchers. The obvious conclusion was that the chimpanzees, despite their capacity for empathy and cooperation, were basically aggressive animals and were 'demonic apes'.

Although these observations are authentic, and well documented, doubt has recently been cast on the 'demonic ape' theory. A study of chimpanzees in Congo has produced a rather different picture. This study is unique in that the chimpanzees in this area, known as the Goualougo Triangle, had never seen a human being. The chimpanzees of Goualougo were like those of Gombe in most respects – they too used tools and had a culture of their own. However, they showed little or no aggression; they did not kill their own species nor were they involved in territorial disputes (Sanz, 2001). These and other findings have pointed out some of the basic weaknesses in the Gombe study that may have led to the overstatement of aggression in those groups.

First, in her pioneering work, Goodall fed the chimpanzees regularly with bananas in order to befriend and study them. No doubt this led to competition for food and brought about a change in their interactions within their group. Second, interactions with humans may have brought about subtle and lasting changes. Third, and most importantly, there had been massive ecological changes in Gombe through cutting down of trees, which had resulted in the chimpanzees being cut off from the rest of the rain forest. Human encroachment and environmental changes are thought to have brought about changes in their behaviour. There is no doubt that chimpanzees, like human beings, have the potential for aggression, and environmental factors play a vital role in its manifestation.

To sum up, we may conclude that animal behaviour, especially that of non-human primates, is the result of complex interactions between genetic potential and biological propensities on one hand and the effects of learning and the environment on the other. Non-human primates exhibit complex behaviour patterns that are broadly similar to those of human beings, including those that reflect culture, cooperation, altruism and conflict resolution as well as a propensity for aggression.

It is tempting to conclude that much human behaviour is not dissimilar from that of animals, especially the chimpanzees, our closest primate relations. However, it is dangerous to extrapolate animal behaviour to human societies. Scientists usually choose specific animal models that suit their favourite theories. For instance, honeybees have been cited as an example of co-operative effort and organisation – the fact that the worker bees die for the queen bee is ignored; the male dominant hierarchy in chimpanzees is cited as an example of the need for strong male leadership – while the more equal relationship between male and female gibbons is forgotten. Undoubtedly there are parallels between animal and human behaviour but the selective use of animal models to 'explain' human behaviour is fraught with dangers as the above account of basic ethology illustrates.

Finally, it is common for both laymen and scientists to attribute human characteristics to animals and animal characteristics to humans. Attribution of human characteristics, usually inappropriately, to animals is called *anthropomorphism*. For example, dogs are said to be intuitive, intelligent and loving. While dogs are loyal and obedient in many aspects, it is not unusual for dog owners to project their feelings on to dogs. The converse, attribution of animal characteristics to humans, *zoomorphism*, is a much more common error. War between nations and groups has been deemed to be the extension of 'territoriality' in animals, aggression in humans is interpreted to arise from 'basic animal instincts' and dominance hierarchies have been used to justify male domination.

REFERENCES

Barlow GW (1977) Modal action patterns. In TA Sebeck (ed.), How animals communicate (pp. 98–134). Bloomington, IN: Indiana University Press.

Bowlby J (1969) Attachment and Loss (Vol. 1). New York: Basic Books.

Cairns RB (1979) Social Development: the origin and plasticity of interchanges. San Francisco: WH Freeman.

de Waal FBM (2000) Primates – a natural history of conflict resolution. Science, 289, 586–590.

de Waal FBM (2001) The Ape and the Sushi Master. Harmondsworth, UK: Penguin.

Goodall J (1990) The Chimpanzees of Gombe: patterns of behaviour. Boston, MA: Bellknap Press of the Harvard University Press.

Hess EH (1973) Imprinting. New York: Van Nostrand Reinhold.

Hinde RA (1982) Ethology. London, UK: Fontana.

Kawai M (1965) Newly acquired pre-cultural behaviour of the natural troop of Japanese monkeys on Koshima islet. Primates, 6, 1–30.

Lorenz K (1971) Studies in Animal and Human Behaviour (Vols. 1 and 2). London, UK: Methuen.

Lorenz. K (1966) On Aggression. London, UK: Methuen.

Moyer K (1968) Kinds of aggression and their physiological basis. In R Buglass & P Bowden (eds), Principles and Practice of Forensic Psychiatry. Edinburgh: Churchill Livingstone.
Noble GK (1939) The role of dominance in the social life of birds. Auk, 56, 263–273.
Rowell T (1972) The social behaviour of monkeys. Harmondsworth, UK: Penguin.
Salzen EA (1998) Imprinting in Comparative Psychology: a handbook. New York: Garland Publishing.
Sanz CM (2001) Curious and naïve responses of *Pan troglodytes* to primatologists in the Goualougo Triangle, Republic of Congo. Project paper.
Sternglanz SH, Gray JL, Murakami M (1971) Adult preferences for infantile facial features: an ethological approach. Animal Behaviour, 25, 108–115.
Strayer FF, Strayer J (1976) An ethological analysis of social agonism and dominance relations among preschool children. Child Development, 47, 980–999.
Strum SC (1987) Almost Human: a journey into the world of baboons. London, UK: Elm Tree Books.
Thorpe WH (1961) Bird Song. Cambridge, UK: Cambridge University Press.
Tinbergen N (1951) The Study of Instinct. London: Oxford University Press.
Whitten A, Goodall J, McGrew WC, Nishida T, Reynolds V, Suglyma Y, Tutin CEG, Wrangham RW, Boesch C (1999) Cultures in chimpanzees. Nature, 399, 682–685.

FURTHER READING

Goodall J (1990) The Chimpanzees of Gombe: patterns of behaviour. Boston, MA: Bellknap Press of the Harvard University Press.

- The original Gombe study with photographs and tables; makes fascinating reading.

Greenberg G, Haraway M (eds.) (1998) Comparative Psychology. New York: Garland Publishing.

- A comprehensive textbook on the subject.

Hayes N (1994) Principles of Comparative Psychology. London, UK: Psychology Press.

- A brief but useful introduction to ethological concepts.

Developmental psychology and lifespan development

12

'Children begin by loving their parents; as they get older they judge them; sometimes they forgive them.'
Oscar Wilde, *The Picture of Dorian Gray*

Often developmental psychology (and psychopathology) is thought to belong to, and be synonymous with, child development, and therefore be germane only to child psychology and child psychiatry. This is a highly misleading and outdated view of development. A developmental perspective is essential in adult as well as in child psychology and psychiatry for a number of reasons. First, development and age-related progression occur throughout an individual's lifetime, from infancy to old age until death (lifespan development). Admittedly the pace of change is rapid in childhood but, nonetheless, normative biological, psychological and social changes continue into adulthood and old age. For example, a 65-year-old man presenting with depressive features raises the question whether he has just taken retirement. The latter event may be viewed as a developmental milestone that may be significantly related to his symptoms. Thus, it is necessary to identify the point that a person has reached in terms of his/her life span development in order to appreciate the relevance of the individual's experiences to psychopathological presentations.

ISSUES IN DEVELOPMENT

Continuities and discontinuities

Second, a developmental perspective takes into account continuities *and* discontinuities in traits, states and psychopathology across the lifespan. It is not suggested that all adult characteristics and personality functioning have their origins in childhood. Rather developmental processes involve normal progression, continuity and stabilisation *and* discontinuity and decline (Figure 12.1). Continuity implies the acquisition (or decline) of functional characteristics as a continuous process. For instance, speech, height, weight and IQ levels show progressive development and remain largely stable over adulthood while aggression and antisocial behaviour show a marked reduction around the age of twenty or so. These characteristics can be conceptualised as undergoing smooth change over time. The development is quantitative and may be represented as 'growth curves'.

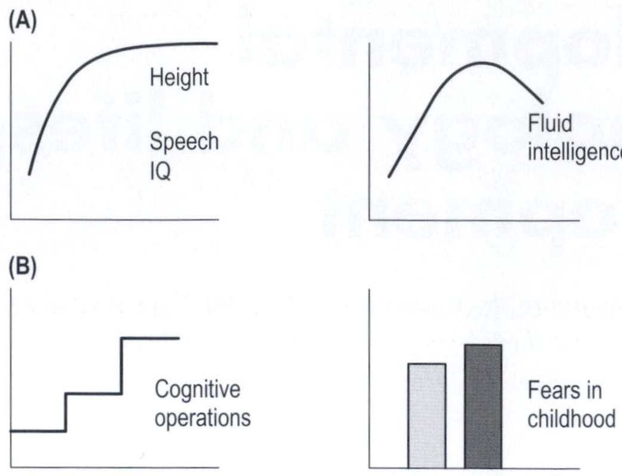

Fig. 12.1 Developmental continuity (**A**); discontinuity (**B**)

Discontinuous development refers to qualitative changes in a characteristic that occur over time. For example, fears in childhood vary with age. Cognitive development, according to Piaget (see later), largely follows a discontinuous, stepwise trajectory and childhood and adolescent anxiety disorders develop into adult depression in a significant proportion of cases (heterotypic continuity). A dramatic example of qualitative change in the animal kingdom is the metamorphosis of the caterpillar into the pupa and, later, into the butterfly. Although such spectacular developmental changes are rare in humans, some of the cognitive changes in childhood described by Piaget are remarkable events in the course of human development.

Third, a developmental approach emphasises the interaction between biological (genetic) and environmental factors. The notion of *maturation* implies that development is biological unfolding that proceeds according to a genetic blueprint. Speech and motor development fit this model where normal acquisition of various 'mile stones' occur in a predetermined order. The second critical factor is learning, the process whereby experience of the environment produces relatively permanent changes. Thus, speech gets better and motor coordination shows improvement with better practice. Thus, developmental changes are the product of both genetic potential and environmental influences: nature and nurture.

Nature and nurture

Current theories view development as resulting from the interaction between an *active* person (nature) and an *active* environment (nurture). In this transactional model of development the individual is seen as the product of the continuous dynamic interaction between the person and the experience provided by the environment and the social context. It emphasises the effect of the person on the environment and the environment on the person, as shown in Figure 12.2. For example, an enthusiastic and conscientious new appointee triggers a different response from the working environment than a diffident and less-competent worker. As a result the former may elicit a more

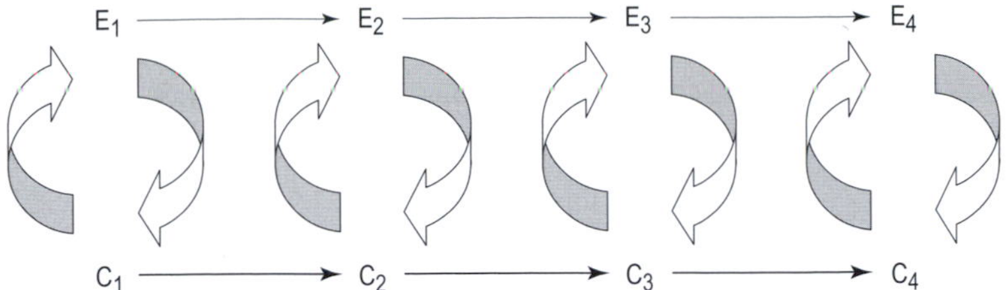

Fig. 12.2 Transactional model of development. E_1–E_4 represent environmental experiences at successive points in time. C_1–C_4 represents the individual's personal characteristic at successive points in time

favourable response and may be promoted thus producing a move to a more congenial environment.

The occurrence and timing of major life experiences and transition points have important developmental implications. Important examples include starting school or university, having a child, family dissolution and loss of a loved one. Many such transitions are irreversible. Some events have been characterised as *turning points*. Turning-point effects involve some form of marked environmental or personal discontinuity that entails a change in direction of future development. Examples include geographical moves, divorce and parenthood.

Research designs for studying development

It should be clear by now that developmental processes are complex and, therefore, research methods that aim to capture developmental changes over time need to be designed accordingly. Three commonly used research designs are cross-sectional design, longitudinal design and cohort sequential design.

Design. More details of research designs and their advantages and disadvantages are beyond the scope of the book. Lawrie, McIntosh, & Rao (2000) have provided an excellent critical discussion of various research designs.

Next we deal with some selected topics on development across the lifespan. The various phases of development are outlined in Table 12.1. First, we begin at the seat of life – in the foetus and the period immediately following it, infancy.

FOETAL AND INFANT CAPABILITIES

One of the surprising findings of prenatal and foetal research is that all senses, with the exception of vision, function remarkably well in the developing foetus. Thus, newborns come into this world well prepared to respond to and interact with their immediate environment, especially with their mother.

Hearing. The foetus responds to sound as early as 24 weeks of gestation. More importantly, the growing foetus is able to discriminate between different spoken sounds while in the uterus. Newborns selectively attend to (and show preference for) their mother's voice compared to those of a female

Table 12.1 The main developmental phases

0–2 years		Infancy	
2–12 years		Childhood	
	2–6 years		Early childhood
	6–12 years		Middle childhood
13–18 +		Adolescence	
20–64		Adulthood	
	18–45 years		Early adulthood
	46–64 years		Middle adulthood
65 +		Old age	
	65–75		Young old
	75 +		Old old

stranger (DeCasper & Fifer, 1980) and, it has been shown that this ability to recognise the mother's voice is acquired before birth. In one experiment, newborns were shown to prefer to hear a story that had been read to them while *in utero* rather than a modified version of the same story (DeCasper & Spence, 1986). Infants as old as two days show a preference for their native language. These findings suggest that sensitivity to some aspects of language develops in the prenatal period.

Between birth and four months infants are capable of distinguishing between each of the 150 basic units of speech sounds (phonemes) that make up universal languages. They are said to be 'universal linguists' at this stage. However, as they grow older they lose most of these abilities and by 10 months they are able to discriminate only the sounds and words of the language that they have been exposed to. In short, within a few months, they are only able to perceive the words of their native language.

Taste. The foetus is able to distinguish between sweet and noxious substances while in the uterus. When sweet substances are introduced into amniotic fluid, foetal swallowing increases while with bitter-tasting substances there is a demonstrable slowing of swallowing movements. Studies on newborns show that their sense of taste is well developed. Newborn infants have been observed making distinct facial expressions when they taste sweet, bitter and sour solutions.

Smell. The foetus inhales and exhales amniotic fluid early in its development and, therefore, experiences odours and smells. Newborns show odour preferences and their sense of smell is highly developed. As well as simply responding to smells, by one to two weeks the newborn is able to discriminate between its mother's breast pads and those of another nursing women.

Learning. The foetus shows habituation to auditory stimuli from about 24 weeks of gestation suggesting that learning begins in the uterus. After birth newborns have been shown to prefer music that they heard in late pregnancy compared with music that they have never heard.

Pain. When touched with the needle during amniocentesis, foetuses show behavioural reactions and it is highly likely that they experience pain.

Vision. At birth, vision is the least developed of the senses, presumably because there is little opportunity for it in utero. Newborns can see faces at a distance of 10 to 20 inches, the distance at which mothers holds their babies. Visual acuity reaches near adult levels by 6 months and is complete by 3 years.

Face perception. Infants as young as 12 hours spend more time looking at their mother's face than those of a stranger. Visual recognition of the mother's face seems to be based on the general contour of mother's head and face such as external features and her hair line rather than on internal features like the eyes and nose. When mothers cover their outer features with a scarf, for example, newborns no longer prefer to look at them. These findings are consistent with those from studies tracking eye movements. Recordings of the eye movements of infants show that one-month-old infants tend to scan the external features of faces, whereas two-month-old babies focus on internal features of faces, such as eyes and mouth. Another constant finding is that one-month-old infants show no particular preference for facial pattern but two-month-olds show a marked inclination for face-like stimuli. When presented with three face-like stimuli – a natural face, an asymmetrical scrambled face and a symmetrical face resembling a normal face – one-month-old infants show no particular preference for any one of them whereas two-month-olds show a marked preference for looking at the normal face. The general conclusion from these studies is that up to the age of one month infants recognise their mother's face based on categorisation of stimuli into faces and non-faces; as the visual system undergoes development the baby starts perceiving the details of faces.

By three months of age infants are able to recognise photographs of their mother's face. At 6 months children can remember a face even after two weeks indicating the development of memory for faces. The various sensory capabilities of the neonate are summarised in Table 12.2.

Infant–mother interactions

The infant is born with the capacity to attract parental care for immediate biological needs, to communicate with the primary caregiver (usually the mother) with expression of feelings and to actively try to engage her in emotional exchanges. This is paralleled by sensitive responding by the mother. For example, infants' sucking has been shown to occur in a burst–pause pattern. Mothers tend to interact (stroke, talk and jiggle) with the infant during the pause phase and be generally quiet during the sucking phase. Thus, the infant and the mother show a turn-taking pattern of communication even when feeding is the primary task. Frame by frame analysis of video footage of infant–mother interaction has confirmed that as early as two months, infants and mothers look and listen to each other in rhythmic patterns. This style of exchange bears a close resemblance to conversations between adults and has been termed *protoconversation.*

Table 12.2 The newborn's capabilities

Hearing	Can discriminate sounds Recognises mother's voice
Taste	Well developed Can discriminate sweet, salty, sour and bitter tastes but prefers sweet solutions
Smell	Shows odour preferences Can discriminate mother's odour, if breast fed
Learning	Shows habituation Prefers to hear music originally heard while in utero
Vision	Least well developed Can see mother's face at 10 to 20 inches (holding distance)
Pain	Sensitive to pain from foetal life

There appear to be two elements to the exchange of emotional communication: (1) the infant's awareness of the mother's subjective state (intersubjectivity); and (2) the mother's readiness to respond to the infant's signals. During the protoconversations, infants look at the eyes and mouth of the person addressing them while listening to the voice; mothers intuitively respond to such communication from the infant by gentle gaze, vocalisations and playfulness.

In experiments where mothers were instructed to show no facial reactions (the still face procedure), two-month-old infants, after attempting to engage the mother by smiling, vocalising and gesturing, avoid eye-contact and show distress or become withdrawn. When healthy mothers assume the depressed facial expression and pretend to be unresponsive, infants too show depressive affect.

A particular form of adults' conversation with infants that has been researched is *motherese* or infant-directed speech. Infant-directed speech has been observed in all cultures and consist of high-pitched, slow speech with long pauses and exaggerated intonations. It has a certain 'musical' quality with rhythmic and melodic features. Three different functions have been attributed to the way adults talk to infants: (1) the speech engages the infant's attention; (2) it communicates feelings and promotes interaction; and (3) it facilitates language development.

As may be expected, maternal psychiatric disorders interfere with early mother–infant interactions. Research into the effects of maternal postnatal depression have shown impaired response to infant cues and lack of sensitivity to the infant's communication by the parent is associated with initial and subsequent apathy on the part of the infant as well as delayed cognitive development (Murray & Cooper, 1997). A more worrying finding is that mothers with borderline personality disorders are not only insensitive to infant's cues but they are also intrusive ('intrusively insensitive') in their speech and behaviour towards their 2-month-old infants. The infant's responses were ones of distress and avoidance. It has been hypothesised that these deviant patterns of early mother–child interactions have subtle but drastic effects on children's emotional and cognitive development.

TEMPERAMENT

Children show remarkable individual variation in the way that they respond to day-to-day changes in the environment. Some are friendly, approach new situations with confidence (such as a new play group and unfamiliar people), are quite active and boisterous in familiar surroundings, while others are shy, reluctant to venture or try new things, fearful, clingy, quiet and retiring. These differences in behavioural tendencies are noticeable in neonates even as early as the first week of life. It is now believed that infants come in to this world with their own intrinsic tendencies for experiencing and expressing emotions. This, of course, influences the response they elicit from caregivers.

These hypothesised behavioural predispositions have been described under the umbrella term *temperament*. It is widely acknowledged that temperament in childhood is an important psychological attribute distinct from such characteristics as cognitive abilities and motivation. Not everyone is in agreement as to the nature, meaning and measurement of temperament. Of the contemporary theories of temperament the best known is that proposed by Thomas and Chess (1977), which is described here. A second theory, put forward by Buss and Plomin (1984) is mentioned in brief.

Thomas and Chess conceptualise temperament as representing the behavioural *style* – the *how* of behaviour. They differentiate the *how* of behaviour from the *why* (motivations or goals) and *what* (abilities and contents) of behaviour of the individual. These variations in style are thought to reflect their temperamental characteristics. Thomas and Chess view temperament as a phenomenological term that describes behaviour tendencies, that has no aetiological implications and as a characteristic that is open to environmental influences and developmental maturation. Their original research, known as the *New York Longitudinal Study* (NYLS), comprised of a sample of children who were studied intensively during their infancy and followed up at 5, 18 and 22 years. Data were obtained by semi-structured parent interviews (except during adolescence and young adulthood) and from nurseries and schools. Based on quantitative and qualitative analysis of the data, they identified and described nine categories of temperament: (1) rhythmicity; (2) activity level; (3) approach/withdrawal; (4) adaptability; (5) threshold for responsiveness; (6) intensity of reactions; (7) quality of mood; (8) distractibility; and (9) attention span. These are described in Box 12.1.

Qualitative analysis and factor analysis of the data led to three temperamental constellations made up of various combinations of the nine individual categories (Table 12.3).

1. *Easy temperament*. Typically this comprises the combination of biological regularity, approach tendencies, rapid adaptability to change and a predominantly positive mood of mild or moderate intensity. This group comprised approximately 40% of the study population.
2. *Difficult temperament*. This, the opposite of easy temperament, namely biological irregularity, withdrawal tendencies to the new situations, slow adaptability to change and frequent negative emotional expressions of

Box 12.1 Infant temperamental characteristics (Thomas & Chess, 1986)

1. *Activity level.* The motor component present in a child's functioning and the diurnal proportion of active and inactive periods
2. *Rhythmicity (regularity).* The predictability in time of functions – it can be analysed in relation to sleep–wake cycle, feeding patterns or elimination schedules
3. *Approach/withdrawal.* The nature of initial responses (smiling, verbalisation, moving away) to a new stimulus, be it food, a new toy or a new person
4. *Adaptability.* Responses to new or altered situations
5. *Threshold of responsiveness.* The intensity level of stimulation that is necessary to evoke a discernible response (to sensory stimuli, environmental objects or social contacts)
6. *Intensity of reaction.* The energy level of response, irrespective of its quality or direction
7. *Quality of mood.* The amount of pleasant, joyful and friendly behaviour, as contrasted with unpleasant, crying and unfriendly behaviour
8. *Distractibility.* The effect of extraneous environmental stimuli in interfering with or altering the direction of ongoing behaviour
9. *Attention span and persistence.* The length of time a particular activity is pursued by the child and the continuation of an activity in face of obstacles

high intensity. This group comprised approximately 10% of the study population.

3. *Slow-to-warm-up temperament.* This category comprises withdrawal tendencies to the new stimuli, slow adaptability to change and frequent negative emotional reactions of low intensity. Such individuals are often labelled as 'shy'. This group comprised approximately 15% of the study population.

It should be apparent from the percentages given for each group that some children do not fit any of these patterns. This subgroup of children showed varying combinations of temperamental traits and failed to conform to the three categories.

In addition to the descriptions of temperament, the concept of '*goodness of fit*' introduced by Thomas and Chess is central to the analysis of psychological development of the child. Goodness of fit results when the opportunities, demands and expectations of the parents and others are in *consonance* with the child's temperament and other abilities. On the other hand '*poorness of fit*' arises out of a lack of consistency between environmental demands, and the child's temperamental and other characteristics. While

Table 12.3 Temperament clusters (Thomas & Chess, 1986)

Easy	*Difficult*	*Slow to warm up*
Positive mood	Negative mood	Slow changes in mood
Regular biorhythms	Irregular biorhythms	Somewhat regular habits
Adaptable	Slow to adapt	Gradual adaptations
Low intensity of emotions	'Fiery' emotionality	Mild intensity
Positive approach to novelty	Negative response to novelty	Negative response to new stimuli

some parents find the child with high levels of motor activity taxing and difficult to manage, others may find it challenging and find ways and means of channelling the child's energy towards constructive ends like sports, outdoor activities and so on.

The original study has been replicated by the authors and other researchers and several temperament questionnaires have been developed for various age groups. The methodology has been applied to different populations, in different cultures and countries. It has also been used in low-birth-weight babies and those with mental and physical handicaps.

Is temperament a stable characteristic? The longitudinal nature of the NYLS and the remarkable follow-up studies carried out from infancy to adulthood (over a period of more than 20 years) have yielded a vast amount of data that have been used to address this question (Thomas & Chess, 1986). In general, studies on continuity and discontinuity of temperamental characteristics show a moderate degree of stability and continuity from infancy to early childhood and from early school years to teenage period. But as the period of follow-up increases, the correlations show a progressive downward trend, so much so that they are near zero when scores between the first two years and adolescence are compared. Between the ages of 5 to 7 the correlations are as high as 0.8 but drop to around 0.3–0.5 between early school years and adolescence. However, consistency for extreme temperamental characteristics is greater. Continuities appear to be greater when the level of analysis is more general than specific. In short the clusters of easy and difficult temperaments may be more stable than the nine temperamental characteristics.

These findings should come as no surprise. The fall in the correlations between temperamental scores on the nine categories reflect the ever increasing influence of two factors. First, the growing child is subjected to various environmental effects in a widening social world and, second, maturational development such as increasing cognition and language abilities together with the changes associated with puberty tend to bring about change and modification in one temperamental characteristic or another.

Another area of temperament research has been the search for the biological origin of temperament. The evidence for a biological basis for temperamental features is overwhelming, so much so that temperament has come to be defined as 'biologically rooted individual differences in behaviour tendencies that are present in early life and are relatively stable across various kinds of situations and over the course of time' (Bates, 1987). Several genetic studies, some using different categorisations of temperament, have shown that monozygotic (MZ) twins show more significant inter-pair correlations on various temperamental parameters than dizygotic (DZ) twins. There is a general consensus that the major elements of temperament are present early in life and that these elements are largely biologically based. As development proceeds, however, their expression becomes increasingly influenced by learning, experience and environment.

How is temperament related to adult personality? Various workers in the field of personality have made attempts to map these childhood traits to the five big personality factors (Shiner & Caspi, 2003) but the results have been unconvincing. Temperament is only one of the factors influencing adult personality development. Personality is a far wider concept than temperament. In the newborn, temperament constitutes the entire 'personality' of the infant. In the course of development and maturation many other factors come to be included. Adult personality includes attitudes, expectations, self-concept, values, standards, and so on. Temperament may be a subset of personality or the two types of constructs may be conceptually distinct.

Clinical implications

The concept of temperament and the three clusters of temperamental characteristics, together with the notion of goodness of fit, have significant practical implications. First, the recognition and identification of the temperamental patterns of children provides a way of understanding their behaviour. This is particularly important in the case of parents whose children show difficult temperament so that they do not blame themselves for being 'bad parents' or label their child as 'bad' or 'evil'. Second, temperament may be a protective or risk factor for development of subsequent psychopathology. It is important to emphasise that difficult temperament *per se* does not lead to psychopathology; it is the combination of temperamental constellation with environmental factors such as maternal depression or poor parenting that lead to maladjustment. Difficult temperament at the age of three is associated with subsequent externalising problems (oppositional defiant disorder/conduct disorder). The link between 'slow-to-warm up' infants and the development of 'internalising' problems (e.g. separation anxiety) is less strong. Infants and children with 'easy temperament' elicit positive responses from family members as well as others. They more readily obtain suitable care and help with coping.

Other theories of temperament

Buss and Plomin (1984) define temperament as a set of emergent personality traits that appear in early life. Further, they hold that they are inherited and are evident in the first year of life. They specify three traits as constituting temperament, referred to as EAS.

1. *Emotionality* – varying from lack of reaction to intense and overwhelming emotional reactions, whether it be fear, anger or distress.
2. *Activity* – the level of tempo, vigour and endurance.
3. *Sociability* – tendency to affiliate with others and social responsiveness.

Temperament is assessed using the *EAS-temperament survey* (EAS-TS). The authors assert that the three EAS dimensions of temperament are: (1) genetically grounded and highly heritable; (2) show high stability over developmental periods; (3) predict adult personality traits (with increasing age they become differentiated); and (4) are of evolutionary importance. The three temperamental traits are said to be evident in other primates. The original theory included impulsivity as a dimension but it was excluded in later revisions because of its poor heritability. The correlations across the three temperament dimensions were 0.66 in MZ twins as compared with 0.14 for DZ twins (Buss & Plomin, 1975).

In summary:

- Temperament refers to basic predispositions that underlie children's behaviours.
- It includes, according to Thomas and Chess, nine categories of disposition. Buss and Plomin describe three.
- The dimensions of temperament are relatively stable in childhood, in fact more consistent than personality traits in adulthood.
- It is thought to be inherent and strongly influenced by biology, but its expression is subject to influences from the environment. It is expressed in its purest form in infancy and becomes increasingly subject to environmental influences with age.
- It is a useful concept in understanding that not all aspects of children's behaviour are due to parental or other outside influences and that the child is an active agent in initiating responses.

ATTACHMENT

In the latter part of the first year of life, infants show a constellation of behaviours indicating the establishment of a close emotional relationship with the primary caregiver, usually the mother. This intense dyadic (two way) affective tie between the infant and the mother is called *attachment*. Attachment became a concept to be studied, researched and applied following the pioneering work of John Bowlby, a psychiatrist and psychoanalyst, who set forth his ideas in his first article on the subject entitled 'The nature of the child's tie to the mother' in 1958. He elaborated his observations and theory in his seminal work, the three volumes entitled *Attachment and Loss* (Bowlby, 1969/1982). He was joined by Mary Ainsworth (a psychologist who, by chance, answered a newspaper advertisement for a postdoctoral researcher with Bowlby) whose innovative experiments on individual differences in attachment relationships broke new ground and laid the foundation for all future attachment research. The combined efforts of Bowlby and Ainsworth laid the foundations for the theoretical framework and research into the field of attachment – an elegant example of how collaboration between psychiatrists and psychologists can prove to be creative and productive.

It is helpful, at the very start, to make a distinction between attachment behaviour and attachment theory. Attachment behaviour refers to the various readily observable dimensions of the child's behaviour with respect to the primary caregiver, whereas attachment theory is a systematised framework that has been advanced to explain and understand attachment behaviour. More recently many workers have shown great interest in extending theory to close relationships in adults (e.g. Holmes, 1993b).

Attachment behaviour

Bowlby emphasised that attachment is distinct and different from other kinds of social ties and behaviours. Three specific characteristics that distinguish attachment behaviour from other behaviour such as play are: proximity-seeking behaviour, secure-base effect and separation protest.

- *Proximity seeking* (comfort seeking) refers to the tendency of the infant to follow and remain in close proximity to the attachment figure. It is increased by fear, discomfort or anxiety. Children seek comfort even from a rejecting or abusing parent and, when parents are not available, from total strangers.
- *Secure-base effect* (exploratory behaviour) is the ability of children to move away, explore and interact with the social and physical worlds in the presence of the person to whom the child is attached. The child uses the mother as a 'secure base' from which to explore the surroundings, using her as a reference figure and continuously monitoring her proximity and availability. If the child senses danger or feels anxious it returns to the mother swiftly, thus using her as a safe haven.
- *Separation distress* (separation anxiety). Separation or threat of separation from the mother induces distress in the child. Young children show signs of protest and distress when separated from the attachment figure. Typically young children separated from parents and admitted to hospital, for example, go through three phases: (1) 'protest' (becoming angry, tearful and distressed); (2) 'despair' (showing quiet misery and apathy); and (3) 'detachment' (becoming sullen and 'cut off'). Descriptions of these effects on infants (Robertson & Robertson, 1971) were largely responsible for changes in hospital policies regarding admission of children.

Achieving a degree of cognitive development is essential before infants can form attachments. The infants need to be able to recognise faces, develop person permanence and, to some extent, predict the adults' behaviour before attachment can occur. Typically these maturational changes have occurred by the time they are six months of age. A wide range of studies has now established that children develop *specific* attachments in the 'third quarter of the first year' (6 to 9 months). There is considerable individual variation ranging from 3 to 15 months. As the infant grows older he is able to tolerate longer distances and longer times away from the mother and attachment behaviour decreases. After about 3 years attachment behaviours start showing decline and become less prominent.

Nature of attachment

Since attachment behaviour exists side by side with other similar behaviours, it is essential to distinguish it from other related behaviours so that one is clear about what attachment behaviour is, and what it is not. The main features of attachment may be stated as follows:

1. *Attachment behaviour is different from feeding relationship.* Proximity-seeking behaviour that is attributed to attachment is distinct and independent of the provision of food or milk. Attachment is not driven by the need for food,

rather it belongs to a different behavioural system in which the need for comfort, reassurance and affection appears to be the central feature. In the famous monkey experiments, Harlow placed infant monkeys in cages with wire 'mothers' that provided milk and another in which the wire was covered with warm terry cloth that did not provide milk. The infant monkeys were seen to spend most of the time with the warm cloth 'mother', although they made occasional visits to the wire 'mother' to feed themselves. Any noise or disturbance made them cling to the cloth 'mother' and not to the wire 'mother' (Harlow, 1958).

2. *Attachment is only one aspect of the infant–mother relationship*. Such actions as play, feeding, controlling and care-giving occur alongside attachment and are thought to belong to other 'behavioural systems'. How these varied aspects of parental care interact with attachment is still unclear.
3. *Attachment is distinct from learned behaviours and is not the result of conditioning or reinforcement*. Abused children are no less attached (though the attachment may be of the insecure type, see later) to the abusing parent than those who are well treated, indicating that the processes in operation are different to those put forward by learning theorists.
4. *Attachment refers to a particular dyadic relationship and is not an attribute of the child or the parent*. For example, a mother may show considerable attachment toward one child and not another.

Security of attachment

Children show considerable variation in their attachment relationships to their mothers. Mary Ainsworth pioneered a method of studying the *quality* of attachment by activating the attachment behaviour through enforced separation of the infant from the mother under controlled laboratory conditions. The *Strange Situation Procedure* (SSP) developed by Mary Ainsworth has become the standard method of assessing the security of an infant's attachment to the caregiver (usually the mother). It is designed for use with children between 1 year and 18 months. The test procedure has remained unchanged since its first description in 1978 (Ainsworth et al., 1978).

Box 12.2 Strange situation procedure (Ainsworth, 1978)

Episode*

1. Observer introduces mother and child to the play room (1 minute)
2. Child plays with mother
3. Stranger enters room and joins play
4. Mother leaves child in company of stranger
5. Mother and baby reunited (stranger leaves)
6. Second separation from mother (baby is alone)
7. Stranger returns to room (mother remains absent)
8. Mother and child reunited (stranger departs)

*Three minutes each.

Table 12.4 Patterns of attachment in infancy and corresponding parental behaviours

Attachment pattern	*Behaviour of child*	*Behaviour of carer*
Secure (B)	Uses caregiver as 'secure base', explores freely, may or may not be distressed at separation but greets positively on reunion, seeks comfort, settles down and returns to exploration	Dependable, available, sensitive to infant's cues, available and warm
Avoidant (A)	Appears normally interested in caregiver, explores busily, minimal distress at separation, ignores or avoids caregiver on reunion	Rejecting, hostile and intrusive
Resistant/ambivalent (C)	Minimal exploration, stays close to carer, both seeks and resists contact on reunion	Insensitive, unresponsive, passive, under involved
Disorganised (D)	Disorganised, disorientated behaviour in the presence of caregiver (freezing, odd postures)	Frightened or frightening, abusive, unresolved grief

SSP is a controlled observation carried out in a comfortable room equipped with toys. The procedure consists of eight episodes, three minutes each, that essentially attempt to simulate naturalistic infant–mother interactions to brief separation and reunion (Box 12.2). The infant's reactions to separations and, more specifically, to reunion are believed to measure the degree to which the mother provides the infant with feelings of security and trust.

On the basis of the findings from SSP, Ainsworth described three main attachment types (Table 12. 4):

Type B – secure attachment. The infant explores the room actively in the presence of the mother and is distressed when the mother leaves. Upon reunion the child greets the mother, actively seeks proximity and bodily contact and accepts comfort easily. In the American samples, 65% of infants showed secure Type B attachment. It is inferred that secure infants anticipate that their caregiver is accessible and available to them for comfort when necessary and their primary carer is sensitive to the infants signals and cues.

Type A – insecure (avoidant/anxious) attachment. The child tends not to protest or be distressed when the mother leaves the room and upon reunion actively avoids the mother, ignoring her and focusing on the environment. Studies in the USA showed avoidant attachment in 20% of infants. Care giving in these infants is thought to be characterised by rejection, covert hostility and intrusive interventions. It is inferred that the avoidantly attached child expects to be rebuffed, rejected or subject to anger and hostility if he makes demands in stressful situations. In order to avoid this, and the distress that would result if his/her needs for comfort go unfulfilled, the child ignores the attachment figure. The child also learns to suppress or falsify the expression of negative affects that are normally used to alert the mother to the child's distress.

Type C – insecure (ambivalent/resistant) attachment. Infants in this group show high levels of distress on separation from the mother. On reunion they approach their mothers but are angry and ambivalent (seeking and avoiding comfort at the same time). They resist comforting and take a long time to settle down, often pushing their mother away. About 10% of children showed resistant attachment patterns in US studies. Resistant attachment is thought to be due to inconsistent care giving where the mother is insensitive to the child's needs. Often the mothers are passive and withdrawn and the child attempts to provoke the mother to meet its needs by angry outbursts. The child finds that it cannot predict the mother's response to its signals of distress and is uncertain whether the mother is available and responsive.

A proportion of cases have been found that do not fit neatly into the three patterns described by Ainsworth. Main and Solomon (1990) have described a fourth category of attachment, the 'disorganised/disorientated' type, or Type D.

Type D – disorganised/disorientated attachment. This refers to a diverse array of fearful, odd, disorganised and overly conflicted behaviours exhibited during the SSP. The child displays contradictory behaviour patterns such as strong initial proximity seeking followed by strong avoidance, distress, anger, freezing or stereotypic anomalous postures when the mother returns.

Studies have shown that, in middle-class, non-clinical groups, around 15% of children show a disorganised/disorientated attachment behaviour pattern. Disorganised infant behaviour is thought to arise from experiencing the attachment figure as frightening (as in physical or sexual abuse) or when the caregiver appears frightened herself (as in severe domestic violence). Fear activates the attachment system but when the child seeks proximity it gets more frightened resulting in incoherent, confused and inconsistent behaviour patterns. In clinical samples, especially in the presence of serious family-risk factors such as unresolved traumatic experiences, manic-depressive illness and alcohol abuse in parents, as well as in the case of abused children, the prevalence of disorganised attachment is significantly increased. Some studies have reported as much as 80% category D attachment behaviour pattern in children subjected to abuse.

Bowlby's assertions have sometimes been misunderstood and subjected to criticism. Some feminists have taken issue with him for assigning the task of parenting primarily to the mother. As research into attachment has progressed his postulates have been clarified. Some of the questions raised by his critics are discussed below.

Monotropy or multiple-attachment figures?

Bowlby has been criticised for emphasising monotropy, the view that the child initially forms attachment to one caregiver, usually the mother. This seems an unfair criticism. Bowlby himself pointed out in the first volume in his trilogy, *Attachment and Loss* (1969/1982), that from the very beginning many children have 'more than one attachment figure towards whom they direct attachment behaviour'. Later studies have confirmed that, by their first birthday, children do form attachments with more than one familiar figure. This includes fathers, siblings, grandparents, and so on. But available evidence suggests that although multiple attachment is the norm, the infant does not treat all attachments as equivalent or interchangeable. Even when several carers are available, infants appear to show a clear preference for the primary caregiver. Bowlby termed this tendency of the infant to form one special attachment 'monotropy'. The primary caregiver may be the mother or father or anyone who provided the greatest interaction with the infant. This is consistent with the view that the infant forms a hierarchy of attachments with a small number of caregivers, some attachments being stronger than others, but these attachments are subordinate to those formed with the primary attachment figure. The 'mothering' could be performed by a male or a female.

Is attachment universal?

Ainsworth's studies included observation of infants in Uganda, which provided confirmatory support for her assertions. Variations have been found when the SSP was carried out in different countries. For example, most Japanese infants are almost never left alone at 12 months, and fewer infants were categorised as securely attached (Type B); there is an excess of Type C attachment in Japanese infants at 12 months. The cross-cultural differences appear to be due to differences in the way that mothers interact with their infants in various cultures. There is no doubt that attachment behaviour is universal, although categorisation of the types of attachment is open to different interpretations.

Critical period or Sensitive period?

Bowlby strongly suggests that attachment develops in the latter part of infancy, in the period from six months to eighteen months. This is one example of sensitive periods in human development. It is likely – although not yet conclusively proven – that parallel neurological changes take place in the developing brain. After this period attachment gets stabilised and disruption of the bond is likely to lead to deleterious effects. This does not imply that disrupted attachment is completely irreversible. Although infancy may be the optimal time to develop attachment, it has been shown that children adopted at four years are capable of developing long and lasting attachment to their adoptive parents (Tizard & Hodges, 1978). Nevertheless, such attachments appear to be vulnerable and at greater risk of disruption and maladaptation. Sensitive period has to be distinguished from critical period, which has an all-or-nothing implication. In all cases of attachment, empirical evidence points to the ability of the child to form later attachments beyond the sensitive period although the age from 6 to 18 months seem to be the most optimal for development of such attachments.

Attachment theory

Bowlby brought together knowledge derived from such diverse fields as developmental psychology, psychoanalysis (object relations theory in particular), evolutionary biology, ethology and control systems theory to formulate the attachment theory. The main features of attachment theory may be summarised as follows:

1. The infant is born with a biological propensity – 'pre-programmed' was the word Bowlby used – to form a specific affectional bond with the primary caregiver.
2. Attachment is not mediated by feeding or physical care taking, it differs qualitatively from dependency. It has adaptive evolutionary value in promoting protection from potential threats from the environment. By increasing the chances of mother–infant proximity, attachment increases the likelihood of protection and survival advantage.
3. A fundamental tenet of attachment theory is that the quality of parenting and the way the caregiver interacts with the baby is crucial in shaping the security of an infant's attachment relationships with parents. Children form attachments more readily with people who are sensitive and responsive to their cues and signals.
4. Attachment theory proposes that, in addition to the attachment system, in normal development, three other behavioural systems are involved: exploratory system; fear/weariness system; and sociable (affiliative) system.
5. Bowlby postulated that what children carried into their future were *internal working models* (IWM), which are internalised mental representations of early relationships with the caregiver. A person's internal working models of close relationships incorporate two discrete yet interrelated cognitive schemas:

   - a *self model* containing perceptions of one's own worth and lovability; and
   - an *other model* embodying core expectations about the trustworthiness and dependability of intimate others in one's social world.

   These early experiences become internalised and create anticipatory images that shape perceptions, attitudes and reactions to individuals encountered later. IWMs affect how we perceive, remember, interpret and react to experiences. Such working models become part of one's personality organisation, which influences perceptions, feelings, thoughts and behaviour unconsciously and automatically. IWMs of self and the attachment figure are, according to attachment theory, stable but open to revision through subsequent development and experience. They operate relatively automatically without need for conscious appraisal. Bowlby postulated that children carried their IWMs into their adult life.

6. Attachment relationship provides the prototype on which future adult relationships are based. It is hypothesised that attachment forms the building blocks for future intimate relationships. Attachment relationship, in short, continues throughout life and to a large degree is shaped by early attachment experience. A basic assumption of attachment theory is that the child's initial relationship with a caregiver, usually the mother, shapes and predicts later relationships. This is consistent with the psychoanalytic concepts of Freud and Melanie Klein.

The theory has been subjected to extensive study. In general, research findings have borne out the main thrust of Bowlby's attachment theory and most key components of the theory have received empirical support. It has important implications for psychotherapy in general and child psychotherapy in particular (Holmes, 1993a).

Attachment in adulthood

For Bowlby, attachment continues through one's entire life course and plays a 'vital role from the cradle to the grave'. The early parent–child relationship is thought to be the template on which later relationships, especially intimate relationships, are built. Hence such relationships influence adult personality characteristics and subsequent family relationships. More importantly, they play an important role in transgenerational transmission of parent–child attachment patterns.

One approach to assessment of adults' attachment to *their* parents is the *adult attachment interview* (AAI) developed by Mary Main and her colleagues (George, Kaplan & Main, 1986). It is a semi-structured interview procedure comprised of 18 questions designed to assess the security of the adults' overall working model of attachment. A few sample questions from the AAI are given in Box 12.3. The answers are analysed according to an accompanying scoring system. In addition to the contents of the narratives provided by the interview, the individual's ability to give a coherent and integrated account of the parenting experience and meaning as well as the language used form the basis of the scoring. The emotional quality, relevance, and the manner in which the experiences are recalled form vital aspects of the assessment. The AAI, it has been emphasised, does not measure security of attachment of the subject to any specific person (spouse or parent), rather it assesses the individual's 'state of mind with respect to attachment' and is intended to 'surprise the person's unconscious'. Based on the findings of AAI four categories of adult attachment have been described:

1. Secure/autonomous (F) – the subject provides a reasonably coherent narrative in a non-defensive manner with sufficient elaboration, whether the experiences described are positive or negative.

Box 12.3 Example of questions in the adult attachment interview (George, Kaplan, & Main, 1986)

- Could you describe your relationship with your parents as a young child, starting as far back as you can remember?
- Could you give me five adjectives or phrases to describe your relationship with your mother/father during your childhood?
- Tell me what memories or experiences led you to choose each one.
- Were there any changes in your relationship with your parents between your childhood and adulthood?
- How do you think your overall early experiences have affected your adult personality?

2. Dismissing (D) – the subject gives brief answers, either 'I don't remember' statements or provides a generalised positive description ranging from favourable to an idealised picture but fail to provide evidence of these descriptions.
3. Preoccupied (E) – the subject shows an outpouring of emotion with lengthy discussion of childhood memories and is often angry, distressed and tearful.
4. Unresolved/disorganised (U) – during the interview subject becomes incoherent or irrational (e.g. talks of the dead person as if he/she is alive).

An interesting finding is that there is an 80% correspondence between a mother's attachment category on the AAI and her infant's attachment pattern. In short, the AAI appears to predict with a high degree of accuracy the infant's response on the SSP (van Ijzendoorn, 1995). An important study by Fonagy and colleagues (Fonagy, Steele, & Steele, 1991) showed that the mothers' adult attachment rating during pregnancy predicted the SSP status of their infants at 12 months. Numerous studies have shown that mothers in the dismissing adult attachment category typically have children who exhibit an insecure/avoidant attachment pattern; those who were classed as preoccupied on the AAI were observed to have insecure/resistant attachments with their children; mothers with unresolved/disorganised attachment are more likely to have children with disorganised/disorientated attachment pattern (Table 12.5). Thus mothers' attachment relationships appear, to a large extent, to predict attachment organisation with her children indicating that mothers' care-giving behaviour towards their child is significantly influenced by their own attachment experience.

Attachment and psychopathology in childhood

Problems in the development of attachment between the child and the primary caregiver may arise from a number of sources:

1. *Early disruption in parenting*. Children are sometimes removed from parents because of neglect, abuse or severe lack of parenting capacity. A proportion of such children are placed with foster parents and, unfortunately, some of them go from one foster carer to another without the chance of forming an attachment to any one of them.
2. *Severe parenting problems*. Children living with parents who are abusive and neglectful typically show disorganised attachment patterns. Another

Table 12.5 Correspondence between mother's attachment and infant's attachment

Mother's AAI category	*Infant's SSP behaviour pattern*
Secure/Autonomous (F)	Secure (B)
Dismissing (D)	Avoidant (A)
Preoccupied (E)	Resistant/ambivalent (C)
Unresolved/disorganised (U)	Disorganised/disorientated (D)

common cause of poor attachment is mental disorder in the mother, especially if the condition is enduring and severe (e.g. borderline personality disorder).

It is important to point out that most children subjected to early parenting breakdown, leading to adoption or permanent foster care, overcome the initial setback of attachment disruption and grow up to become relatively well adjusted. The chances of forming new attachments are better when the child is adopted or placed with a substitute parent during early childhood. Research shows that the earlier the age of adoption the better is the outcome for the child. For this reason early adoption is recommended as a matter of social policy. Children adopted before the age of four or five have been shown to do well provided there are few other risk factors such as further disruption in their placement.

It has been shown that late adoption, after the age of eight, does not necessarily lead to problems in adjustment but such children are more vulnerable and are at risk of developing future problems. Tizard and Hodges (1978) followed up a group of children who had been in institutions from early infancy and were adopted at the age of four. The children had been looked after by a number of carers who changed often. Follow-up of the children showed that:

- *At the age of eight* most of the children had formed reasonably good attachment with their adoptive parents. But many were seen to show behaviour problems at home and school and to experience problems in peer relationships.
- *At the age of sixteen* the adolescents appeared to be functioning rather well. But on closer examination showed a constellation of features termed 'ex-institutional syndrome'. These young people related better to adults than to their peers, were less likely to have a special friend, were less likely to be selective in choosing their friends and turned to peers less often for emotional support (Tizard & Hodges, 1989).

These findings are matched by the results of Harlow's studies on infant rhesus monkeys separated from their mothers at birth. These primate studies showed that:

- Infants reared away from their mothers turned out to be socially incompetent when placed with their peers. They were aggressive and fearful and, in adolescence, were unable to mate satisfactorily (for example, they did not know how to mount a female). If such a female monkey later had a baby, she subjected the baby to abuse. Later work has shown that if the infants were placed individually with a younger monkey (therapist monkey) over time, their social behaviour in the peer group improved a great deal (Harlow & Harlow, 1962).
- When the separated monkeys are raised with peers instead of their mothers, they exhibit aggressive behaviour, showed less grooming behaviour and dropped to the bottom of their dominance hierarchies. These behaviour patterns persisted into adolescence (Suomi & Harlow, 1978).

Taken together, these findings from studies of children and primates who had suffered early separation from their caregivers point towards the conclusion that separation in the first year of life does indeed lead to insecure attachment, which in the medium term, is linked to impaired interpersonal functioning. These deficiencies in relationships are not completely irreversible and may be ameliorated by good-quality care received after separation. Confounding factors often associated with parenting breakdown (e.g. child abuse, marital conflict, parental psychopathology) make it more difficult to draw direct inferences.

How is attachment related to psychopathology in childhood? A number of studies show an association between insecure attachment during early childhood and behaviour problems (mainly oppositional defiant disorder) at school age. But the links between the two variables are far more complex. It is doubtful that insecure attachment *alone* leads to a disorder. The aetiology and the developmental trajectory of most childhood mental health problems are multifactorial and the same disorder may arise out of a combination of different factors and through different pathways (the principle of equifinality). Insecure attachment in early childhood is best conceptualised as a *risk factor* for a number of childhood disorders which, in combination with other vulnerability factors such as family dysfunction, poor parental management or difficult child temperament, may give rise to later childhood psychopathology. Secure attachment, on the other hand, appears to be a protective factor against the development of childhood disorders.

Attachment and psychopathology in adulthood

There is little empirical data linking attachment insecurity and later adult psychopathology, although poor quality of early caregiving – neglect, abuse, rejection and disrupted parenting – is associated with most forms of psychopathology ranging from depression to personality disorders. Deficient parenting is often accompanied by a variety of other adversities so that it is difficult to single out the role of attachment difficulties in the genesis of the disorder. Borderline personality disorder (BPD) is a case in point. Up to three quarters of persons diagnosed as showing BPD report physical and sexual abuse and prolonged separation from parents in early childhood. While it is tempting to conclude that the factor common to all the above situations is insecure attachment or dysfunctional IMWs, there is little evidence to support such an assertion. The same is true of antisocial personality disorder, depression and anorexia nervosa.

Maternal deprivation is an outdated concept and is mentioned here purely for historical reasons. In one of his early studies, *Forty-four Juvenile Thieves*, Bowlby (1944) noted that a subgroup who had experienced prolonged separation from parents after six months of age exhibited features of 'affectionless psychopathy'. Later, in a report he prepared for the WHO on the effects of institutionalisation on children after the Second World War he described a similar behaviour pattern. His finding was that institutionalised children grew up to be unfeeling, angry and hostile, showing superficial relationships and antisocial tendencies. These observations led

Bowlby to overestimate his case. In 1951 he wrote, 'mother love in infancy and childhood is as important for mental health as are vitamins and proteins for physical health' (Bowlby, 1951).

In a major review and reassessment of Bowlby's work, Rutter (1972) objected to the use of the words 'maternal' and 'deprivation' and the other aspects of Bowlby's assertions and concluded that:

- The effects of separation from the mother described by Bowlby were due to privation (lack of something) rather than deprivation (loss of something).
- The long-term effects described by Bowlby were due to the lack of attachment formation with *anyone*, not just the mother.
- Attachment formation is not always with the mother; attachment may form between the child and any primary caregiver with whom the child has continuous interaction.
- Adverse family circumstances, neglect and abuse were factors as important as disruption of parenting in leading to childhood difficulties.
- What matters is whether the child experiences a safe, secure and stable placement *after* separation from the parent. In such conditions *most* children develop normally and form secure attachments with their new carers, especially if the move occurred in the first few years of the child's life.

Attachment disorders

DSM-IV and ICD–10 refer to pervasive disturbance in social relatedness arising in early childhood (usually before the age of five years) as *attachment disorders*. Two types of attachment disorders have been described: (1) inhibited type; and (2) disinhibited type. In the former the child is withdrawn and avoids social interactions or is hypervigilant, while in the latter children show a lack of selective attachment together with indiscriminate over-sociability. Attachment disorder is associated with pathogenic caregiving as seen in repeated change of caregivers, emotional, sexual and physical abuse, severe neglect, institutional upbringing and severe parental psychopathology, such as severe and prolonged maternal depression. There is general agreement that the description and classification of attachment disorders in DSM-IV is rather simplistic and it is bound to be revised in the next edition.

DEVELOPMENT OF PLAY, EMOTIONS AND LANGUAGE

Children's play

During infancy, children spend much of their time exploring the environment than playing with it. Exploration dominates infants' behaviours for the first nine months of life. By 18 months play accounts for more and more of the child's interaction with the environment. Different aspects of play have been described:

- Sensorimotor play – the infant plays with objects (e.g. shaking a rattle); occurs around six months.
- Pretend or symbolic play – here one object is understood to stand for another (e.g. a piece of stick stands for a cigarette) or pretending something exists where it does not (e.g. speaking to grandma over a toy phone); evident by two years.

Children's play has also been categorised according the quality of interaction with peers:

- *Solitary play* – the child plays on its own.
- *Parallel play* – the child plays along side other children carrying out the same activities.
- *Cooperative play* – child interacts with others in complementary ways, sharing, turn taking and negotiating with other children. This is usually evident by three years.
- *Rule-governed play* – children understand the rules of games; starts around five years.

Drawing and copying

Copying is a skill that the normal child learns from three years and gets consolidated as the child starts attending nursery. It forms an important aspect of developmental assessment.

Figure 12.3 shows the progression of copying abilities in a highly simplified form. Children's ability to draw human figures has been used as a nonverbal method of assessing their general cognitive abilities. A standardised form of this is the *Goodenough draw-a-man test*. Here the children are asked to draw a man as best as they can. The drawing is scored according to guidelines provided in the test. The greater the details in the drawing the greater the score. For example, a four year old's drawings usually consist of two body parts, the head and arms ('the tadpole stage') whereas a six year old is able to draw a person with a head, neck and hands.

Emotional development

The newborn shows a surprising capacity for emotional expression. Most emotions and feelings are evident in the first three months. The primary emotions of joy, sadness, anger, fearfulness, disgust and surprise are present within the first six months of life and develop over the next three years. Fearfulness of strangers peaks at around 18 months.

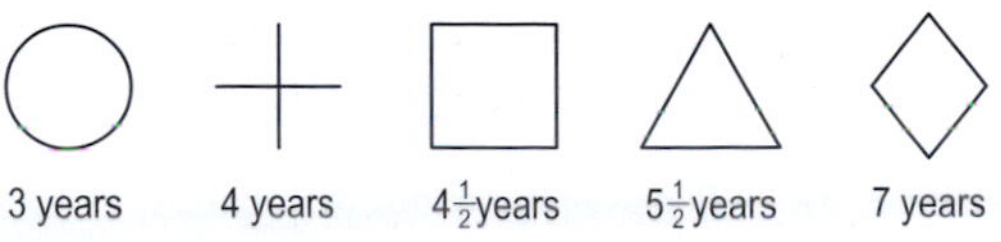

Fig. 12.3 Copying abilities of children according to average age of attainment

The infant's capacity to understand the emotional expressions of others, especially those of the mother, is highly developed. As mentioned above, newborns as young as two days can discriminate facial expressions such as those of happiness, surprise and sadness. Moreover, they have been observed to mirror such expressions. For example, when mothers pretend to be depressed, the infant adopts a sad face soon after. Self-conscious emotions (empathy, jealousy, guilt and shame) arise later, around three years. These emotions require a sense of self, a capacity that develops after 24 months.

Sense of self and self-recognition, the ability to experience ourselves, has been clearly demonstrated by the *rouge test*. In this test a spot of rouge is placed on the infant's nose and he is then placed in front of a mirror (Lewis & Brooks-Gunn, 1979). Up to the age of 24 months children do not show self-recognition, they appear to view the image as if it was another child. But about the age of two years a dramatic change seems to occur. Most 24-month-old children reach for their nose. This has been demonstrated in different cultures.

Fear in children

The prevalence of fear in children is markedly different compared to adults and follows two developmental trends from infancy to late childhood. In general, the overall frequency and intensity of fear declines between late childhood and adolescence. Specific fears peak around three years and decline thereafter. The specific content of fears undergo change as the child gets older. That is, the type of fear varies with age (Table 12.6).

Children appear to show innate fear of some stimuli from infancy. At birth, the newborn infant shows an innate startle reflex to sudden or loud noises. They show a similar reaction to a sense of falling or sudden loss of physical support. They show a fear of any intense, sudden or unexpected stimulus. Between the ages of 6 and12 months (that is as soon as they can crawl) they show fear of height and depth. This was convincingly demonstrated by the classic experiments known as the 'visual cliff'.

The 'visual cliff' consists of an elevated glass platform divided into two sections by a centre board. The 'shallow' side has a checker-board pattern directly under the glass. On the 'deep' end the pattern is placed several feet below the glass creating the illusion of a sharp drop or 'visual cliff'. The child is placed on the centre board and persuaded by the mother to cross both the

Table 12.6 Normal fears in childhood

0–6 months	Loss of support, falling, loud noises
7–12 months	Strangers, sudden and unexpected objects
1 year	Separation from parents, strangers
2–3 years	Dark, animals, thunder
5–8 years	Supernatural things (e.g. ghosts, monsters, TV creatures)
9–12 years	Bodily injury, disasters

shallow and deep sides. Most infants six months or older cross the shallow side but not the deep side, showing that, by the crawling age, most infants: (1) perceive depth; and (2) are afraid of heights (Gibson & Walk, 1960).

Infants develop a fear of strangers when they are around six months of age and stranger fear peaks at around twelve months. This coincides with the ability of the infants to recognise faces of familiar figures. Fear of strangers declines after the age of three years. Around the age of one year children become fearful of animals despite previous familiarity. Fear of animals peaks at around three years before declining after four years. Children develop a fear of darkness, ghosts and imaginary creatures about the age of five years. In middle childhood fear of bodily harm and disasters are more prominent. Thus, fear is universal in children (and adults), the contents of fear appears to follow a discontinuous developmental course. It should be noted that there is great individual variability in the tendency of children to show fear or timidity.

Between middle childhood and adolescence two trends have been observed: (1) fears concerning physical danger (fear of injury, danger, death, medical situations and fear of the unknown) and punishment show a distinct decline; and (2) social-evaluative fears (fear of failure and fear of criticism) show a marked increase. The latter observation has lead to the suggestion that social anxiety disorders, seen in adolescence, are related to this increase in normally occurring fears. It is worth noting that the average age of onset of social phobia is in the mid-teens.

Speech and language development

Research into language development has identified four basic elements that are thought to underlie all linguistic abilities:

1. *Speech sound production*. The smallest unit of sound that make up words is called a *phoneme*. Phonemes roughly correspond to letters in the alphabet. The English language has about 40 phonemes. Phonemes combine together to form *morphemes*, the smallest unit of language that has meaning (e.g. do, un-, dog). Words are made up of one or more morphemes.
2. *Syntax*. This refers to the conventions about combining words according to grammatical rules.
3. *Semantics*. This refers to the meaning conveyed by words and sentences.
4. *Pragmatics*. This is the conversational use of language in real social situations and different contexts.

Learning to communicate involves acquisition of the above expressive language skills as well as comprehension of speech and language. Moreover, the ability to understand and interpret non-verbal signals such as gestures and facial expression is an important aspect of communication.

Several phases of language acquisition have been described (Table 12.7):

- *Cooing*. By two months infants start producing sounds composed predominantly of vowels such as 'ooo' and 'aaa'.
- *Babbling*. The first speech sound that resembles ordinary speech such as

Table 12.7 Development of speech in infants and children

Babbling	6 months (4 to 10 months)
One-word stage ('mamma', 'doggie')	1 year (10 to 18 months)
Two-word stage ('mummy go')	2 years (18 to 24 months)
Basic adult grammatical sentence	3 years

'gaga' and 'dada' begin at about six months. Babbling at this stage is a universally observed phenomenon and is seen in all cultures. Babies who are deaf make the same speech-like sounds.

- *One-word stage*. At about 12 months babies start to make understandable one-word utterances such as 'mama', no, cat, and so on.
- *First sentences*. At around 18 months children start putting together two words to produce meaningful sentences, for example, 'daddy go' and 'mummy come'. This condensed form of speech has been referred to as 'telegraphic speech'.
- *Complex sentences*. By three years children start using three-to-four-word sentences with verbs that are generally understood by all adults. At this stage the 'wh' questions (who, why, where) are common.
- *Adult speech*. By five years of age the child starts speaking in fully formed grammatical sentences similar to adult speech.

The rapidity with which linguistic skills are acquired is one of the most remarkable feats of the human species. Within a short span of four to five years the child has achieved mastery of phonology, syntax, grammar and pragmatics. This unique ability is achieved seemingly effortlessly and without systemic instruction. How children attain this spectacular achievement is unclear and controversy surrounds all theories of language acquisition. Reinforcement and modelling by parents and others do play a part, but this does not provide a complete explanation. Chomsky (1965) has proposed that human beings are born with a *language acquisition device* (LAD) that enables children to gather information about the rules of language usage.

Specific developmental disorders of speech and language in children (SDLD)

This is a group of disorders in which children exhibit isolated deficits in language development that are not due to other conditions like autism or mental retardation. In SDLD impairment of language acquisition is usually evident by early childhood, usually by two years. These children are of average intelligence but their verbal abilities are significantly below other cognitive abilities and non-verbal IQ. SDLD is a heterogeneous group that includes three clinical categories: (1) articulation disorder (persistent difficulties in articulation); (2) expressive language disorder (limited speech output); and (3) receptive language disorder (language comprehension below expected levels). It is necessary to exclude other causes of speech and language delay

Box 12.4 Causes of impaired speech and language in children

1. Hearing impairment and neurological conditions
2. Extreme psychosocial deprivation
3. Mental retardation (learning disability, global)
4. Specific developmental disorders of speech and language (SDLD)
   - Specific speech articulation disorder
   - Expressive language disorder
   - Receptive language disorder
5. Autism and other pervasive developmental disorders
6. Elective (selective) mutism

before diagnosing SDLD (Box 12.4 provides a list of conditions in which language delay may occur).

Psychosexual development

Before discussing psychosexual development it is important to distinguish between three related concepts:

1. *Gender identity* is the person's concept and awareness of themselves as male or female.
2. *Sex-typed behaviour* refers to the behaviour that is thought to be associated with members of each sex within a culture. Gender or sex role is a closely related concept that includes attitudes and roles in society.
3. *Sexual orientation* refers to sexual object choice (i.e. homosexual or heterosexual).

Children develop an understanding of whether they are male or female (i.e. gender identity) by about three years of age. They also become aware that it is permanent and will not change. Although there is considerable individual variation, gender identity is well established before children develop full awareness of the genital basis of sex differences. About the same time, around the age of three to four years, there are considerable observable differences in the behaviour of boys and girls: boys show preferences for rough and tumble play, choose toys like guns and trucks and fire engines; girls typically like doll play and dressing up. Whether these reflect existing cultural practices and expectations or biological predispositions is open to debate.

From the foregoing account it should be clear that by the age of three most children show remarkable development in various spheres. The main developmental landmarks that occur at the age of three years are summarised in Box 12.5.

Box 12.5 Developmental capabilities of an average three-year-old child

- Copies a circle
- Uses basic grammatical sentences
- Shows cooperative play
- Has sexual identity
- Has fear of animals and dark

COGNITIVE DEVELOPMENT

Cognition is the general term used to designate all the processes involved in 'knowing'. Cognitive activities are largely non-observable and have to be inferred from behaviourally observable phenomena. The distinction between the *contents* of human cognitions and the nature of cognitive *processes* is a useful one. The content versus process distinction is an important one in cognitive psychology for psychology is concerned more with processes (*how* mental activities occur) than the contents of cognitions (*what* the activities are), which are rightfully the domains of linguists, mathematicians and the like.

Thus, while developmental psychology seeks to provide descriptions of *what* develops, it goes beyond characterisation to attempt to understand *how* mature ways of thinking emerge. While observations are sufficient for the former purpose, the latter requires developmental theories to explain the processes that drive development. This section deals with how children's abilities to think and reason change from infancy to adulthood and the factors that influence them. There are three major theories or approaches to the study and understanding of cognitive development:

1. Piaget's cognitive theory.
2. Social constructionist theories (e.g. Vygotsky).
3. Information processing theories.

Of all the models and theories Piaget's theory is the most popular and influential. It is discussed in some detail, while others are mentioned in outline only.

PIAGET'S THEORY OF COGNITIVE DEVELOPMENT

Jean Piaget was a zoologist by training. He was a precocious child who published his first scientific article, about an albino sparrow, at the age of ten. By the age of 15 he had several publications (about shellfish) to his credit. When he took to studying children's thinking he used two basic methods: observations and clinical interviews. Often this involved presenting children (including his own) with tasks to test their ways of thinking. Piaget was struck by the finding that the mistakes children made on cognitive tasks were systematic – most children of a given age range made the same mistakes. He concluded that children were not just less knowledgeable than adults but how they thought was qualitatively different.

Piaget's explanation of cognitive development rests on two conceptual pillars: cognitive structures and adaptation. *Cognitive structures* are understood in terms of schemes and operations. *Schemes* (or schema) are basic units of knowledge, organised patterns of thoughts and actions consisting of internal representations and generalisations. The other structure identified by Piaget is *operations*, which refers to mental actions that develop later in life (around the age of seven) as the child begins to understand the logical rules of how the environment 'works'. This invariably involved an understanding of rules such as reversibility and classification or grouping. Schemes and operations undergo change, modification, become more complex and sophisticated as children develop.

Adaptation. This refers, as in biology, to the process of adjustment and modification to the demands of the environment. Adaptation of cognitive schema, according to Piaget, is achieved through two processes: assimilation and accommodation.

Assimilation. This is the process by which new experiences, (new ideas or objects) are understood by incorporating them into already existing schemas. It refers to 'taking in' experiences and making them a part of what already exists (akin to assimilation of food). Thus, a child who has a grasping schema for the mother's finger eventually generalises it to grasping other objects. When a child encountering a horse for the first time calls it a 'doggie' he is applying the general schema that he already has for a four-legged animal (doggie) to the new four-legged creature that he has just encountered.

Accommodation. This is the complementary process in which the schema is modified to fit new experiences into it. Taking the above example, where the child encounters a horse, when the child begins to call the bigger four-legged animal 'horsie' a fundamental change has occurred in his or her thinking. Here new information has been fed back to the schema and, consequently, the schema has been modified. In real life, both assimilation and accommodation occur with every interaction with the environment – some knowledge is simply added on and existing units of knowledge altered, leading to growth and change.

According to Piaget, as development proceeds through the various stages, schemas undergo change and underlying each stage is a new category of schema. The motivational force that drives the child's cognitive development on to a higher and more flexible level is known as *equilibration*.

Piaget's stages of development

Piaget held that, through a process of continuous accommodation and assimilation, children progress through a series of stages of cognitive development

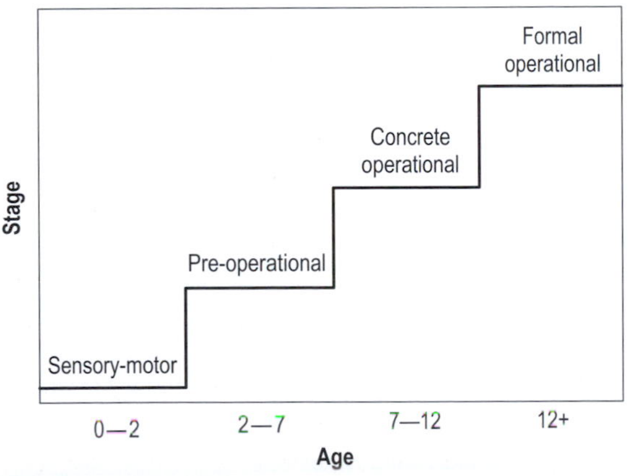

Fig. 12.4 The Piagetian stage model

(Figure 12.4). Intelligence and thinking do not develop on a quantitative basis (i.e. a change in the *amount* of knowledge held), but rather the changes that occur during development are qualitative. That is, cognitive development is discontinuous. Although Piaget associated age ranges with each stage, these were intended as averages and variations have been acknowledged. More important is the fact that although the rate at which a child moves through each stage may vary from child to child, the order in which they progress is fixed or invariant. Each stage has to be achieved before proceeding to the next one.

Piaget described four stages, each subdivided into several substages. Only the four main stages are described here (Table 12.8).

Stage 1: Sensorimotor stage (approximately 0–2 years, corresponding to 'infancy'). During this period the infant's mental efforts are focused upon sensory experiences (hearing, seeing and motor skills – grasping and sucking). Infants discover that they can make things happen (circular reactions), they begin to distinguish between themselves and other objects. Towards the end of this stage, the child begins to acquire the ability to represent objects and people symbolically. The achievement of *object permanence* is the highlight of the sensorimotor stage – infants learn that objects exist even when they are no longer visible. Around 18 months, and not until then, they look for a hidden object in places other than where they last saw it, thus providing proof that they have capacity for mental representation.

Stage 2: Preoperational thinking (approximately 2–7 years). This stage is characterised by development of language and the capacity for symbolic thought. At this stage the children are capable of pretend play and of understanding that one may be represented by another. But their thinking is typically dominated by egocentrism, centration and irreversibility. Piaget's

Table 12.8 Summary of Piaget's stages of cognitive development

Stage (average age)	*Important tasks*	*Experiment*
Sensorimotor (birth–2 years)	Circular reactions Development of Object permanence (18 months) Beginning of symbolic thought	Hiding objects
Preoperational (2–7 years)	Egocentrism Centration Irreversibility	Mountain task Conservation tasks
Concrete operational (7–11 years)	Attains most conservation operations Unable to use abstract concepts	Classification of objects according to rules (seriation)
Formal operational (11 + years)	Capable of abstract thought, e.g. deductive reasoning, hypothesis testing	Pendulum experiment

experiments with children illustrating these features have become the most famous in developmental psychology.

Egocentrism refers to the tendency to view the world from one's own perspective and the inability to understand the world from other people's point of view. Piaget illustrated egocentric thinking with his famous *mountain task*. In this the child is presented with a model of a mountain scene consisting of three mountains (remember Piaget is Swiss) and asked what an observer would see from a vantage point different from that of the child. This is usually carried out by placing a doll in different positions and getting the child to describe what the doll would see (e.g. a hidden church, cows and so on). Typically children under the age of eight years assume that others share their viewpoint and find it impossible to take a perspective different from their own.

Centration is the bias towards focusing attention on only one aspect of a situation and the inability to attend to other features. Piaget's famous *conservation tasks* strikingly demonstrate the deficiencies in preoperational reasoning. The aim of these experiments is to get the child to judge quantities that remain the same in spite of changes in appearances. A typical example involves showing two identical glasses with equal amounts of liquid and then pouring the liquid from one glass into a taller thinner glass. The preoperational child would say that the taller glass has more liquid because the level has risen higher. The child has difficulty understanding that despite appearances the quantity remains the same because none has been added or taken away. By a series of experiments Piaget showed that during this stage the child has not grasped the concept of conservation of volume, mass, number, length, area and weight (see Figure 12.5).

Stage 3: Concrete operational stage (7–11 years; primary school years). From 7–11 years children start achieving conservation. They are successful in

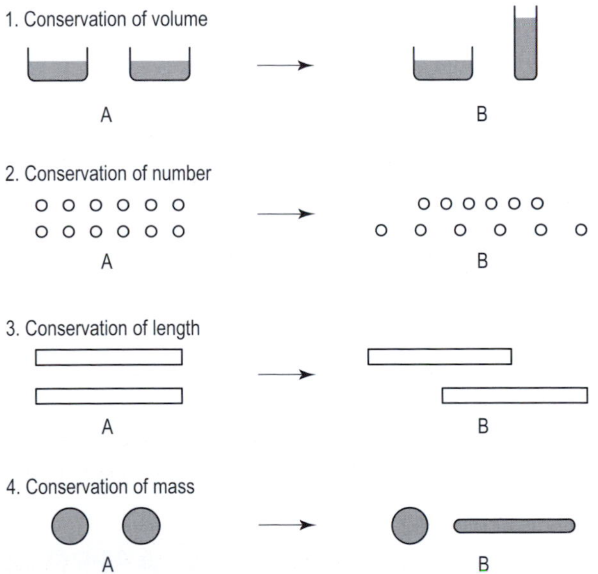

Fig. 12.5 Piaget's conservation tasks: the preoperational child (2–7 years) does not realise that certain properties of objects, e.g. volume, number, length and mass, remain unchanged when the objects' appearances are altered

conservation tasks involving numbers, quantity and volume by 7 to 8 years. Thus, they are operational and are able to work out complex logical and mathematical rules. But there is an important limitation. These operations are successful only as long as they concern real objects. For example, they are able to *classify* objects into categories according to rules, size, weight, and so on (seriation). These operations are concrete insofar as they are concerned with real objects. However, they are unable to apply strategies to abstract situations (like 'A is taller than B, B is shorter than C, who is the shortest?') although they have no difficulty in accomplishing the task when given dolls named A, B and C. Conservation of weight is attained much later, about 9 or 10 years for the same reason.

Stage 4: Formal operational stage: (11 years onwards; secondary or high school years). This stage is characterised by the emergence of abstract reasoning, logical thinking and hypothesis testing. Children at this stage are able to solve abstract problems (such as the height of A, B and C above) and can reason purely verbally. They can hypothesise and proceed to test hypotheses systematically. The *pendulum task* illustrates this ability. Given a set of weights and a string that can be shortened or lengthened, the subject is asked to work out what determines the time taken to complete one oscillation of the pendulum. The child in the formal operational stage proceeds systematically to test all the factors that may affect the frequency of oscillations, length of string, weight of the object, the force of the push and so on. Thus at this stage the individual is able to think about many possible eventualities, thereby promoting deductive reasoning and hypothesis testing. Moreover they are able to think about thinking – an activity known as metacognition. (Piaget's stages of cognitive development are summarised in Table 12.8.)

Piaget's claims have been subject to retesting and reinterpretation. Although Piaget's findings have been largely confirmed, it is now believed that Piaget underestimated the capabilities of children in the sensorimotor stage. In the preoperational stage, children have been shown to perform better in the mountain experiment when the experiment is redesigned as 'the naughty boy and the policeman' task. It has been argued that the latter task was more child-friendly (Donaldson, 1978). As for the formal operation stage, it is now known that only about 30% of adolescents and some adults reach this stage at all. A second criticism that has been made of Piaget is that he was concerned with cognitive development and that he ignored social factors in development. His experiments rarely or never involved people from the social world of the child, such as the mother, peers or even teachers. He treated the emergence of social knowledge as no different from other forms of knowledge. His theory is based on the assumption that the individual child constructs his or her own knowledge. In spite of the many criticisms of Piaget's theory, his influence in the field of developmental psychology has remained undiminished, especially in the field of education.

VYGOTSKY: THE SOCIOCULTURAL APPROACH

Working independently, Vygotsky, a Russian psychologist, came to the conclusion that the child, as an active agent, constructs knowledge by interpersonal activity, most notably by interaction with other more knowledgeable people in the environment. Vygotsky assigned a central role to social processes in intellectual development. The sociocultural approach goes further than the Piagetian constructionism, by stating that although the child arrives in the world through activity (as Piaget suggests) the nature of the activity is primarily one of social exchange embedded in the social context from the very beginning of life. Vygotsky's theory is an elaborate one and only some aspects of it are mentioned here.

Zone of proximal development. A fundamental tenet of Vygotsky's theory is the *zone of proximal development* (ZPD). Vygotsky defined ZPD as 'the distance between the actual developmental level, as determined by independent problem solving, and the level of potential development, as determined through problem solving under adult guidance or in collaboration with more capable peers'. It refers to the area between actual ability in any one domain and the potential level of ability that could be achieved with assistance from an adult. Vygotsky holds that what children can do with the assistance of others might in some sense be even more indicative of their mental development than what they can do alone (Vygotsky, 1978). This has two important applications: (1) assessment of the child's abilities should include both the actual developmental level and the ZPD; and (2) the caregivers need to fashion their interventions to keep the task within the child's ZPD for them to be effective.

Scaffolding. Vygotsky emphasised the role of instruction as providing a framework (scaffolding) within which children's thinking and learning development. The more able person is seen as providing the scaffolding within which the child works to build its understanding. Therefore, the more assistance that it has from adults and peers the better the accomplishments of the child. Thus, parents and teachers play an important role in the child's intellectual growth.

Speech and 'inner speech'. Piaget insists that language plays no role in the development of thinking. For Vygotsky, thinking is a social process mediated by signs and language plays a central role in development of thinking. Signs are employed by individuals as psychological tools to mediate between higher mental activity (thinking) and action. Although thoughts originate in the child's biological development, language originates in social interactions with the adults in the external world. An important aspect of Vygotsky's theory is the evolution of 'inner speech' (conversations that do not take others into account). Used originally for communication with others, later they become directed internally.

MORAL DEVELOPMENT

Morality is a fundamental and pervasive aspect of human functioning. It involves both interpersonal and intrapersonal components. In its interpersonal sphere it involves other people's rights and welfare, while in the intrapersonal domain it is concerned with basic ethical standards. Morality entails dynamic interaction of emotions (feelings associated with guilt and trust), cognitions (distinguishing right from wrong) and behaviour (acting on the beliefs about right and wrong). The study of moral development has been dominated by the cognitive approach and Kohlberg's (1984) moral stage theory in particular.

A prerequisite for moral reasoning is the cognitive ability for abstract thought. As children grow up they come to rely less on external discipline and more on deeply held beliefs. According to Kohlberg they go through six stages (grouped into three levels) of moral reasoning. In a long-term study of young men interviewed periodically over two decades their moral development was judged on how they analysed hypothetical dilemmas. The most famous of these was the *Heinz dilemma,* in which the subjects had to judge whether a man named Heinz should steal an expensive drug to save his wife who is suffering from cancer. It was not their decision that was important; rather, what mattered was how they justified it. Based on answers to such stories from people of all ages and socio-economic backgrounds, Kohlberg identified three levels of moral development, each consisting of two stages. According to Kohlberg, people proceed through these invariant stages in the same order (Table 12.9).

Kohlberg's theory singles out adolescence (conventional level) as the phase during which moral reasoning undergoes a qualitative change by internalisation of parental and societal rules. Research findings largely support Kohlberg's stages. Cross-cultural studies have confirmed the universal applicability of Kohlberg's stages. But few, if any, people reach the sixth and most advanced stage in which their view is based purely on abstract principles.

Does moral reasoning lead to moral behaviour? The key issue is what makes people live up to their ideals, or not. Recent studies have focused on situational dilemmas (e.g. reward) and hypothetical morality (as predicted by

Table 12.9 Kohlberg's six stages of moral development and typical answers to Heinz dilemma

	Level 1: Pre-conventional (7–12 years to middle childhood)	
Stage 1	Obedience and punishment orientation	'I will not do it, because I don't want to get punished'
Stage 2	Individualism and Exchange	'I won't do it because I want the reward'
	Level 2: Conventional (approximately 13–16 years)	
Stage 3	Maintaining good interpersonal relationships; being a good person	'I won't do it because I want people to like me'
Stage 4	Maintaining social order and law	'I won't do it because it would break the law'
	Level 3: Post-conventional (approximately 16–20 years)	
Stage 5	Social contracts and individual rights	'I won't do it because I am obliged not to'
Stage 6	Universal principles of justice	'I won't do it because it is not right, no matter what the others say'

Kohlberg's stages). There appears to be a moderately positive link between the two. Admittedly, the relationship between rational thinking and behaviour is a complex one and is subjected to various influences.

DEVELOPMENT OF SOCIAL COGNITIONS AND THEORY OF MIND

Cognitive psychologists make a distinction between object cognition and social cognition. *Object cognition* is that pertaining to our thinking about inanimate physical objects. Most of Piaget's experiments are related to object cognitions. *Social cognitions*, on the other hand, embrace all cognitive processes involved in understanding the social world and social environment, especially the behaviour of other people and oneself. Moral reasoning, perception of others (person perception), empathy and comprehension of others' emotions belong to the realms of social cognitions. Social cognitions form an important part of day-to-day social interactions, personal relationships and interpersonal functioning, and are, therefore, vital to the study of human behaviour. Only one particular area of interest, the theory of mind, is dealt with here.

Theory of mind

Understanding other people's minds is a fundamental human skill that is acquired early in life, around four years of age. Since other people's mental states – beliefs, desires and intentions – are not directly observable, the child is seen as one who forms a hypothesis, or a theory of mind. Simply stated, theory of mind refers to the child's understanding of thoughts, beliefs, desires and intentions of others. Acquisition of 'theory of mind' is central to interpersonal understanding. Before understanding other people's minds the child has to understand that different thoughts can be held by different people about one and the same thing. These insights into the mind of others help the child to acknowledge that people hold factual beliefs about reality and that these beliefs determine their behaviour. Since testing a child for true beliefs does not help us to test the theory of mind (for it tests reality rather than belief) a test of theory of mind has to be based on a task that dissociates belief from reality. *False-belief tests* are designed to achieve precisely this. First-order false-belief tests are designed to infer what someone else is thinking. Second-order tests are about understanding what one character thinks another character is thinking.

Wimmer and Perner's (1983) experiment with young children's ability to appreciate that other people can have false beliefs is considered to be a seminal piece of work in developmental psychology and has paved the way for other false-belief tests. In this study, a boy called Maxi puts his chocolate in a blue cupboard in the kitchen. He leaves the scene and his mother who comes in later transfers the chocolate to a green cupboard in the kitchen. Children were asked what Maxi would *do* when he came to look for the chocolate. Most older children said that Maxi would look in the place where he left his chocolate (blue cupboard), while children under four judged it to be in the place where they knew it was (green cupboard). Thus, older children seem to understand about false beliefs, while the young ones do not.

Several variations of Wimmer and Perner's original false-belief tests have been employed with groups of children. Baron-Cohen, Leslie and Firth (1985) employed a false-belief test called the *Sally–Ann test*. It consists of the following scenario:

Scene: There are two dolls, Sally and Ann. Sally has a basket and Ann has a box. As the child watches, the experimenter makes Sally put her marbles into her basket and makes her leave the scene. In her absence, Ann transfers the marbles to her own box. A little later, Sally comes back into the room.

Question to the child: Where were the marbles in the beginning? (Reality and memory question.)

Correct answer: In the basket.

Question to the child: Where will Sally look for the marbles? (Belief question.)

Correct answer: In the basket.

All studies have unequivocally demonstrated that children below the age of four years fail the test and that, by implication, they lack a 'theory of mind'. More than 85% of four-year-old children give the correct answer. Tests carried out with children in different cultures, including those living in preliterate societies, show that these findings are universal.

Acquiring a 'theory of mind' during the course of development appears to serve at least two important functions:

1. To make sense of social behaviour. The ability to attribute intentions and desires to people's actions helps one to understand and predict the behaviour of others.
2. To make sense of communication. Non-verbal communication is understood through interpretation of what the person has in mind, including beliefs, desires and intentions.

Autism and deficits in theory of mind

There is a considerable body of evidence to demonstrate that children with autism have a specific theory-of-mind deficit. They exhibit significant deficiencies in attributing beliefs, desires and intentions, as shown by results of false-belief tests. In the Sally–Ann test 80% of autistic children (five years and over) fail to answer the question correctly, while the majority of a control group of five-year-old normal children and children with Down's syndrome, having a mental age of five years, had no difficulties in passing the test. The inevitable conclusion is that the autistic child's lack of understanding of the mind cannot be explained on the basis of any learning difficulties that they may have. This circumscribed, but pervasive, cognitive deficit is hypothesised to account for the social and communicative dysfunction in autism, as well as deficits in empathy and pretend play (Baron-Cohen, 1989).

ADOLESCENT DEVELOPMENT

Adolescence is considered to be a transitional phase between childhood and adulthood. It lasts approximately from 10 to 20 years but it is the teenage years that are thought of as typical adolescence. The early years from approximately 10 to 13 years are dominated by pubertal changes, the middle phase from 14 to 16 by issues of identity and the late teens from 17 to 20 by transition to adulthood. There is wide individual variation in the timing of these phases. For the young person this is a period of dramatic change and challenge. It requires adjustment to biological, psychological and social changes in self.

Psychological changes

One way of approaching the issues that the adolescent is faced with is to look at the tasks that he or she has to achieve during this period.

Developmental tasks of adolescents

The number of 'tasks' that the adolescent has to achieve during the short period from 13 years to 18 years are many and varied – the mastery of some of them extends into early adulthood. Some of the more important developmental tasks facing adolescents are to:

- Adapt to bodily changes and cope with sexual development and drive.
- Establish a firm sense of personal identity.
- Strive for autonomy and separation from their family.
- Develop appropriate peer relationships.
- Develop career focus.
- Develop appropriate moral standards.
- Prepare for mature sexual relationships.

Development of identity

In Erik Erikson's eight-stage model of psychosocial development, adolescence is seen as a pivotal period (Erikson, 1968). He considered the formation of identity the essential and fundamental task of adolescence. According to him the young person goes through a stage of psychosocial development in which the crisis is characterised as 'identity versus role confusion' which occurs around 12 to 18 years of age. During this period creating and consolidating ones own personal identity is seen as the major task facing the person. Establishment of a strong sense of self or ego identity is thought to be the central goal of adolescents. Erikson held that the adolescents try out various roles and 'identities' in different domains before finally committing themselves. In each of these domains the adolescent would first experience identity diffusion, followed by experimentation, and culminating in identity formation involving integration and consolidation.

Erikson's formulations have gained general acceptance over the last 30 years. His theory, based mainly on clinical observations, has been expanded and clarified by James Marcia (1980). Marcia developed a semi-structured interview to assess the identity status in such domains as occupation, political belief, sexual attitudes and religion. Studies have shown that 'identity status' is broadly age related.

'Adolescent turmoil'

Contrary to popular conception of adolescence as a period of 'storm and stress', of high anxiety and turmoil, empirical studies into the world of adolescents paint a different picture. The vast majority of adolescents go through adolescent years without great misery, sadness or turmoil. Both parent and self-reports provide little support for the 'storm and stress' theory. In the Isle of Wight study (Rutter, 1976), involving over 2300 adolescents between the ages of 14 and 15 years, definite psychiatric disorders were present in roughly 10% of the sample. (In 11 year olds the figure was about 7%). Numerous researches carried out since the Rutter study attest to the fact that adolescent turmoil is not the rule although a significant minority show evidence of it in the form of distress, depression and confusion. In the words of Rutter, 'Adolescent turmoil is a fact, not a fiction, but its psychiatric importance has probably been overestimated in the past' (Rutter et al., 1976).

Biological changes

The onset of puberty and its effects on the body are a major challenge for the adolescent. Puberty is not an event but a process that begins before the onset of menstruation in girls (or the time of first ejaculation in boys) and lasts for variable periods thereafter. The appearance and progression of secondary sexual characteristics occur in a predictable sequence. The physical changes of puberty are usually described in line with Tanner's stages of growth of breasts and pubic hair. This ensures that descriptions are uniform and standardised (Tanner, 1990).

In western countries, menarche in girls occurs approximately at 12.5 years. There has been a decline in western countries in the age of menarche over the last hundred years from sixteen in the 1860s to around thirteen in the 1960s. This secular trend is thought to be due to the improved nutritional status of society in general.

An interesting finding that has emerged in recent studies is the causal link between pubertal development and relationships within the family. Several studies have shown that the quality of family relationships affect the timing and course of puberty, with faster maturation observed among adolescents raised in homes characterised by less closeness and more conflict (Kim & Smith, 1998) and among girls from homes in which the biological father is not present.

There have been attempts to link adolescent moodiness with pubertal changes and changing hormone levels. The evidence for such correlation is quite weak and studies indicate that puberty is not characterised by 'raging' hormones. The relationship between changing hormone levels and variations in adolescent mood is rather slim.

Social changes

Adolescents and their peers

Peer groups is a term that refers to a limited number of similar-aged adolescents who develop close relationships and identify with one another. (Friendships, in contrast, are close two-person relationships.) During adolescence peer relationships are on the increase as the young person spends more time interacting with those of his/her own age, both at school and outside.

In a typical week, secondary school children spend twice as much time with peers as with parents or adults. For this reason peers have been called the 'second family'. In childhood and early adolescence the peer group typically consists of children of the same sex. A distinct change occurs in middle and late adolescence in the composition of the peer group as the groups tend to be made up of both males and females. Forming successful peer relationships is a crucial aspect of development. Peer influences on adolescents can be both negative and positive. Adolescents in dysfunctional and less cohesive families are more influenced by peers than by parents, i.e. peer factors are more important in less adaptive families or problem families. Peer groups serve several important functions. Peers are important in the establishment of identity of the young person and the reaffirmation of values. They provide emotional support and facilitate exploration and adaptation to a social world that is less structured than the family.

The importance of peer influence in the development of social and personal competence was most powerfully demonstrated by Harlow in one of his experiments with rhesus monkeys. Harlow and his co-workers bred groups of young monkeys with their mothers but in isolation from their peers. The peer-deprived monkeys failed to develop normal patterns of socialisation and when exposed to same-age monkeys they tended to avoid them. When they did interact with them they were aggressive and antisocial. Such social impairment and peer-directed behaviour problems continued into their adult life (Suomi & Harlow, 1978).

Parent–adolescent relationships

Research into adolescent–parent relationship patterns has demolished the myth of adolescence as being the period fraught with tension, hostility and conflict between teenagers and parents. Several large-scale studies and surveys of adolescents and parents have reported that approximately 75% of families enjoy warm, caring and pleasant relations with adolescents (Offer, 1969). Nevertheless, a small proportion, between 5% to 10%, experiences dramatic deterioration in the quality of parent–child relationships. In the Isle of Wight study (Rutter, 1976) only one in six families reported regular arguments with adolescents. The so-called 'generation gap' has been shown to be a misnomer.

Adolescence as a period of vulnerability and risk

Adolescence is also a period of relatively high risk. A substantial minority of adolescents carry an increased risk of physical and psychiatric disorders. For example:

- The commonest cause of death in this age group is accidents. Adventure-seeking behaviour and rebelliousness against authority often account for such deaths.
- The onset of HIV and other sexually-transmitted diseases resulting from unprotected sex is more common in teenagers than in adults.
- Delinquency or offending behaviour reaches a peak in late teens (around 17 years) and declines thereafter (Farrington, 1995).
- Psychiatric disorders with specific onset in adolescence include major depression, anorexia nervosa and panic disorder. One in five cases of schizophrenia begins before the age of 18 years.

Child psychiatric disorders

In keeping with the philosophy of current classificatory systems, DSM-IV and ICD-10, the classification of childhood psychopathology is based on symptom clusters or syndromes, irrespective of presumed aetiology or causation. The broad outline framework of child and adolescent psychiatry is described briefly in the following paragraphs. The reader would benefit from reading the relevant sections from the excellent textbook by Goodman and Scott (1997).

The criteria for diagnosis of child and adolescent psychiatric disorders are two-fold:

1. Emotions or behaviour outside the normal range; *and*
2. Impaired functioning or development, *or* significant suffering to the child/family.

Most symptoms encountered in child mental health work are quantitative variations from normality – deficits or excesses that are inappropriate for the developmental stage. Some of the common misconceptions regarding childhood mental problems are:

1. Mental health problems are uncommon in childhood.
   - No, they are common. Most studies show that about 10–15% of children and adolescents fit the criteria for mental disorders.
2. Children and adolescents who have mental health problems grow out of them.
   - Not true. Up to 45–50% of problems persist into adulthood.

For practical purposes the main disorders can be placed in one of four groups:

1. Disruptive behaviour (externalising) disorders. These account for more than half the referrals to child mental health services and include conduct disorder, oppositional disorder and hyperkinetic disorder.

2. Emotional (internalising) disorders specific to childhood. These include attachment disorder and separation anxiety disorder.
3. Developmental disorders. This is a diverse group consisting of at least two clusters of conditions:
   a. Developmental delays. Here developmental pattern is normal but it has been arrested or retarded. It may be further divided into general (global) developmental delay (mental retardation) and specific developmental delays (e.g. specific reading retardation).
   b. Abnormal or deviant development. In certain conditions the developmental trajectory is abnormal or deviant. This is best illustrated by autism and other pervasive developmental disorders.
4. Disorders that are broadly similar to adult psychiatric disorders. Many disorders such as depression, eating disorders, various forms of anxiety and somatisation disorders occur in childhood and adolescence. A significant proportion of psychotic disorders have their onset in adolescence. Generally, they show similar features but there may be subtle adolescent variations.

ADULT DEVELOPMENT

Adopting a developmental perspective is the norm in dealing with mental health problems in children and adolescents. However, when it comes to adults, the tendency among most psychologists, psychiatrists and allied professionals has been to treat the whole of adult life from early adulthood to old age as a fixed and static phase of life. Adulthood is not the end point of development. Development does not stop with the cessation of physical growth. Psychological development continues throughout life until death. The course of adult life is punctuated by milestones that mark particular transitions, such as leaving home in late adolescence, courtship and marriage, parenting, and old age, to name but a few. At some of these nodal points in their life course individuals are more prone to physical illness, psychological distress and psychiatric disorders than at other times.

Two terms commonly used in life-span development are ‘transitions’ and ‘crisis’. *Transitions* imply gradual change from one stage to the other; the term *crisis* refers to turmoil resulting from rapid change. Transitions may or may not lead to crises. Two types of transitions have been described:

1. Normative changes. These are age-related changes common to all individuals. These events are shared by everyone and are, therefore, predictable. Getting married, securing an employment and having children are examples of normative changes that occur in most, if not all, people’s lives.
2. Non-normative changes. These are non-shared events that are unique to the individual. Illnesses, divorce, migration and loss of employment are non-normative life events. Such transitions are unexpected and tax the potential of the individual and are experienced usually as more stressful.

In addition, changes that have an effect on whole societies such as war and natural disasters affect people’s lives in a deep and profound way.

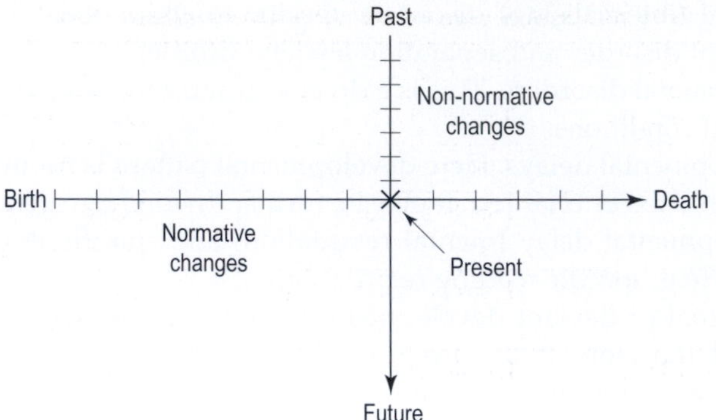

Fig. 12.6 The 'slide ruler of life' plotting the normative and non-normative life changes of individuals. Plotting the person's life course along these two dimensions is a useful exercise when answering the question, 'Why is this person presenting with these features at this particular point in time?'

Transitions, by their very nature, demand change but often they may go unnoticed and unacknowledged by the individual. Recognising transitions and making appropriate adjustments is a necessary part of life. Individuals can become 'stuck' at transitional moments and may present with psychological distress or symptoms. In clinical encounters a useful question to ask oneself is: 'what normative and non-normative life-cycle changes are being experienced by this person at the moment?' Figure 12.6 shows the 'the slide ruler of life'

Erickson's stages of psychosocial development

Of the several theories of adult development the 'eight stages of man' formulated by Erikson (1963, 1968) is the best known. Erikson was a psychoanalyst who, in the Freudian tradition, was interested in the development of the ego. But, unlike Freud, he applied the insights gained from his psychoanalytic knowledge to adult development. He differed from Freud in two important aspects. First, for Erikson development continued throughout life. Freudian emphasis on early childhood experience, important as that was, was not the only factor that shaped life. Second, Erikson held that intrapsychic factors alone were not sufficient to explain the course of development of the ego and any theory of development had to take the powerful role of the environment into consideration. Hence, he named the stages of development psychosocial stages in contrast to the psychosexual stages of Freud.

According to Erikson, psychological development continues throughout life and through eight stages (Table 12.10). Each stage is characterised by a crisis during which the individual has to achieve certain developmental tasks. For Erikson 'crisis' refers, not to a catastrophe, but to a turning point during which there is increased vulnerability as well as heightened potential for change and development. How well the individual negotiates these tasks determines their psychological well-being at any given point in time. Erikson proposed that psychological growth occurs in a sequence of invariant stages.

Table 12.10 Erikson's stages of psychosocial development (Erikson, 1968)

Age	*Life crisis*	*Outcomes*
Birth to about 18 months	Trust vs. mistrust	Hope/insecurity
18 months to 3 years	Autonomy vs. shame	Self-certainty/self-doubt
3–5 years	Initiative vs. guilt	Experimentation/fear of punishment, guilt
6–11 years	Industry vs. inferiority	Sense of achievement/inadequacy
Adolescence 12–18 years	Identity vs. role confusion	Strong personal identity/identity confusion
Young adulthood, 20–40 years	Intimacy vs. isolation	Love and commitment/superficial relationships
Middle adulthood, 40–60 years	Generativity vs. stagnation	Concern about public good/lack of growth
Late adulthood, 65 + years	Integrity vs. despair	Satisfaction/regret over omissions, fear of death

Each person is thought to go through the stages in the same order and, although each individual does it in ways that are unique to him or her, the tasks that are to be completed remain the same. In keeping with Freudian tradition he believed that each maturational task is never completely achieved and that subsequent events may trigger old developmental crises.

The main features of the eight stages of psychosocial development as propounded by Erikson have received broad support from research studies. There is general agreement that developmental changes continue to occur in one's personality and mental life throughout one's lifetime and, in particular, that identity formation during adolescence is pivotal to the development of later personality. A particular criticism of Erikson's theory is that it is heavily based on male identities, especially in the adult stages, and that for some women, relationships, and not careers, are more important. The various stages during adulthood are briefly mentioned below. Table 12.11 provides a comparison of the stages of development as described by Piaget, Freud and Erikson.

Early adulthood (intimacy vs. isolation, 20–40 years)

The inherent strength of this early stage is love and the major task is intimacy and the formation of a bond with a future partner. To accomplish this the individual needs to have, to a large extent, achieved a degree of separation from his/her parents and formed an identity in the preceding stage (identity vs. role confusion) of adolescence.

Early adulthood entails several developmental tasks and roles:

- Leaving home and the gradual physical and emotional separation from parents.

Table 12.11 Comparison of the stages of development as described by Freud, Erikson, Piaget, Kohlberg.

Age	*Freud*	*Erikson*	*Piaget*	*Kohlberg.*
0–18 months	Oral phase	Basic trust vs. mistrust	Sensory-motor (0–2 years)	
18 months–3 years	Anal phase	Autonomy vs. shame		
3–7 years	Phallic phase (3–5 or 6 years)	Initiative vs. guilt (3–5 years)	Preoperational stage (2–7 years)	
7–13 years	Latency phase (6–11 or 13 years)	Industry vs. inferiority (6–11 years)	Concrete operational stage (7–11 years)	Preconventional morality. Stage 1 and 2 (7–12 years)
13–20 years	Genital phase (13–adulthood)	Identity vs. role confusion (12–18 years)	Formal operational stage (11–adulthood)	Conventional morality Stage 1 and 2 (13–16) Post-conventional morality. Stage 1 and 2 (16–adult hood)
Young adulthood (20–40 years)		Intimacy vs. isolation		
Middle adulthood (40–65 years)		Creativity vs. stagnation		
Late adulthood (65 + years)		Integrity vs. despair		

- Finding a partner and formation of new attachments.
- Parenthood.
- Finding and 'settling down' in a career.
- Forming a network of friends and companions.

Forming romantic relationships, choosing a partner and committing oneself to a long-term relationship, in the form of marriage or living together, is one of the foremost tasks of early adulthood. Interpersonal attraction, love and marriage are areas that have been studied in some detail.

Interpersonal attraction and mate selection

Attraction towards a potential mate has been shown to be influenced by several factors. The most important factors are (Argyle & Henderson, 1985):

Attractiveness. Within a given culture there is a general agreement as to which individuals are most attractive. Men and women vary in what features they find attractive. Most studies have found that men rate physical attractiveness, sensuality and affection high, while females considered achievement, leadership and assertiveness more attractive.

Similarity. Contrary to the popular belief that 'opposites attract', all studies have shown that people are attracted to those who are *similar* to themselves in age, social class, height, intelligence, values and some personality traits. Dominant individuals tend to select dominant partners and submissive persons prefer submissive mates, but the overall correlations are rather small.

Support. Support from parents and family enhances romantic relationships.

Contact. Interpersonal attraction usually develops in the context of frequent contact between the two potential partners. Regular and repeated contact, socially or at work, sets the stage for self-disclosure and expression of love. Increase in time spent with the other person leads to intimate conversations and eventual sexual intimacy. Premarital sexual activity is determined by cultural norms.

Marriage and marital satisfaction

Dating, love affairs and courtship culminates in a more or less permanent relationship with a partner. In western countries, the great majority of people go out on dates and have affairs with a number of members of the opposite sex before eventually selecting a partner. A period of 'living together' or cohabitation precedes marriage in some cases.

Marital satisfaction

Marital and family therapists have drawn attention to closeness/distance differences between partners whose marriage is under strain. One way in which distance is regulated may be by the development of 'symptoms' in either of the partners or in a child. (Byng-Hall, 1980).

Marital satisfaction or happiness is a multidimensional concept and a number of questionnaires have been constructed to measure it. One of the best-known rating scales are the *Golombok–Rust inventories* of *sexual satisfaction* and *marital satisfaction* called the GRISS and GRIMS, respectively (Rust & Golombok, 1985; Rust et al., 1988). These are self-reported measures of sexual and marital satisfaction respectively and have been used extensively in research.

Two independent aspects of marital satisfaction have been highlighted by research:

1. Satisfaction – happiness, affection, sexual satisfaction, acting as confidant; and
2. Lack of criticism, argument and rows.

It is the sum total of these two factors – 'good times' spent together minus the frequency of rows that determines marital satisfaction. In short, frequent rows can ruin a marriage that is perceived as otherwise satisfying.

Marital conflicts

The very factors that promote intimacy and closeness – close contact over long periods of time, sharing finances, chores, and a life together – inevitably lead to conflicts. The common subjects (content) of marital conflicts are money ('he is not earning enough'; 'she spends too much'), sharing household duties ('he does not help with housework'; 'he is too tired all the time'), sex ('he only wants sex'; 'she always has headaches') and how to manage children ('she is too lenient'; 'he does not spend time with them').

Diversity of the 'family'

So far we have assumed that the 'family' is formed of a heterosexual couple with two or more children. This idealised version of the family ignores the varied forms of family relationships and does no justice to other adult–adult relationships that are seen in society. Prime examples of non-conventional forms of family are homosexual couples, childless couples and single parents and adults. There is a real danger of marginalising these groups by stereotyping the 'Dick and Jane' nuclear family with a working father, housewife mother and two or three children (Hill, 1987).

Feminists have challenged the earlier version of the family as 'a stable and universal institution composed of heterosexual parents and children living in complete harmony'. Certainly the structure and functions of the family have changed from the stage of hunter-gatherer society to the present one and will continue to change in future. The family needs to be studied and treated as it is, rather than what it should be. Next we consider divorce before discussing family functioning.

Divorce and separation

Rates of divorce have doubled over the last 25 years and one in three marriages now end in divorce in the UK. The rates are even higher in the USA. It is estimated that 20% of children experience the divorce of their parents before they reach the age of 16 and that 2.5 million children grow up in step-families. Divorce is now so common that some argue that it needs to be recognised as a normative event rather than an aberration of normal marital relationship.

Divorce is more common in some groups than others:

- People in the lower social classes (III and IV).
- People in the first five years of marriage – the most vulnerable period is the first two years.
- People in a second marriage – 50% of second marriages end in divorce.
- People who marry in their teens – teenage marriages are twice as likely to end in divorce as those of people marrying in their 20s.

Divorce has its costs and benefits. It is rated as the second most stressful life event, second only to death of a spouse. On the other hand it comes as a welcome relief to one or both partners when they have been locked in intense conflict or where there has been domestic violence. It can also be a time for maturation and growth.

It has been pointed out that divorce is not a single event but a process in which stress is often ongoing and persistent (Robinson, 1991). The effects of divorce on the partners and their children are a combination of a number of factors:

- Loss and bereavement – like most losses the individuals go through the phases of protest, anger and depression.
- Loss of income – 70% of families experience economic decline; income drops by 40% in the first year. Of children living in poverty, 75% come from families that have experienced separation and divorce.
- Change in parenting roles – for the non-custodial parent there is a diminution in their parenting role and contact with their children. For the parent who has care of the children there is increased responsibility, lack of support and reduced capacity to parent children, at least initially.
- Continuing conflict – in a significant proportion of families the conflict continues for years. It takes many forms, women who have separated from violent husbands are at risk of being murdered by their ex-husbands in the first few months. Legal battles centre around custody and contact with children and property issues and may go on for years.

Effects of divorce on children

Research in this field is relatively recent and the evidence is controversial. The problems faced by the child, called the '3Ls', include (Visher & Visher, 1996):

- Loss and change – it is not only the loss of one parent that the child is faced with but also the loss of friends, home and grandparents, together with a change of school, residence and, often, the introduction of a new step-parent.
- Loyalty conflicts – children have an overwhelming wish to remain loyal to *both* parents, and may find it difficult to maintain their loyalties against demands placed on them by each of the parents.
- Loss of control over their lives – children realise that things happen to them and that they have little choice in these, such as contact visits and remarriage of the parent with whom they live.

All studies on the effect of divorce on children show that, in spite of the increased demands made on the children, the majority weather divorce without adverse psychological sequelae but a significant number have difficulties, some of them lasting into adult life. The Exeter study of 152 children of divorce (Crockett & Tripp, 1994), found the children of divorcees to be low in self-esteem, to have special educational needs, to experience friendship difficulties and to encounter health problems more often than a control group. In the long term these children are more likely to leave home early and experience serious relationship problems.

Parental separation appears to have differential impact on children depending on their age and gender. For example:

- It has a more marked effect on children of school age than pre-school children.
- Boys respond to the separation of parents more adversely than girls. Often this manifests as disruptive behaviour, poor school performance and behaviour and low self-esteem.
- Girls appear to cope with the disruption relatively well but in adolescence girls from 'broken homes' experience turmoil, poor relationship with their mothers and are more likely to have short-term sexual relationships (Wallenstein, 1991).

The family

The function of an individual, in the context of family relationships and family life, has a major impact on that individual. An extensive body of research has confirmed that, in general, those who have intimate family relationships are healthier (less likely to suffer from a wide range of diseases from asthma to coronary heart disease), recover better from illnesses and operations, have a lower mortality rate, enjoy better mental health, are happier, and have fewer psychological symptoms than those who are single, widowed or divorced. The benefits to the individuals in a marriage are considerable when the marital relationships are especially good.

The overall positive effect that the family has on the individual, however, conceals the considerable suffering that some individuals experience. The 'darker side' of the family includes:

- Marital violence, usually perpetrated by the husband against the wife.
- Physical and sexual abuse of children.
- Depression in the wife – while marriage is a protective factor against depression for males, many studies have shown that it is a risk factor for women.

The family as a system

One approach to thinking about families is to consider the family as a system. The *general systems theory* developed initially by von Bertalanffy (1968), a biologist, has been profitably applied in both engineering and biology and, later, to organisations, small groups and, of course, the family.

A system is a set of elements that interact with one another over a period of time. Change occurs in the system by feedback, which leads to a new stability or homeostasis. A system has a number of subsystems but the 'whole is more than the sum of its parts' because it is made up of all the parts *plus* their relationships. It is demarcated by a boundary, the permeability of which is variable. Systems are governed by rules that may be overt or covert. A prime example of a system is the human body, which is formed of various subsystems (cardiovascular, respiratory, and so on), each consisting of elements (heart, arteries, veins, etc., in the case of the cardiovascular system), each of which functions in relation to both one another and the larger system, the human body.

The systems theory, as applied to the family – loosely called systems or systemic approach or thinking – has had an enormous impact on the way that the complex processes occurring in families have been conceptualised. More importantly, it has lead to the development of therapeutic interventions, particularly family therapy. The main features of the family system are:

Structure. The family system (Figure 12.7) consists of a parental subsystem bound by a marital bond, and a sibling subsystem. The family system itself is a subsystem of a wider system. The boundary between it and the wider system is usually permeable (hence called an 'open system') and is responsive to the environment. There are also boundaries between the subsystems, which differentiate the different generations. Change in one part of the system necessitates change in other parts of the system. One person in the family cannot experience a difficulty without having some effect on other members of the family. The system maintains its stability (homeostasis) through feedback loops. When a child reaches adolescence, for example, a greater degree of autonomy is permitted by the parents to maintain the cohesiveness of the family.

Rules and power roles. Families, like other systems, are rule governed. Often the rules in the family are taken for granted and not explicit. Implicit rules about power and authority (who makes decisions and how they are made) and roles (who makes dinner or who takes young Johnny to school) help regulate the behaviour of individual members within the system. Belief systems are fundamental to the way the family functions.

Pattern of interactions. Between family members these are often recurring, characteristic and observable. Repetitive interactive processes occur over a long time through overt and covert negotiations and are based on shared beliefs or rules. Some of these behaviour patterns may be identified as 'routines', 'habits' or 'rituals'.

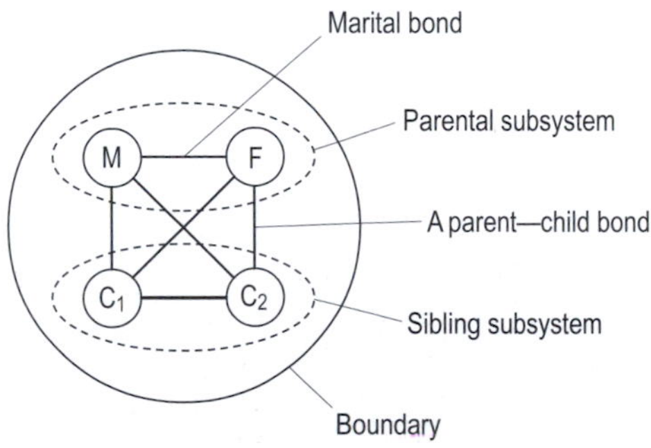

Fig. 12.7 The family system. m = mother; f = father; c1 and c2 = children

Box 12.6 Definitions of common terms used in family therapy

Alliances. Close relationships based on interests.
Coalition. Two members uniting against a third person (usually pathological).
Circularity. Interdependence of action and reaction (A leads to B leads to A), as opposed to linear causality which implies A leads to B.
Context. The interpersonal milieu that surrounds and influences the behaviour of individuals, families and larger groups.
Disengagement. Emotionally uninvolved or too distant; psychological isolation.
Enmeshment. Loss of autonomy due to a blurring of psychological boundaries; emotionally too close or overinvolved.
Reframing. Describing the family's version of the behaviour to make it more amenable to therapeutic change; for example, describing someone as 'discouraged' rather than 'depressed'.
Scapegoating. Blaming a convenient, but innocent, person for problems and conflicts among other members of the family.
Triangulation. A pattern of relationship in which a third person is recruited to bypass the conflict between two people thus stabilising the relationship between the original two people.
Hypothesis. An initial supposition about family functioning that can be tested out in the session; the starting point for further investigation.
Family life cycle. Transitions that occur in then lifetime of families; unattached young person, married couple, family with children or adolescents, children leaving home and family in later life.

Detailed consideration of systemic principles (which forms the basis of family therapy) is outside the remit of this book. A few of the terms that are used in systemic family therapy are defined in Box 12.6. The interested reader is referred to an introductory book on family therapy, for example, the book by Jones (1993).

Parenting

A major task of adulthood is the bringing of children into this world, nurturing them, fostering their development and competence and passing one's beliefs and values on to them. With the arrival of children the quality of the relationship between a couple undergoes a radical change as most of the couple's energies are directed towards bringing up children. Parenting is a complex task, the main aim of which is to meet the needs of the child in an appropriate and sensitive way.

The main needs of children are:

1. *Safety and security*. The most fundamental of needs, this is met by consistent care from one or both parents. Attachments develop in the context of a secure relationship with the parent(s). The ability of parents to contain the child's anxieties reassures the child and provides the basis for later self-regulation of affect.
2. *Love*. The most striking feature of parental love is that it is unconditional. This is communicated to the child in many ways. Feeling loved is the precursor to feeling worthy of being loved.

3. *Control and discipline*. Consistent discipline and supervision in the context of a loving relationship helps the child to internalise the rules of society with regard to what is acceptable and unacceptable behaviour.
4. *New experiences*. Exploration is a prerequisite for mental and social growth. Stage-appropriate tasks like play, socialisation and education lead to the mastery of skills and experiences.
5. *Praise and recognition*. Encouragement enhances performance and is a recognition of the achievements of the child.
6. *Responsibility*. Entrusting the child with responsibility permits autonomy and encourages independence.

No parent can provide all these needs all the time or be 'superparents'. Those who manage to meet most of the above conditions for the developing child are considered to be 'good enough' parents. Various dimensions of parenting have been studied. Two dimensions are emotional warmth/acceptance and control/discipline. Three styles of parenting have been identified (Baumrind, 1971).

1. *Permissive*. Parents are caring and nurturing but demand less in terms of control and discipline.
2. *Authoritarian*. Parents demonstrate high degree of demand and control but less warmth and nurturance.
3. *Authoritative*. Parents exhibit high levels of appropriate control and make appropriate demands on the child.

The three parenting styles have been shown to be associated with distinct patters of socialisation in children and adolescents (Baumrind, 1971). Children of permissive parents have been shown to be immature, dependent, unhappy and demanding. Authoritarian parenting have been associated with withdrawn and isolated children. Authoritative parenting produced optimal development – the children were confident, friendly and sociable.

A fourth, but important, category has been added recently (Maccoby & Martin, 1983).

4. *Neglecting*. Parents are psychologically not available to the child and there is little parenting. It has also been shown that neglected children have the worst outcome.

After this rather lengthy consideration of early adulthood, it is time to get back to adult development. The next stage is middle adulthood.

Middle adulthood (generativity vs. stagnation, 40–64 years)

Generativity refers to the contribution that the individual makes to the wider society. It is concerned with one's role in transmitting skills and knowledge and wisdom. This in turn fulfils the individual's need to feel wanted and valued. Erikson made a study of the Indian leader, Ghandi, and his most productive and creative years in middle age, when he led the Indian independence movement.

Many authors have written about '*mid-life crisis*' around the age of 40 when individuals become acutely aware of their limitations, comparing their achievements with their previous goals and re-evaluating their life. Research has not confirmed this view of the 40s as a period of inner turmoil and crisis.

During this period cognitive functioning declines differentially. Fluid intelligence begins to decline after 40 years, while crystallised intelligence (verbal abilities and skills) remains intact. On novel tasks and those requiring speed, performance shows a gradual downward trend. Short-term memory (digit span) remains largely intact under normal conditions but a brief delay or distraction impairs recall. Long-term memory usually shows some impairment but only after about the age of 60 years.

Children usually leave home around latter part of middle age but there is no evidence to support the mythical concept of 'empty nest syndrome'. The parenting role continues to be important, albeit in a changed form. Grandparenting roles emerge and more demands are made by the individual's parents. Often the role of caring for parents falls on the female. For this reason this has been called the 'sandwich generation'. There is some sex role cross over. Females become more assertive and take more responsibilities while males tend to step back a little!

On the whole, middle adulthood is less stressful and more enjoyable, with greater marital and vocational satisfaction, but this period also marks the beginning of disease and disability for most people. Heart disease, cancers and cerebrovascular accidents are common, and depression in women peaks at this age.

Adaptation to illness is a crucial task that is encountered. The way that individuals perceive, appraise and deal with illness (including mental disorders) and disability differs from person to person. Illnesses, particularly when chronic or life-threatening, are experienced as a loss – loss of health – thus provoking a grief reaction (see later). Illnesses limit and restrict one's independence and autonomy, and provoke primitive anxieties. Defence mechanisms are called into action to guard against the mental pain and discomfort. Maladaptive responses may aggravate the original medical condition, as when a person in denial ignores medical advice. Three common responses to illness ('3Ds') are:

1. Denial. Denial is a common response to illness, ranging from ignoring a minor physical symptom to outright dismissal, for example, of a serious chest pain as 'heartburn or indigestion'. Whilst denial has undoubted adaptive value in the early stages of some conditions, thus permitting the person to continue to function unhindered by fear and anxiety, persistent denial is both maladaptive and potentially dangerous.

2. Depression. Depressive reactions to illnesses are common especially when the individual begins to understand the significance and consequences of the illness. It may range from depressive symptoms to a depressive illness. Depression that accompanies a physical illness often increases functional impairment and, when extreme, the patient may give up the will to live (the 'giving up, given up' syndrome).

3. Dependency. Regression is a feature of all illnesses. We take to bed, and we expect to be served and cared for by others when we are ill. Excessive dependency, on the other hand, is pathological and counterproductive in the long term. It often involves secondary gain, such as avoidance of work and attention from loved ones.

Old age (integrity vs. despair, 65 to death)

The main task at this stage is acceptance of one's life experiences as 'givens' that are 'permitted of no substitutions'. The ultimate goal is acceptance of death. It is interesting to note that in his 70s Erikson set himself the task of studying the lives of octogenarians (parents of his cohort of children) thus completing his study of the human life cycle.

Two subgroups have been described: the young old (65–75) and the old old (> 75). The central feature of old age can be summed up in one word – losses. The succession of gradual and sudden losses that old people suffer makes old age 'the age of losses', which the individual has to cope with and adjust to. The main areas where 'losses' occur are:

Physical health. Impairment of hearing, presbycusis (impairment of hearing of higher frequency sounds), tinnitus and deafness. Impairment of vision and smell. Poor mobility and sense of balance, resulting in falls.

Mental health. Poor short-term and long-term memory but good abilities of recognition. Onset of dementia. Surprisingly, rates of depression are lower than in young people (2–3% in people over 65 compared to 10–12% in the young). Fear of dependency, illnesses, suffering and death is common.

Social. Loss of spouse and friends, loss of home, loss of independence. Retirement results in loss of role and income. Isolation from family is common as is marginalisation by society where the elderly are ignored and considered a burden.

The prospect of facing death can no longer be postponed. Fear of dependence and suffering usually outweighs fear of death.

Death and dying

Everyone meets with death sometime or other – that of family members, friends, patients and, ultimately, their own. Death comes in many ways – suddenly and unexpectedly like a thief at night, insidiously and surreptitiously creeping in little by little, progressively and inescapably. Death, for most people, is not an event but a process. It involves strong emotions for both the dying person, his or her family and carers, including professionals. Elisabeth Kubler-Ross' (1969) observations and groundbreaking work on dying patients opened the way for people to think and talk about the experiences of death and dying. She described five phases that patients with terminal illnesses pass through:

1. *Denial* – the initial 'Not me' response.
2. *Anger* – the 'Why me?' reaction. Anger is directed at oneself, family

members and often towards professionals involved in the patient's care.

3. *Bargaining* – the 'Yes me, but ...' process involving generous promises in the hope of extending life.
4. *Depression* – a 'Yes' response in recognising the reality of the situation brings despair and despondency.
5. *Acceptance* – after going through the previous stages, the patient accepts and is ready to embrace death.

The terminally ill do not go through the five phases in the sequence proposed by Kubler-Ross. Patients with terminal cancer, for instance, move in and out of the phases quite rapidly, for example from denial to acceptance and then back to denial again. Many do not reach the stage of acceptance at all.

The predominant feeling states that people close to death experience are fear and grief (Parkes, 1998). Curiously, fear of dying comes lower down in the list. Fear of separation from loved ones, fear of becoming a burden to others and fear of losing control are more important to the dying person than fear of death itself. Grieving one's own death (anticipatory grief) is unavoidable as the person begins to acknowledge the various losses he faces, including the loss of a future.

Normal grief

The first systematic study of grief following the loss of a loved one was carried out by Lindeman (1944). This pioneering study involved 101 bereaved individuals who lost their loved ones in a fire at a night club in Boston called The Coconut Grove. This study described the symptoms and course of grief and established grief as a distinct syndrome. Numerous studies have been carried out since and have confirmed the validity of the descriptions. It is now generally accepted that people go through four stages when grieving. These are:

Stage 1 – numbness. Shock and disbelief last for a number of days.

Stage 2 – pining and 'pangs' of grief. Sadness, yearning for the lost person, anger (directed at the deceased or those who cared for the deceased, e.g. hospital, doctors) and guilt accompanied by intense anxiety are common features at this phase. Often there is also loss of appetite and weight. Physical symptoms are common, some of these may be similar to those experienced by the deceased. The bereaved person becomes irritable and depressed.

Stage 3 – disorganisation and despair. Ruminations of events surrounding the death, preoccupation with thoughts of the loved one and general despair characterise the third stage. Transient pseudohallucinations (e.g. hearing the deceased call one's name) may occur.

Stage 4 – reorganisation. In due course the bereaved persons regains control over their emotions. Grief tends to get less but may return on anniversaries and special occasions like Christmas.

The course of the grief reaction may not follow the four stages strictly in the order outlined above, rather the bereaved person often oscillates between stages 2 and 3 before recovering from it. Uncomplicated grief lasts from 1 to

2 years and by the middle of the second year most people have come to terms with the loss, mourned the loss and started reinvesting their emotions in other people, activities and duties. In some, however, grief may take a more complicated course.

Complicated (morbid) grief

Occasionally the grieving and mourning process does not progress toward reorganisation. This is more common in high-risk situations. Two pathological grief syndromes have been described (Parkes, 1998):

1. Delayed or inhibited grief. Failure to mourn and denial of the loss often produce depression, sleep problems and somatic symptoms. This category of people has been called 'avoiders'. They 'put on a brave face'.

2. Chronic grief. Here the person is stuck at stage 2 or 3 of the grieving process and is unduly preoccupied with thoughts of the deceased. The grieving process extends for years. This group, called 'sensitisers' have difficulty 'letting go' and have mixed feelings of guilt and anger. Preserving the deceased clothes, keeping the dead person's room as it was and the inability to talk about the deceased without an outpouring of excessive emotion are common features of chronic or unresolved grief.

A number of studies have identified factors that are associated with morbid grief. They include the following:

- Unexpected and sudden death (particularly if associated with traumatic circumstances).
- Death by suicide or homicide.
- Ambivalent attachment to the deceased.
- Dependency on the deceased or looking after the deceased for a long time.
- Not having had the opportunity to see the body of the deceased.

A variety of psychiatric syndromes may be associated with bereavement and grief, the commonest being depression, anxiety states and panic disorder. Often morbid grief and psychiatric disorders coexist and both may need treatment.

REFERENCES

Ainsworth MDS, Blehar MC, Walters E, Wall S (1978) Patterns of Attachment : assessed in the strange situation and at home. Hillsdale, NJ: Lawrence Erlbaum.

Argyle M, Henderson M (1985) The Anatomy of Relationships. Harmondsworth, UK: Penguin Books.

Baron-Cohen S (1989) The autistic child's theory of mind: a case of specific developmental delay. Journal of Child Psychology and Psychiatry, 30, 285–297.

Baron-Cohen S, Leslie AM, Firth U (1985) Does the autistic child have a 'theory of mind'? Cognition, 21, 37–46.

Bates JE (1987) Temperament in infancy. In JD Osofsky (ed.), Handbook of Infant Temperament Concepts (2nd ed.). New York. Wiley.

Baumrind D (1971) Current patterns of parental authority. Developmental Psychology Monographs 4(1) Part 2.

Bowlby J (1944) Forty-four juvenile thieves: their characteristics and home life. International Journal of Psychoanalysis, 25, 19–52, and 107–207.
Bowlby J (1951) Maternal Care and Mental Health. WHO Monograph No. 2. Geneva: World Health Organization.
Bowlby J (1958) The nature of the child's tie to the mother. International Journal of Psychoanalysis, 39, 350–373.
Bowlby J (1969/1982) Attachment and Loss. Volume 1, Attachment and loss; Volume 2, Separation; Volume 3, Loss. New York: Basic Books.
Buss A, Plomin R (1975) A Temperament Theory of Development. New York: Wiley.
Buss AH, Plomin R (1984) Temperament: early developmental personality traits. Hillsdale, NJ: Lawrence Erlbaum.
Byng-Hall J (1980) Symptom bearer as marital distance regulator: clinical implications. Family Process, 19, 355–365.
Chomsky N (1965) Aspects of the Theory of Syntax. Cambridge, MA: MIT Press.
Crockett M, Tripp J (1994) The Exeter Family Study. Exeter, UK: University of Exeter Press.
DeCasper AJ, Fifer WP (1980) Of human bonding: newborns prefer their mother's voice. Science, 208, 1174–1176.
DeCasper AJ, Spence MJ (1986) Prenatal maternal speech influences newborns' perception of speech sounds. Infant Behaviour and Development, 9, 133–150.
Donaldson M (1978) Children's Minds. London, UK: Fontana.
Erikson EH (1963) Childhood and Society. New York: Norton.
Erikson EH (1968) Identity: youth and crisis. New York: Norton.
Farrington DP (1995) The development of offending and antisocial behaviour from childhood: key findings from the Cambridge study of delinquent development. Journal of Child Psychology and Psychiatry, 36, 929–964.
Fonagy P, Steele H, Steele M (1991) Maternal representation of attachment during pregnancy predicts the organisation of infant–mother attachment at one year of age. Child development, 42, 891–905.
George C, Kaplan N, Main M (1986) Attachment Interview for Adults (Unpublished manuscript). Berkeley, CA: University of California.
Gibson EJ, Walk RD (1960) The 'visual cliff'. Scientific American, 202(April), 64–71.
Harlow HF (1958) The nature of love. American Psychologist, 13, 573–685.
Harlow HF, Harlow MK (1962) Social deprivation in monkeys. Scientific American, 207, 5, 136.
Hill P (1987) Research on adolescence and their families past and present. In CE Irwin (eds), Adolescent Social Behaviour and Health. San Francisco, CA: Jossey-Bass.
Holmes J (1993a) John Bowlby and attachment theory. London: Routledge.
Holmes J (1993b) Clinical implications of attachment theory. British Journal of Psychiatry, 163, 430–439.
Kim K, Smith PK (1998) Childhood stress, behavioural symptoms and mother–daughter pubertal development. Journal of Adolescence, 21, 231–240.
Kohlberg L (1984) Essays on Moral Development: the psychology of moral development (Vol. 2). New York: Harper and Row.
Kubler-Ross E (1969) On Death and Dying. London, UK: Macmillan.
Lewis M, Brooks-Gunn J (1979) Social Cognition and the Acquisition of Self. New York: Plenum Press.
Lindeman E (1944) Symptomatology and management of acute grief. American Journal of Psychiatry, 44, 2–23.
Maccoby EE, Martin JA (1983) Socialisation in the context of the family: parent–child interaction. In EM Hetherington (ed.), Handbook of Child Psychology. Vol. 4 Socialization, personality and social development (pp. 1–101). New York: Wiley.
Main M, Solomon J (1990) Procedures for identifying infants as disorganised/disorientated during Ainsworth's strange situation. In MT Greenberg, D Ceccheti, M Cummings (eds.), Attachment in Preschool Years: theory, research and interventions. Chicago, IL: Chicago University Press.
Marcia JE (1980) Identity in adolescence. In J Anderson (ed.), Handbook of Adolescent Psychology. New York: Wiley.

Murray L, Cooper PJ (eds) (1997) Postpartum Depression and Child Development. New York: Guilford Press.
Offer D (1969) The Psychological World of the Teenager. New York. Basic Books.
Parkes CM (1998) Coping with loss: bereavement in adult life. British Medical Journal, 316, 856–859.
Robertson J, Robertson J (1971) Young children in brief separations: a fresh look. Psychoanalytic Study of the Child, 26, 264–315.
Robinson M (1991) Family Transformation During Divorce and Remarriage: a systemic approach. London, UK: Routledge.
Rust J, Golombok S (1985) The Golombok–Rust Inventory of Sexual Satisfaction (GRISS). Windsor, UK: NFER Nelson.
Rust J, Bannum I, Crowe M, Golombok S (1988) Handbook of the Golombok–Rust Inventory of Marital State (GRIMS). Windsor, UK: NFER Nelson.
Rutter M (1972) Maternal Deprivation Reassessed (2nd ed.). Harmondsworth, UK: Penguin Books.
Rutter M (1976) Isle of Wight studies, 1964–1974. Psychological Medicine, 6, 313–332.
Rutter M, Graham P, Chadwick O, Yule W (1976) Adolescent turmoil: fact or fiction? Journal of Child Psychology and Psychiatry, 17, 35–56.
Shiner R, Caspi A (2003) Personality differences in childhood and adolescence: measurement, development and consequences. Journal of Child Psychology and Psychiatry, 44(1), 2–23.
Suomi SJ, Harlow HF (1978) Early experience and social separation in rhesus monkeys. In ME Lamb (ed.), Social and Personality Development. New York: Holt, Rhinehart & Winston.
Tanner JM (1990) Foetus to Man: physical growth from conception to maturity (2nd ed.). Cambridge, MA: Harvard University Press.
Thomas A, Chess S (1977) Temperament and Development. New York: Brunner Mazel.
Thomas A, Chess S (1986) Temperament in Clinical Practice. New York. Guilford Press.
Tizard B, Hodges J (1989) IQ, behavioural adjustment of ex-institutionalised adolescents: social and family relation. Journal of Child Psychology and Psychiatry, 30(1), 53–97.
Tizard B, Hodges J (1978) The effect of early institutional rearing on the development of eight year old children. Journal of Child Psychology and Psychiatry, 99, 119–118.
Van Ijzendoorn MH (1995) Adult attachment representations, parental responsiveness and infant development: a meta-analysis on the predictive validity of the adult attachment interviews. Psychological Bulletin, 117, 387–403.
Visher EB, Visher JS (1996) Therapy with Step Families. New York: Brunner Mazel.
von Bertalanffy L (1968) General Systems Theory: foundation, development, application. New York: Brazillier.
Vygotsky LS (1978) Mind and Society: the development of higher psychological processes. Cambridge, MA: Harvard University Press.
Wallenstein JS (1991) The long-term effects of divorce on children – a review. Journal of the American Academy of Child Psychiatry, 30, 349–360.
Wimmer HG, Perner J (1983) Beliefs about beliefs: representation and constraining function of wrong beliefs in young children's understanding of deception. Cognition, 13, 103–108.

FURTHER READING

Cassidy J, Shaver PR (eds) (1999) Handbook of Attachment: theory, research and clinical applications. New York: The Guilford Press.
- A comprehensive text on attachment.

Goodman R, Scott S (1997) Child Psychiatry. Oxford, UK: Blackwell Science.
- An outstanding textbook that is both concise and clear. If you wish to read just one book on child psychiatry, this is the one. Highly recommended.

Jones E (1993) Family Systems Therapy: developments in Milan systemic therapies. Chichester, UK: Wiley.
- A very readable and lucid account of systemic ideas.

Lawrie SM, McIntosh AM, Rao S (2000) Critical Appraisal in Psychiatry. Edinburgh: Churchill Livingstone.

- A remarkably informative book on critical appraisal that provides a lucid account of various forms of research study designs.

Slater A, Lewis M (eds) (2002) Introduction to Infant Development. Oxford, UK: Oxford University Press.

- An excellent book that provides a clear account of current research findings in the area of infant research.

Psychoanalytic concepts

13

'Psychic reality is a particular form of existence not to be confused with physical reality.'
Freud (1900)

Psychoanalysis is an all-embracing theory of human nature and the working of the mind in the tradition of Darwin's theory of evolution. Its scope wider, its utility infinitely greater, and its influence immensely more far-reaching than that of 'scientific psychology'. Freud's ideas permeate culture, art, literature, and anthropology, in short any field in which human beings are the subject of enquiry, study or description. Psychoanalytic concepts, such as the unconscious and 'Freudian slip', have become part of our thinking and daily language. His ideas have radically changed the way we think about ourselves. Freudian thought has established itself as one of the most significant and lasting intellectual achievements of the twentieth century. Even those theories that vehemently disallow Freudian underpinnings almost always have some elements of Freudian thinking embedded in them.

Freudian ideas have evoked strong reactions from overwhelming adulation and unqualified admiration to outright condemnation and vilification as evidenced by the vast number of books about him and his works, which bear titles such as *What Freud Really Said* (Stanford-Clark, 1988) and *Why Freud Was Wrong* (Webster, 1995).

It is important to emphasise that psychoanalysis refers to the theoretical description of the human mind and its associations that provides a framework for thinking about clinical and non-clinical situations. Freud was the first to admit that his ideas were assumptions. Describing the paradigm of the psychic apparatus he wrote, 'We *assume* that mental life is the function of apparatus ... being made up of several parts, i.e. id, ego and superego' (Freud, 1940). Taken as a body of theories and ideas about psychic processes, Freudian teachings and their later developments provide us with ways of observing, thinking and conceptualising mental and interpersonal processes that are invaluable for the clinician who encounters the human condition in his or her day-to-day work. It is made all the more significant to the psychiatrist by the fact that, first and foremost, Freud was interested in understanding psychopathology and his primary data were things that patients told him about themselves during clinical encounters

To the beginner, psychoanalytic terminology can be off-putting and confusing. Freudian use of phrases such as castration anxiety, Oedipal complex and penis envy need to be understood as metaphors and be translated into their everyday equivalents. Castration anxiety, for example, refers to invoked feelings of impotence in the face of life's demands and the fear engendered by authority figures. Similarly, penis envy refers to the sense of deficiency, inferiority and a desire to have the superior potency supposedly possessed only by men. As in other technical fields of study such terms are used as short hand to communicate complicated ideas and should not be taken literally. Also some of the words carry different connotations. For example, the word sexuality is used to refer to all phenomena that pertain to pleasure and therefore has non-sexual dimension as well.

Freud was a prolific writer. His professional life covered a period of nearly forty years during which he wrote a large number of essays, which have been collected into twenty-four volumes published as *The Standard Editions of the Complete Psychological Works of Sigmund Freud* (SE) by the Hogarth Press and the Institute of Psychoanalysis (now also published by Penguin Books in 15 volumes). Any attempt to summarise his work necessarily impoverishes the richness of clinical details and takes away the power inherent in all his writings. Often such outlines can appear absurd and unbelievable. Nevertheless, a brief account of classical psychoanalysis is given here and it is hoped that the student will then sample a work by Freud, such as the *New Introductory Lectures on Psychoanalysis* (Freud 1933a), which provides an overall picture of psychoanalysis whilst giving a taste of the elegance of Freud's style and the richness of his thinking.

Psychoanalysis, or the classical theory, as is sometime called, includes most of Freud's formulations about the human mind. Sometimes the word 'psychodynamics' is used in place of it. Strictly speaking psychodynamics refers to the interplay between the conscious and unconscious forces and the working of the three parts of the mind as postulated by Freud but it is often used as a term to denote some aspects of Freudian thinking. Therapy based on Freudian and post-Freudian concepts but which does not adhere strictly to the classical analysis is often referred to as psychodynamic psychotherapy.

Freudian psychoanalysis consists of two distinct but related aspects of his work:

1. It is a theory of organisation and functioning of the mind (the psyche and psychic processes).
2. It is a method of treatment (psychoanalytic psychotherapy).

The rest of the chapter provides a very brief outline of both of these aspects, followed by a short account of the significant developments of his theories made by other psychoanalysts. Any attempt to summarise psychoanalytic concepts runs the risk of making the subject uninteresting and almost meaningless. The reader is urged to read a short text on the subject (see Further Reading for examples of suitable works).

FREUD'S MODELS OF THE MIND

Freud put forward various models of the mind at different stages of his career. His theoretical formulations kept changing and developing over his working life. Freud's theories of the structure, organisation and processes of the mind (known as metapsychology) comprises a number of separate but interlinked working models. These are given below in the chronological order in which he described them together with the major essays in which he first described them:

- *The topographical model* (1900, *The Interpretation of Dreams*), which divides mind into the conscious, preconscious and unconscious systems.
- *The developmental (genetic) model* (1905, *Three Essays on the Theory of Sexuality*), which signifies the psychosexual stages of development.
- *The dynamic (drive–instinct energy model)* (1915, *The Instincts and their Vicissitudes*), which deals with the concept of mental energy variously described as libido, psychic energy and drive energy.
- *The structural model* (1923, *The Ego and the Id*), which sees the mind as tripartite psychic apparatus consisting of the Id, Ego and Superego.

The topographical model

The topographical model, the first of Freud's models of the mind, was elaborated in his work *The Interpretation of Dreams* (1900). He postulated three regions metaphorically arranged in the 'psychic apparatus' on a vertical axis from the surface to the depths. According to this model, mental processes are divided into three different systems: the conscious (Cs); the preconscious (Ps); and the unconscious (Ucs).

The unconscious mental contents and activities are those that are beyond awareness. The Ucs consists of primitive desires, wishes and urges that are primarily sexual or aggressive. The system consists of two parts: (1) the unconscious proper made up of primal thought processes, which are primitive in origin; and (2) repressed conscious material that consist of actively disavowed (repressed) impulses together with associated memories. Freud placed much emphasis on the role of the unconscious postulating that it occupied the largest area of the psyche and determined behaviour in various ways.

The preconscious refers to those processes that can be made aware and which are therefore available to be made conscious. The Ps imposes rigorous censorship on the Ucs and keeps its mental contents away from the Cs.

The Cs is synonymous with what the person is aware of at the moment.

The conscious and unconscious operate according to different rules and laws. The Ucs is governed by *primary process thinking*, which by its very primitive nature lacks logic and has no sense of time or space. It is dominated by the pleasure principle and seeks immediate gratification with no thought or delay. There is no organisation of thought and often opposites are held together in illogical and uncoordinated ways. The manifestations of unconscious mental functioning are evident in dreams, selective forgetting, neurotic symptoms and slips of the tongue (parapraxes). It is the earliest and most primitive form of mental activity. It is freely mobile in form and allows condensation and displacement (see later). Many aspects of religions, artistic creations, dreams, fantasies and even political institutions are seen as manifestations of primary process thinking. The conscious part of the psyche operates on the basis of *secondary process thinking*. The latter is governed by the reality principle and is capable of logical problem solving and delayed or modified gratification.

Although Freud described the Ucs, Ps and Cs as separate entities, he emphasised that no such separation exists and that they work together in a dynamic way to produce behaviour. For example, retiring to one's usual bed when tired or sick can be traced to unconscious (comfort of 'return to the womb'), preconscious (seeking attention from a loved one) and conscious (getting some rest) motivations.

Dreams

Freud considered dreams to be psychologically meaningful and to reflect unconscious mental activity. He held that dreams represented unconscious wishes and repressed conflicts that cannot find expression in waking life. Freud called the underlying unconscious content of dreams as the *latent content*. The *manifest dream content* refers to the dream as experienced by the subject. The mental process involved in the conversion of latent contents into manifest contents is known as *dream work* (Figure 13.1). Dream work involves several archaic modes of thinking, particularly *displacement*, *condensation*, *symbolism* and *substitution*. In condensation, several objects or people are combined into a single image. For example the mother becomes an unrecognisable figure and then the wife. Symbolism is the transformation of thought into sensory or symbolic images. Pointed objects are thought to represent the penis, home the womb and travel a journey through life. In addition *secondary elaboration* is said to occur during the conversion linking together the separate elements of the dream into a coherent story that makes the manifest content more realistic and acceptable.

Whilst emphasising the unconscious and infantile nature of dreams, Freud added two here-and-now experiences that affect the content of manifest dreams. One was the role of sensory stimuli at the time of dreaming, such as hunger, thirst and a full bladder. For example a full bladder produces images of urination and seeking out of toilets. The other was the effect of *daily residues*. Daily residues are ideas, feelings and experiences from everyday life in the recent past that contribute to the formation of the dream. They link the unconscious infantile drives, wishes and conflicts to create images that replace thought. Freud described dreams as 'the royal road to the unconscious'. Analysis of dreams is an important aspect of psychoanalysis. Interpretation of dreams is thought to help discover underlying unconscious mental processes, infantile fantasies and defences.

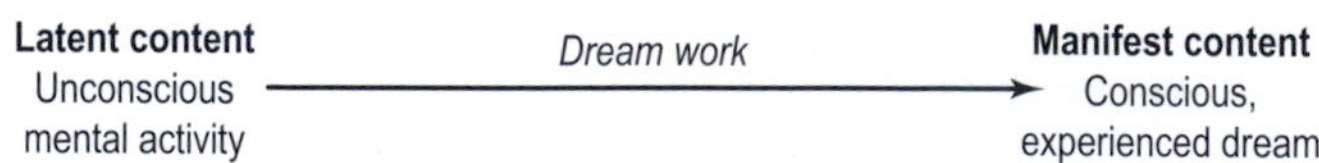

Fig. 13.1 The development of dreams

The developmental (genetic) model and the stages of psychosexual development

Freud made two bold assertions about human development. One was that the first few years of life were the most important years for the development of personality. All psychoanalytically orientated practitioners are unanimous in claiming that early experience is crucial to later personality organisation and functioning. The other assertion is that this development takes place through psychosexual stages. It is interesting to note, however, that Freud never saw children and his formulations were made mostly on the basis of accounts of what his adult patients told him of their early experiences.

During development, from infancy to adulthood, libidal energies become invested in various 'erotogenic zones'. Freud hypothesised that such psychosexual development occurred in an orderly fashion from the oral stage in the infant to the genital stage in the young adult (Table 13.1). It is important to note that Freud's idea of stages of development is different from those of others like Piaget. In the Freudian scheme one stage does not completely replace the other and remnants of the earlier stage are always present. Thus, a child in middle childhood may start sucking his thumb after a traumatic experience indicating regression to the oral stage.

Oral stage (0–18 months). In the first months of life, the most intense activities of the infant are centred on the mouth and the act of feeding. At this stage the mouth is the main source of pleasure. The first awareness of object (in psychoanalysis the term object is used as the opposite of subject; it refers to any emotionally significant person, part of a person or object) arises from the need to satisfy hunger and thirst. The object (the mother) is experienced by the baby as satisfying his needs and providing pleasure. In addition to providing oral pleasure, the infant also exhibit aggressiveness towards the object by biting, spiting out and rejecting. This is the first *object relationship* experienced by the infant. The mother thus becomes the primary love object in the infant's life. Freud claimed that the mother is 'unique, without parallel, established unalterably for a whole lifetime as the first and strongest love-object and as the prototype of all later love-relations' (Freud, 1940). The major task for the infant at this stage is to establish a trusting and dependent relationship

Table 13.1 Stages of psychosexual development

Stage	*Age*	*Characteristics*
Oral	0–18 months	Establishment of trust
Anal	18 months–3 years	Strive for control
Phallic	3 years–5 or 6 years	Castration anxiety, penis envy Resolution of Oedipal complex
Latency	5 or 6 years–11 or 13 years	Period of quiescence
Genital	11 or 13 years–young adulthood	Establishment of mature object relationships

with the object. Fixation at the oral stage is said to result in 'oral character' characterised by greed, dependency and demandingness.

Anal stage (18 months–3 years). During the anal stage the anus and defaecation are the major sources of pleasure for the infant. For the first time he realises that he has mastery over his physiological activities without the assistance of an outside object. Exercising control becomes the major preoccupation for the child. The 'anal character' resulting from fixation at this stage shows as the triad of obstinacy, orderliness (including bodily cleanliness and conscientiousness) and parsimony (frugality, miserliness).

Phallic stage (3–5 or 6 years). During this stage, the penis becomes the central focus of the child. Children become aware of their gender identity and their activities focus on sexual stimulation and excitement. The main preoccupation is centred around the wish to penetrate and possess. It differs from the other stages in two aspects: (1) the drive is not directed towards one's own body, but towards outside objects; and (2) the relationship moves from a dyadic one to a triadic one as evidenced by the Oedipal complex.

Oedipal complex. With the investment of libidal energies in the genitals, the mother becomes the boy's first love object. He falls in love with her and wants to possess her (in Greek mythology, Oedipus killed his father and married his mother), but this brings him into conflict with his father whom he considers his rival. He would like to get rid of his father and have the mother for himself. The murderous feelings that the boy develops towards his father produce fear of retaliation from his father. Freud called this perceived threat and the fear that it engendered, *castration anxiety*. The boy overcomes this anxiety by employing the defence mechanism of *identification with the aggressor*. He renounces his hopes of possessing his mother and identifies with his father. The most important outcome of the Oedipal complex is the boy identifying with the father. The resolution of the Oedipal complex by introjection of parental inhibitions marks the beginning of the formation of the superego. The Oedipal complex thus resolved, the son is free to seek gratification outside the close family.

Electra complex. Girls face a similar, but less intense, conflict during the phallic stage. The father is the object of the girl's sexual desire. This has been called the *Electra complex*. Freud held that part of this longing involves penis envy, which arises out of her realisation that he possesses a penis that she does not have. She feels that she has been castrated and blames the mother for having borne her without a penis.

Latency stage (5–6 years to 11–13 years). Following the resolution of the Oedipal complex there is a period of emotional quiescence. Instinctual impulses are controlled by the superego. This period begins about 5 to 6 years and ends with the onset of puberty. It corresponds to the fourth of Erikson's eight stages of man, industry vs. inferiority.

Genital stage (13 years to young adulthood). The sexual impulses repressed during the latent stage make their appearance in full force as a result of puberty. The instinctual impulses are directed towards the opposite sex. The major task during this period is separation from the parents and the establishment of personal identity, with investment of libidal energies in objects outside the family.

The dynamic (drive–instinct and energy) model

Throughout his career, Freud attempted to conceptualise the nature of motivational forces, their source and effects. He was single minded in asserting that these were endogenous, inborn and biologically derived. His drive–instinct and energy models are described here as a single model, which really consists of two related ideas. The first of these postulates that mental processes are driven by psychological energy that resides within psychic structures and that these must follow certain laws. Although the concept of *psychic energy* has been a recurring theme in Freud's writings it is considered to be the weakest of his formulations. Two types of psychic energy have been proposed: sexual energy, or libido, and aggressive energy. Freud's notion of libido encompasses everything that is included under the word 'love' – pleasure seeking, sexual desire and love of others. Investment of psychic love in an object or idea is known as *cathexis*.

Closely related to the idea of psychic energy is the concept of *instinctual drive*. Unfortunately it is often mistaken for instinct, a biological concept. Freud used the word *Trieb*, which was mistranslated as instinct. Freud's concept of *Trieb* postulates a motivational force that originates in somatic processes. Instinctual drives are said to have a source, an aim and an object. He emphasised two basic drives: sexual and aggressive, which he considered to be innate and inborn but subject to developmental changes. Psychological energy was considered to be analogous to physical energy and, in the same way, transformed, distributed or discharged. Thus, psychic energy may be transformed into anxiety, displaced into the body and manifest as a somatic symptom, like paralysis, or be converted into a thought, such as an obsession.

During the latter part of his life, Freud put forward a *dual theory of instincts*. According to this theory there are two general classes of instinctual drives: (1) libido (Eros) or life impulses, which serve to preserve and unite; and (2) aggression or death instincts (Thanatos), which seek to destroy and kill. Freud explained it thus: 'The death instinct is said to work in every living creature, striving to bring it to ruin and reduce life to its original condition of inanimate matter, while the erotic instinct (Eros) represents the efforts to live ... the organism preserves its own life, so to say, by destroying an extraneous one'. Eros is involved in all healthy relationships and constructive activities of man, while Thanatos represents the aggressive side of humans that brings self-destruction and ruin upon them.

Freud's writing on civilisation and human groups is an extension of his theories on individuals to society as a whole. Given the inborn aggression in man, he said, the object of civilisation is to inhibit human aggressiveness. In his words, 'Aggression is an original, self-subsisting instinctual predisposition in man ... and it constitutes the greatest impediment to him'. An interesting correspondence between Albert Einstein and Freud is worth quoting. Appalled by the destructiveness and atrocities of the Second World War, Einstein wrote to Freud with the question, 'Is there any way of delivering man from the menace of war?' In reply, Freud (1933b) painstakingly elaborated his theory of Eros and Thanatos in his characteristic and powerful way. According to Freud war was an extreme expression of the death instinct, which had escaped modification by the process of civilisation. A pessimistic Freud replied, '... of the psychological characteristics of civilisation two appear to be the most important: strengthening the intellect ... and internalisation of aggressive impulses'.

The structural model

In his later years, Freud put forward a structural model in which he conceptualised the mind (psychic apparatus) as consisting of three interacting components, the id, the ego and the superego. This is sometimes known also as the *tripartite division of the mind*. These structures mediate between drive and behaviour.

Id. The id (meaning 'it') represents the primitive unorganised part of the mind and is the source of innate desires. It embodies the mental representation of the instinctual drives and contains some, but not all, of the contents of the unconscious (of the topographical model). Freud described the id as the 'dark, inaccessible part of our personality'. It is driven by the primary process and operates under the pleasure principle, hence it avoids pain and tension. It has no sense of time, space or contradictions. Id continues to operate even in adulthood, especially in dreams, imagination, and impulsive and pleasure-seeking behaviour.

Ego. The ego (meaning 'I') occupies a position between the primal instincts and the demands of the outer world. It is the organised part of the mind. It mediates between the demands of the id and the constraints of reality and the superego. The ego has some conscious component, but is to a large extent unconscious; many of its operations are automatic and beyond consciousness. It operates on the reality principle and secondary process thought, reconciling, postponing or denying gratification. The ego is responsible for the thinking that occurs between impulse and action. The ego is not the same as self (self refers to the individual's experience of themselves) but embodies the concept of self within it. Ego serves 'three tyrannical masters': id, superego and external world. Freud compared the ego's relation to the id to that of a rider and his horse. The horse supplies the energy while the rider decides on the goal and guides the powerful animal's movements. But there also arise situations when the rider takes the path along which the horse wants to go.

The ego performs many functions, which may be grouped as follows:

- Control and regulation of instinctual drives.
- Reality orientation.
- Establishment object relationships.
- Defence against anxiety.

Assessment of the ego strength of the individual is an important part of psychoanalysis. The main elements that go to make up ego strength include the individual's ability to tolerate frustration, the capacity for impulse control, appropriate use of ego defences and the ability to use abstract thinking. The constant threats from the id and the external world cause anxiety. Whenever possible the ego deals with this in a rational and practical way. However, when the anxiety is strong and threatens to overwhelm the ego, it defends itself by using one or more of the defence mechanisms.

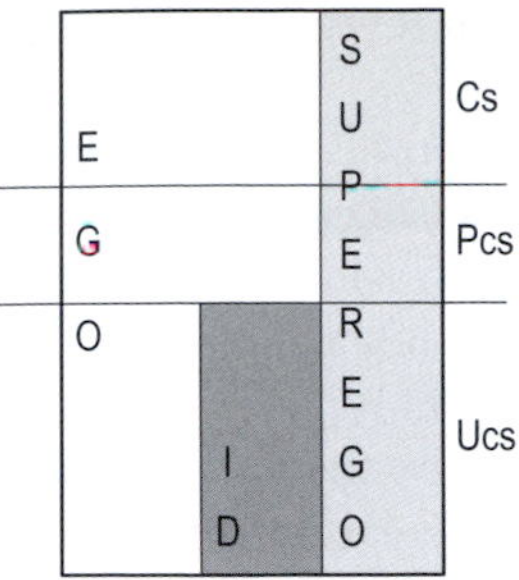

Fig. 13.2 A diagramatic representation of Freud's topographical and structural models (Cs = conscious, Pcs = preconscious and Ucs = unconscious)

Superego. Superego emerges in the course of attempts to resolve Oedipal conflicts. It is partly the result of identification with parents, and the internalisation (introjection) of parental prohibitions. It manifests as guilt, the 'inner voice' and, in lay terms, as the conscience. It differs from conscience in that it is largely unconscious. It is responsible for self-criticism and self-reflective thinking. Conflicts between the superego and the ego often produce shame, guilt and a sense of inferiority. Figure 13.2 depicts Freud's structural model superimposed on to the topographical model.

Defence

One of Freud's lasting contributions to psychology is his 'discovery' of defence. He described defence as 'all the techniques the ego makes use of in conflicts'. According to Freud, when the defences fail, or are overwhelmed, neuroses result. Threats to the ego may arise from three sources: (1) instinctual impulses of the id; (2) the superego; and (3) the outside world. In trying to mediate between the impulses of the id and the demands of the superego the ego employs a number of defences to achieve control and mastery over them, and protect the ego.

Some defences are characteristic of certain stages of development but may persist into adult life. People are often seen to utilise certain defences repeatedly and habitually. So much so, in fact, that it becomes a character trait of the person. Ego defences operate at an unconscious level beyond one's awareness. Often they protect the person from anxiety and mental pain, but may also produce psychopathology. Freud described many defences, especially repression, which he articulated in some detail, but it was his daughter, Anna Freud, who was the first to use the phrase defence mechanism. In her classic work, *The Ego and the Mechanism of Defence* (1936), she described ten defence mechanisms:

1. *Repression*. Described by Freud as the 'master of all defences', repression refers to the process by which impulses, thoughts and memories are pushed out or excluded from the conscious mind. Repression is considered to be the main defence in hysteria.
2. *Reaction formation*. This is the transformation of unacceptable thoughts and feeling into their opposite.

3. *Regression*. This refers to the reversion to an earlier state of ego functioning.
4. *Isolation*. Separation of a significant experience from its affects and associations 'so that it remains isolated and is not reproducible in ordinary thought'. It is typical of obsessional states.
5. *Undoing*. In this the subject relates to a prior thought or action as though it had not occurred. It occurs typically in obsessional neurosis, 'in which one action is cancelled out by the second so that it is as though neither action had taken place, whereas, in reality, both have'. Obsessional rituals are a result of undoing.
6. *Projection*. The process by which aspects of self (impulses, feelings, wishes and objects) are 'put into' another person. It is typical of persecutory delusion and paranoid states.
7. *Introjection*. This refers to 'internalisation' or 'taking in' of the functions of another object. For example, the superego is formed by the introjection of parental figures. It may be followed by identification with the introjected object.
8. *Turning against self*. Here the impulse to harm another is directed towards self. It is said to be a feature of masochism.
9. *Reversal*. This is the capacity to reverse an instinct into its opposite and is similar to reaction formation.
10. *Sublimation*. Transformation of instinctual energies to socially acceptable goals. Considered to be one of the mature defences, it is thought to underlie many humanitarian and altruistic activities.

Many other defence mechanisms have been described and will not be enumerated here. Two other important defence mechanisms described by Klein, splitting and projective identification, are discussed later. Splitting, projection and projective identification are considered to be primitive defences.

PSYCHOANALYTIC TECHNIQUE

One of Freud's greatest contributions to the practice of psychotherapy is his formulation of certain fundamental phenomena encountered during the process of psychoanalytic treatment. First and foremost he was a clinician and his observations of what the patient brought to the analytic situation and what he, the therapist, contributed to it made him describe various phenomena that occurred in such clinical encounters. Initially applied only to psychoanalytic settings, these ides are now seen as relevant to all therapeutic situations, including all doctor–patient contacts, and are therefore particularly relevant to psychiatric practice. The way that these concepts have been understood has constantly changed over time as new theorists have modified the original version. Each of the phenomena described below can, therefore, be viewed as having two definitions, the classical version, as intended by the original author, and a more extended one created by modern or contemporary workers. The following descriptions of psychoanalytic techniques and processes are of particular importance:

Psychoanalytic setting. Freud paid meticulous care to the time and space he made available to the patient. Each psychoanalytic session took place in the same place and lasted usually 55 minutes and was without any interruptions. Sessions were prearranged and therefore predictable. In psychoanalysis the client is seen twice a week, though in most forms of psychodynamic psychotherapy they are seen less often, usually weekly.

Free association. For Freud the technique of free association was the corner stone of psychoanalysis. The basic rule of free association is that the patient tells the analyst everything that comes into his mind spontaneously and without reservation, even if the thoughts are felt to be unimportant, irrelevant or disagreeable. The assumption here is that in a therapeutic setting, thinking is never 'free' but is guided by conscious and, more importantly, unconscious forces. It promotes regression, minimises resistance and brings forth significant material. Freud set certain arduous tasks for the therapist: (1) maintaining neutrality while paying 'free floating' attention; (2) acting as a 'mirror'; and (3) abstinence (denial by the therapist of any temptations to satisfy his/her own needs such as satisfaction, admiration or love).

Resistance. This refers to the powerful forces that oppose the psychotherapeutic process. It is pervasive and occurs at every step. Failed appointments, silences during sessions, not being open about one's thoughts and feelings are manifestations of resistance. The analyst's approach to resistance is not to overcome it, but to subject it to analysis and make the patient aware of his resistances. Freud described various forms of resistances, two of the more important ones are:

1. Transference resistance – here the resistance involves impulses, feelings and fantasies that emerge in relation to the therapist.
2. Repression resistance – this arises from the need of the patient to defend him/herself from feelings that produce pain and suffering if they are made conscious.

Transference. The displacement on to the therapist of feelings, attitudes, ideas and fantasies that were previously experienced in relation to past figures is known as transference. Repetition of the past in the analyst–patient relationship was described by Freud as 'repetition compulsion'. This tendency to re-enact past relationships in the present is unconscious, specific and intense. It is a recreation or re-enactment of the past in the present, which appears quite appropriate to the client. Initially Freud considered the emergence of transference a hindrance to the therapeutic process. Later he came to see it as an essential part of the therapist's work.

Transference is ubiquitous and is not confined to the analytic situation. It occurs in most interpersonal transactions in every-day life. But, in the psychotherapeutic setting it provides the analyst with the opportunity to make interpretations that link the present experience with the therapist with the patient's past relationships (transference interpretation). Not all aspects of the therapist–client relationship are due to transference and a distinction has to be made between transference and non-transference elements.

Countertransference. The concept of countertransference has undergone modification since it was first described by Freud. Initially it was used to signify the analyst's response to the patient's transference. In its current usage, the term countertransference refers to all the analyst's emotional reactions towards the patient (e.g. anger, feelings of impotence, hate). While countertransference can lead to difficulties in the therapeutic process, self-scrutiny of the reactions provoked by the client in the therapist is considered to be a powerful tool in the analytic process. It reflects the analyst's own unconscious reaction to the patient, although some aspects may be conscious. Psychoanalysts in training are expected to undergo personal analysis to make them, among other things, aware of their own 'blind spots' and conflicts (e.g. need for vicarious gratification) so that they are better able to reflect on their reactions to clients.

Interpretation. Interpretations are verbal interventions made by the therapist, which make conscious the unconscious meaning, origin or cause of a given thought, feeling or behaviour. In broad terms, the aim of interpretation is to make the patient aware of some aspect of his/her psychological functioning of which he/she was not previously conscious. It is a construction (or reconstruction) based on material made available to the therapist. Interpretations are well-thought-out statements made with the intention of promoting insight and self-awareness. For example, a patient who has experienced frustration in their previous dealings with another service (e.g. social services) may be found to be hostile towards the clinician. In order to overcome the 'institutional transference' it is important to bring forth and acknowledge the previous disappointment that the patient had experienced. Two types of interpretations have been described:

1. Transference interpretations – these are aimed at linking patient's current attitudes, behaviours and feelings towards the therapist with past significant relationships. In psychoanalysis and psychodynamic psychotherapy, transference interpretations are considered to be the most useful, if not essential, means of producing self-awareness, insight and change (Figure 13.3).
2. Extratransference interpretations – interpretations that do not refer to transference relationships are the commonest in any therapeutic encounter and are as important as transference interpretations.

Acting out. Often, past events that are brought to the surface during analysis are enacted rather than remembered. This may happen within the treatment setting (acting out in transference) or outside it.

Working through. The processes involved in gaining insight as a result of analysis is usually termed working through. It involves reconstruction of the past and deepening of understanding, thus facilitating change.

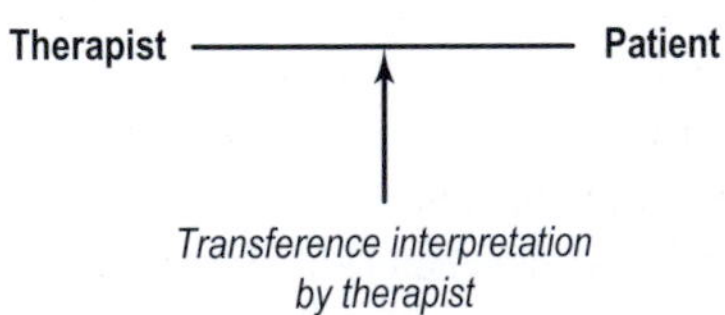

Fig. 13.3 Transference interpretation

OBJECT-RELATIONS THEORY

Object-relations theory, which grew from Freudian concepts, has been developed by Melanie Klein, Ronald Fairburn and Donald Winnicott, among others. It had been particularly popular in the UK, especially among child psychotherapists. The term 'object' is rather misleading. Freud used it to mean 'that towards which an instinct or impulse is directed'. It is an unfortunate choice of word, for it does not mean an inanimate object but refers to persons or part of persons (part objects). The defining feature of the object-relations school is that it sees relationships as the cornerstone of human existence. This is in contrast to the classical theory, which gives primacy to biological drives and instinct. A fundamental tenet of object-relations theory is that people operate in an interpersonal world of subjective relationships and the drive towards relationships with objects is as basic as instinctual drives. Nevertheless, object-relations theory is not an interpersonal or interactional theory. It is concerned not with the relationship *between* the object and the subject, but that of the subject *to* the object.

Klein believed that the infant is born with a predetermined capacity to relate to his mother or part of his mother and this object relationship comes into existence immediately after birth. Thus, the first object relationship that the infant experiences is the one between himself and the mother, particularly the mother's breast or nipple. As the infant develops he internalises (introjects) his experiences with the mother. Klein held that the prototype for the first object relationship was the feeding experience. These early and primitive experiences are introjected so that, in the infant's mind, it comes to be represented and experienced as 'internal objects'. Initially the infant experiences the mother as two separate objects: the 'good object', which feeds, nurtures and is need-satisfying on the one hand, and a 'bad object', which is withholding, harsh and malevolent (when not available to him) on the other. Klein considered internal objects to have an almost concrete existence and to be an integral part of the ego.

Klein postulated two stages in the development of object relationships. She called these phases 'positions' to emphasise the fact that these phases of development may be revisited in later life. The two main positions are:

1. The paranoid–schizoid position. This occupies the first three months of life and is the result of the infant's attempt to master its fear and anxiety immediately after birth. Soon after birth the infant is terrified that it is falling apart, fragmenting and disintegrating. In the face of such terror the infant experiences objects as persecutory and threatening its very existence. The infant deals with these paranoid anxieties through two primitive defences: splitting and projection. Splitting, the division of the object (mother) into a good one and bad one enables the infant to bring order into the chaos it experiences and helps it feel safe. By separating everything bad from everything good the baby experiences good and loving feelings. The infant takes in the good object, i.e. introjects it. The bad object, which contains feelings of hate and badness, are projected on to the object in an attempt to get rid of them. The mother thus comes to contain the disowned bad parts of the self.

2. *The depressive position.* In the course of development, about the age of four to six months, the infant is able to integrate his experiences of the mother, not as separate good and part objects, but as a whole object. He comes to realise that the mother he loved and the mother (the object) he hated is the same person. Klein considered this to be a major developmental step. This new, and more realistic, relationship to the mother is deeply painful for the infant. This causes intense depressive anxiety in the child. The infant becomes concerned for the welfare of the mother and fears that its aggressive impulses may destroy the object that it now recognises as important and loved. The result is grief rather than anger.

The main defences against depressive anxiety at this stage are: (1) to regress to the paranoid–schizoid position; or (2) to invoke manic defences.

Manic defences. This term, which was first described by Klein, refers to a group of defence mechanisms, the central feature of which is the denial of the importance of the good object in an omnipotent way in an attempt to avoid the intense pain and guilt. Alternatively, the anxiety and depression may be modified and dealt with by *reparation*. Reparation arises out of real concern for the whole object, remorse and love. It forms the cornerstone of the maturational process, channelling instinctual impulses into constructive and altruistic goals.

Projective identification

Klein's formulation of the defence mechanism of projective identification is a complicated piece of work and there are different versions of it. Klein defined projective identification as follows: 'Together with these harmful excrements, expelled in hatred, split-off parts of the ego are also projected onto the mother, or, as I would rather call it, into the mother. These excrements and bad parts of the self are not only meant to injure but also control and take possession of the object. Insofar as the mother comes to contain the bad parts of the self, she is felt to be a separate individual but is felt to be *the* bad self. Much of the hatred against the parts of the self is now directed towards the mother. This leads to a particular form of identification which establishes the prototype of an aggressive object relation. I suggest for these processes the term 'projective identification' (Klein, 1952).

Projective identification is best explained as occurring in three steps:

1. Splitting off of an intolerable (e.g. bad or hated) aspect of self from its complementary partner (e.g. love).
2. Projection of the disowned part of self on to the object.
3. Identification with the recipient who received the disowned part, such that what happens to the recipient is experiences as though happening to self. The object is now felt not to be separate but is experienced as part of self.

Projective identification differs from projection in that in the latter there is distancing or isolation of the self from what is projected rather than identification. Later workers like Bion have broadened the phenomenon of projective identification to include the effect on the object. Thus, the recipient unconsciously identifies with what is projected and is induced to think, feel and behave differently. In clinical encounters the therapist is drawn into thinking and doing according to the patient's wishes. For example, the experience of a feeling of intense depression in the therapist after seeing a very depressed patient could be seen as part of projective identification where the clinician has now come to identify with aspects of the depression that the patient has projected on to him/her. Similarly, in the analytic situation, an aggressive patient will induce the therapist to act in an aggressive manner, while a masochistic patient will act in a manner that unconsciously tries to get the analyst to make slightly sadistic interpretations.

It is important to remember that projective identification is an unconscious process and occurs in fantasy (instinct attached to objects, the basic unit of mental activity). It involves subject and object *representations* rather than real self and external objects. Projective identification may be seen to serve two functions. First, it may serve a defensive purpose, such has ridding the self of unwanted parts and painful states of mind (evacuation) and bringing relief. Second, it can be used as a form of communication (of the state of mind by the subject to the object). In psychoanalytic and other clinical encounters patients transmit on to the therapist experiences and feelings that they cannot manage. Awareness of this happening in a therapeutic setting enables the therapist to empathise with the patient. This forms a major part of countertransference. Recognition of the projected origins of the feelings experienced by the therapist is an extremely useful tool in the hands of the therapist. The therapist may or may not choose to interpret it to the patient. In the course of therapy, the therapist receives the projections from the patient, modifies them to a degree and returns them to the patient in a form that they can assimilate. This is usually done by various forms of interpretation. In this respect the therapist functions somewhat like a mother bird that digests food in its own system and then regurgitates it to the chick.

Winnicott

Donald Winnicott was a paediatrician who turned to psychoanalysis in the course of his work with children. In orientation he was an object-relations theorist but he emphasised the role of the environment to a much greater degree than others of the same school. His most famous comment, 'there is no such thing as the baby' stressed the need to take the mother–baby relationship as the unit of analysis rather than the baby alone. Winnicott used the phrase *primary maternal preoccupation* to describe the identification of the mother with the baby during infancy, which provided the latter with *the primary experience* of safety, security and oneness with the mother.

As the baby develops, the mother begins to separate herself from it while providing loving care, enabling the infant to form a personal identity. Winnicott called a mother who was attuned to the mental state and emotional needs of her infant a 'good enough mother'. When the mother does not provide the emotional 'holding', the infant tends to envelop its true self within a 'false self' in order to hide its inner state of anxiety and vulnerability.

Transitional object or *phenomena* is a Winnicottian concept that refers to items such as blankets, rags, and teddy bears that children use to cope with being alone and separated from their mothers and which help them manage their anxiety by themselves. Such items stand for the mother but do not replace her. According to Winnicott (1953), to qualify to be called a transitional object they:

- Must belong to the child.
- The child must be able to treat them any way he/she likes.
- Must have features that symbolise the mother–child relationship (e.g. texture).

As the child grows up, the object is not given up but commonly becomes less and less imbued with meaning and is often forgotten.

For Winnicott, the therapeutic setting represented transitional phenomena in which the patient experienced safe and dependent feelings. Patients with borderline personality organisation are known to use appointment cards, letters and other objects belonging to the therapeutic setting as transitional objects.

Wilfred Bion

Bion is known for his work with groups (not discussed here) and the concept of *container–contained*. According to Bion, the infant's first relation to his first object can be described as follows.

When the infant experiences intolerable anxiety, he deals with it by projecting it into the mother. Normally the mother's response is to acknowledge the anxiety and do whatever is necessary to relieve the infant's distress. The infant perceives this as having projected something into the object, but the object was able to contain it and deal with it. Thus, the mother acts as the container for the child's uncontrollable feelings. The containment of anxiety by an external object is fundamental to the infant's emotional development. It may be disrupted under two situations: (1) when the mother is unable to bear the infant's projected anxiety (or is not attuned to the child's emotions); and (2) when the infant's distress is excessive and extreme. In the former instance, the infant gets more terrified than before and has to resort to primitive defences to protecting himself.

The concept of *container–contained* has been applied to clinical situations where the therapist acts as a safe container for the painful emotions that the client brings into the session. A similar phenomenon is evident in day-to-day interactions between parents and children. For example, children show more distress and disturbance to bereavement or trauma in families when the parents themselves are overwhelmed by the events and take too long to recover. Their own distress (and possibly psychopathology) prevents them from acting as containers for the children's distress and anxiety.

REFERENCES

Freud A (1936) The ego and the mechanism of defence. London, UK: Karnac.
Freud S (1900) The interpretation of dreams, SE 4 and 5. London, UK: Hogarth Press.
Freud S (1905) Three essays on sexuality, SE 7. London, UK: Hogarth Press.
Freud S (1915) Instincts and their vicissitudes, SE 14. London, UK: Hogarth Press.
Freud S (1923) The ego and the id, SE 19. London, UK: Hogarth Press.

Freud S (1933a) New introductory lectures on psychoanalysis, SE 22. London, UK: Hogarth Press.
Freud S (1933b) Why war? SE 22. London, UK: Hogarth Press.
Freud S (1940) An outline of psychoanalysis, SE 23. London, UK: Hogarth Press.
Klein M (1946/1952) Notes on some schizoid mechanisms. In (1975) The Writings of Melanie Klein, Vol. 3. Envy and Gratitude and Other works (pp. 1–24). London, UK: Hogarth Press.
Stanford-Clark D (1988) What Freud Really Said. London, UK: Penguin Books.
Webster R (1995) Why Freud Was Wrong. London, UK: Harper Collins.
Winnicott DW (1953) Transitional objects and transitional phenomena. International Journal of Psychoanalysis, 34, 89–97.

FURTHER READING

The literature on psychoanalysis is vast and there is no alternative to good and sound supervision of the different types of cases that one undertakes to treat. The following books provide a good introduction to the subject.

Bateman A, Holmes J (1995) Introduction to Psychoanalysis: contemporary theory and practice. London, UK: Routledge.

- A masterful but concise piece of work outlining most psychoanalytic concepts in an interesting and clinically relevant way.

Casement P (1985) On learning from the patient. London, UK: Routledge.

- An outstanding book that provides a moving insight into analytic technique.

Freud S (1933) New Introductory Lectures on Psychoanalysis, SE 22. London, UK: Hogarth Press.

- A book well worth reading for a taste of the master's eloquence and sweep of writing.

Segal H (1964/1973) Introduction to the Work of Melanie Klein. London, UK: The Hogarth Press and The Institute of Psychoanalysis.

- A lucid account of Kleinian theory by one of the foremost authorities on her work.

Mental disorders (abnormal psychology)

14

'Science is built up with fact, as a house is with stone. But a collection of fact is no more a science than a heap of stones is a house.'
Jules Hendri Poincare

Defining abnormality

In the previous chapters, for most part, we have discussed various aspects of normal mental functioning. Although references to abnormal mental states were made, what constitutes abnormality was not made explicit. The concept of abnormal psychological functioning or mental disorder is fundamental to both theory and practice in the field of mental health. But the issues remain contentious and provoke heated debates (defining normality is even harder and is outside the scope of this chapter). Some of the main ways of conceptualising abnormality are as follows:

Disorder as deviation from statistical norms. Conditions or behaviours that are rare have been considered to be abnormal. The benchmark in this approach is the statistical norm. Thus, low IQ, dwarfism, hypertension and hallucinations may be considered abnormal by these standards. But, so are giftedness, being seven-feet tall and undertaking space travel, conditions that would hardly be called disorders. In spite of its simplicity and ease of measurement, in the statistical approach any behaviour that is unconventional, and therefore rare, would be deemed abnormal. It is worth noting that it is this statistical approach that is employed in most psychological measurements.

Disorder as distress or suffering. Experience of distress has been considered a hallmark of disorders. Most often it is personal distress and suffering that makes individuals seek help. But the distress or suffering criterion is neither a necessary nor sufficient condition for establishing the presence of abnormality. Suffering is common in society (e.g. bereavement, imprisonment) and many people do not report distress even in the presence of obvious disorders (e.g. asymptomatic cancer, hypertension, hypomania).

Disorder as impairment or disability. Difficulties that result in impairment of social, occupational and personal functioning have sometimes been upheld as the defining feature of disorders. Sometimes such dysfunction has been called maladaptive behaviour. However, although the person with agoraphobia who cannot go out and the patient with hypertension are clearly dysfunctional, they may manage life reasonably well with help from their family.

Disorder as deviation from societal norms. In the past, violation of social standards (e.g. criminality) has been considered to be abnormality. It is not uncommon to hear the same argument today. For example, school refusal in children and recidivism are considered by some to be abnormal. Similarly, the proposed category of 'persons with severe and dangerous personality disorder' would be a clear example of creating a disorder category by legislation, presumably to protect the public.

It should be clear from the foregoing account of abnormality that none of the above criteria on their own are capable of consistently establishing what abnormality or disorder is. A cursory examination of various mental and physical disorders such as agoraphobia, hypertension and cancer would make it clear that the criteria used to define disorder are inconsistent and variable.

A fundamental issue in the analysis of the concept of mental disorder is whether disorders are scientific terms or value judgements. The terms psychological abnormality, mental disorder, disease and illness are used interchangeably here; more accurate definitions of the terms are provided in Box 14.1. Recent scholarship on the subject has helped to verify the issues surrounding the usage of the term mental disorder. In a well-argued analysis of the concept of mental disorder, Wakefield (1992) has defined it as *harmful dysfunction*. His definition combines the scientific (biomedical) and the value (sociopolitical) components and is stated as follows:

> *A disorder exists when the failure of a person's internal mechanisms to perform their functions as designed by nature impinges harmfully on the person's well-being as defined by social values and meanings. The order that is disturbed when one has a disorder is thus simultaneously biological and social: neither alone is sufficient to justify the label disorder.*

The harmful dysfunction approach, as advocated by Wakefield, appears to be closest one could get to clarifying the concept of mental disorders. It appears to have both simplicity and the power of logic. Although there is no unanimity, there is now general agreement that the definition of both physical and mental disorders are based on two essential criteria as proposed by Wakefield:

1. *Personal dysfunction (biomedical criterion)*. The condition arises from behavioural, psychological, or biological dysfunction in the person; it is clinically recognisable as a set of symptoms and behaviours and is often associated with biological disadvantage for the person or species.
2. *Harm (value criterion)*. The condition should cause some harm as judged by the standards of the person's culture. This includes any personal

Box 14.1 Definitions of Disease, Illness and Disorder (the terms are used interchangeably in this chapter)

- **Disease** – disorder of structure or function; deviation from a biological norm; a pathological process concerning cells and tissues
- **Illness** – the subjective interpretation by the patient of experience of problems as related to health
- **Sickness** – the role negotiated by society
- **Disorder** – 'harmful dysfunction'

impairment, handicap, maladaptation, suffering and disability resulting from the condition.

The main point to note is that it is naïve to think that disorders are the same as biological abnormalities of structure or function, i.e. disorders are different from diseases. Most currently recognised disorders are no more than symptom clusters. They are also social constructions, and, to that extent, determined by the prevailing culture. For example, a person showing extreme agoraphobic behaviour may be quite content to be confined to the house (behavioural and psychological dysfunction) but at the same time not be regarded as fulfilling the normative expectations of society (value judgment). Even in the field of physical medicine, for some diseases no objective criteria of dysfunction are demonstrable (e.g. fibromyalgia).

'Being sane in insane places'

Defining what constitutes psychological or mental disorder is all the more difficult because in psychiatry and clinical psychology abnormality has to be inferred mostly from accounts of subjective experiences (and observations) without the benefit of laboratory or other technological information.

These difficulties are illustrated by a remarkable, yet controversial, study by David Rosenhan. In the study (Rosenhan, 1973) eight normal people (five men and three women) tried to get admitted to 12 different psychiatric hospitals in the USA. The pseudopatients complained of hearing 'voices'. They claimed that the 'voices' were unclear but seemed to be saying, 'thud', 'empty' and 'hollow'. Seven of them were admitted to hospital with a diagnosis of schizophrenia even though they did not complain of any other symptoms. After admission they behaved normally apart from writing down their observations (as instructed by the author of the study). On average the length of hospitalisation was 19 days (range 7 to 52 days). At the time of discharge their diagnosis was of 'schizophrenia in remission'.

In a second part of the study, a psychiatric hospital was told that some people would try to get admitted to hospital by pretending to have schizophrenic symptoms. Although no pseudopatients actually presented themselves, of the 193 patients who were examined during this period, 23 were suspected of fabricating their symptoms by at least one psychiatrist. From these studies Rosenhan concluded that, 'it is clear that we cannot distinguish the sane from the insane in psychiatric hospitals'.

The study has been taken to mean that: (1) psychiatric diagnoses are unreliable even at the level of mental illness and no mental illness; and (2) the very act of psychiatric hospitalisation produces a labelling effect that becomes a self-fulfilling prophecy. The first assertion has been challenged on the grounds that the real diagnosis in all the subjects was malingering (and not insanity as claimed by the author). It is not uncommon in medicine to diagnose diseases on the basis of symptoms alone. For example, the diagnoses of migraine and epilepsy are made primarily on clinical symptoms. In such cases it is easy for patients to deliberately mislead professionals by fabricating symptoms. Psychiatry is unique as a discipline in that it relies heavily on the patient's account of the symptoms and signs to diagnose a mental disorder. In many psychiatric conditions observational measures and other objective tests add little to the clinical picture. (It is worth noting that the study was carried out at a time when DSM-II was in use in North America and there were few agreed criteria for diagnosing mental disorders; American psychiatrists were shown to be twice as likely as their British counterparts to make a diagnosis of schizophrenia.)

The second conclusion from the study, that the consequences of admission to a psychiatric ward itself has negative consequences including labelling and loss of power for the patient, is a telling indictment of the effects of psychiatric hospitalisation. Although current hospital practices have changed and care in the community and user involvement have, to a large extent, reduced some of the adverse effects of psychiatric hospitalisation, the study is still a salutary reminder of the potential adverse effects of psychiatric hospitalisation.

Apart from the practical considerations highlighted by the Rosenhan study, in the case of mental disorders we are faced with the added problem of defining the term 'mental'. Mind is not the same as the brain, although it includes some of the functions of the brain. The cerebral mechanisms involved in psychological functions described in the preceding chapters are poorly understood and the little we know about them does not correspond to the abnormal states of mind that psychiatrists are interested in. The brain is an immensely complex organ and psychological functions are even more complex. Given the difficulties in defining what constitutes each of the two words 'mental' and 'disorder', it is evident that we need a more complex science than that available at the moment in order to study, understand and manage the complexities of mental disorders.

Current methods of psychiatric diagnosis of mental disorders are based primarily on symptoms and signs and, at best, the course of the disorder, i.e. the level of description of disorders is mainly at the syndrome level. The two commonly used classificatory systems, DSM-IV and ICD-10 are explicit about what constitutes a disorder: According to ICD-10: 'disorder is an inexact term, but it is used here to imply the existence of a clinically recognisable set of symptoms or behaviour associated in most cases with distress and with interference with personal function' (WHO, 1992). In DSM-IV a mental disorder is: 'conceptualised as a clinically significant behavioural or psychological syndrome or pattern that occurs in an individual and is associated with persistent distress or disability (impairment) in one or more areas of functioning ...' (APA, 1994).

Thus, in psychiatry, at present the definitions of disorders are based on clinical descriptions (and presume no particular aetiology, physiological dysfunction or lesion). No matter how assiduously we use scales to estimate patients' symptoms, we are still using pattern recognition of symptoms – we are making empirical diagnoses based on descriptions of symptom clusters.

Psychiatric classification (nosology)

Having described what a disorder is, the next question that arises is: how does one distinguish one disorder from another, i.e. how are psychiatric disorders

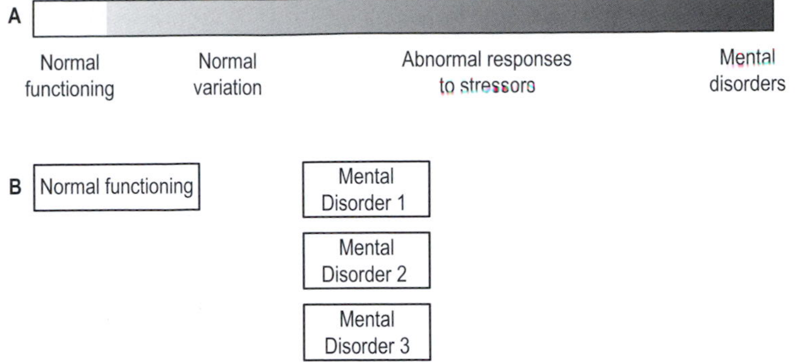

Fig. 14.1 Mental disorder: A, dimensional model; B, categorical model.

classified? There are at least two ways of approaching any classificatory system. The first is a categorical approach that attempts to divide the entities into groups on the basis of common properties or characteristics and the other is the dimensional view that sees them as belonging to one class but as showing a gradation in characteristics (Figure 14.1).

Dimensions and categories

Categories refer to discrete groups with some common characteristics (e.g. birds, furniture, languages, nations). In biology, classification of the animal kingdom into mammals, birds and reptiles, for example, is based on the presence or absence of certain defining characteristics. The process of classification involves the creation of mutually exclusive and jointly exhaustive categories. In a classificatory system, for categories to be mutually exclusive it is assumed that a hypothetical boundary exists between the subpopulations.

In an ideal classificatory system there should be no overlap in the features that are considered to be salient, i.e. the classes should be homogeneous. But this is never the case, even in biology and chemistry where classification forms the very basis of scientific knowledge (e.g. waves and particles). In the case of psychiatric syndromes the assumption is that each syndrome is *qualitatively* distinct from all others, and has its own unique clinical features, course and natural history. This means that in the search for a putative boundary between syndromes it has to be demonstrated that the clinical features that go to form conditions X and Y, for example, show little overlap. Since it is extremely uncommon to see pure forms, in practical terms, we should be able to show that the distribution of the features of the two conditions are bimodal rather than unimodal, thus indicating that a discontinuity exists between them (Figure 14.2). The presence of 'mixed' forms (e.g. features of depression and anxiety) does not necessarily invalidate the assertion that two categories are demonstrable as long as such conditions are relatively infrequent (Kendell, 1975). Cluster analysis of clinical features is one of the common statistical techniques used to identify categories.

In the case of psychiatric disorders, there is the further assumption that a similar discontinuity exists between the normal and the abnormal. Thus,

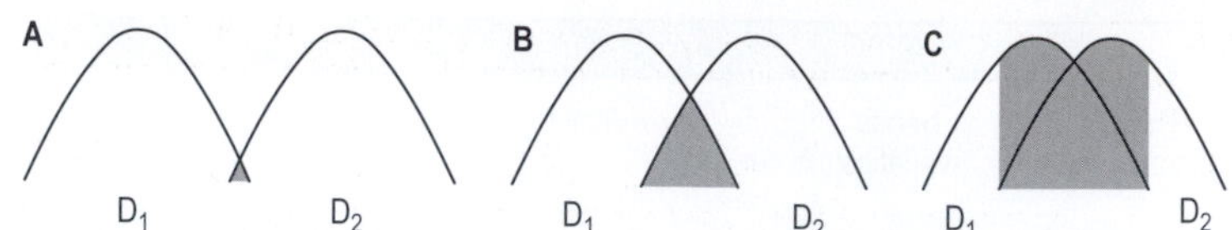

Fig. 14.2 Hypothetical distribution of clinical features of two disorders D1 and D2: A, bimodal distribution with 'point of rarity'; B, bimodal distribution with some overlap of symptoms; and C, bimodal distribution with considerable overlap and a large proportion of 'mixed forms'

'cases' need to be differentiated from 'non-cases' and partial syndromes have to be shown to be uncommon. Pathological presentations are thought to be distinct and qualitatively different from normal functioning. For example, while normal, and even extreme, dieting is quite common in the West, in order to be classified as anorexia nervosa certain features (body weight below 85%, a distinctive psychopathology and amenorrhoea) need to be present.

In contrast, *dimensional approaches* to classification hold that psychiatric conditions are essentially exaggerations of normal psychological processes and the differences are *quantitative* rather than qualitative. The patient's condition is depicted as points on a series of fundamental dimensions of psychopathology. In the case of the eating disorder mentioned above, one could argue that subclinical or atypical forms of eating problems are common and form a bridge between 'normal' dieting and extreme forms of dieting that result in severe weight loss and consequent amenorrhoea. According to this view the difference between normal and abnormal is a matter of degree and abnormal is a variation of normal. It should be noted that in a dimensional system a clinical condition would have to be represented along multiple dimensions. For example, symptoms of schizophrenia have been subjected to factor analysis to yield at least four factors: negative symptoms, hallucinations, formal thought disorder and delusions and, using a dimensional model, the patient can be characterised along each dimension, each with its own presumed aetiology, pathophysiology, and clinical course. A detailed discussion of the advantages and disadvantages of the two systems of classification are beyond the remit of this chapter. Kendell (1975) has provided an in-depth discussion of the issues for psychiatry.

There is no inherent contradiction between the two systems. Some disorders may fit dimensional descriptions better than categorical dichotomies. For example, recent work has made it abundantly clear that there is no point of discontinuity between normal personality and personality disorders and that a dimensional view of the range of conditions is a more accurate reflection of reality (Tyrer & Johnson, 1996). Thus, in the system proposed by Tyrer (2003), a continuum of personality functioning from normal personality, through personality difficulties, simple personality disorder, complex personality disorder to severe personality disorder makes more sense than the categories described in DSM and ICD (Table 14.1).

The differences between the two approaches may be considered complementary than contradictory. Although natural light consists of a spectrum of colours (dimensional view of light) we talk of violet, indigo, blue and other

Table 14.1 Dimensional system of classifying personality disorders (Tyrer, 2003)

Normal personality	–
Personality difficulty	Meets subthreshold criteria for one or more PDs
Simple PD	Meets criteria for one or more PDs within the same cluster
Complex PD	Meets criteria for one or more PDs within more than one cluster
Severe PD	Meets criteria for severe disruption to both individual and society

colours (categorical view) and find them convenient descriptions for understanding and communicating information (Table 14.2). In physics, light is understood as both particles and waves, depending on how we look at it. Even dimensional systems have to consider thresholds and cut-off points for characteristics to be deemed abnormal (e.g. IQ). The issue is not, which of the two systems is a 'true' representation of reality but, more importantly, which of the two is *useful* in a given situation. As our knowledge advances, concepts and approaches are bound to change as well. For instance, the classical view of time and space as different entities has been transformed by Einstein's demonstration of the space–time continuum. Although not as momentous as Einstein's findings, we can expect that, as a result of research, important changes to the way that we think about psychiatric disorders are bound to occur in the near future.

DSM and ICD

It is not the intention to describe the two commonly used classificatory systems DSM-IV and ICD-10 here, rather the purpose is to outline the main principles on which they are based (the reader is referred to standard textbooks on psychiatry for details of DSM and ICD). Both classificatory systems are categorical systems of classification based on clinical descriptions. The DSM is considered in greater detail because most field research has been carried out using it, but the principles underpinning the two systems are almost identical.

The main principles of DSM-IV may be stated as follows:

1. It is theory-neutral (atheoretical) regarding the causes of mental disorders. For example, it does not subscribe to any models of causation of disorders such as learning theories, cognitive theories or psychoanalytic theories.

Table 14.2 Examples of dimensions and categories contained within them

Dimension or spectrum	*Categories within the dimension*
Time	Day, night, 12 o' clock
Temperature	Hot, 17°C
Blood sugar	Hyperglycaemia, hypoglycaemia
Attachment	Insecure, secure
Life span	Adolescence, old age
Sciences	Psychology, psychiatry

2. It takes a descriptive rather than an aetiological approach. This is not to say that aetiology is unimportant, but it is an acknowledgement of our current ignorance of aetiology and pathogenesis.
3. It specifies the operational diagnostic criteria that must be present for a diagnosis to be made.
4. Its diagnoses are non-hierarchical, that is, more than one diagnosis can be made. This was a radical departure from DSM-II, which followed the 'one disease, one diagnosis' approach.
5. Its classification is based on a multiaxial system (see later).

The ICD-10 follows broadly similar principles except that, instead of diagnostic criteria, we are provided with 'diagnostic guidelines' (in the research version of ICD-10 clear criteria similar to those of the DSM-IV are given); the multiaxial classificatory system is optional.

It should be pointed out that both systems of classification were developed through extensive discussions and consultation within the professions and represented a consensus statement at the time of publication. DSM has undergone numerous revisions and has been meticulously and painstakingly researched. In DSM-IV specific mental disorders (Axis I) are separated from personality disorders and mental retardation (Axis II). The classificatory system is polythetic in that not all symptoms or diagnostic criteria are necessary for making a diagnosis. The inclusion of medical disorders under Axis III and psychosocial factors in Axis IV were intended to make the system more comprehensive. Social and personal impairment, called global assessment of functioning, is coded under Axis V. Altogether DSM-IV has 16 clinical conditions under Axis I, and 11 personality disorders are included under Axis II. Chapter V of ICD-10 has 10 major classes of mental and behavioural disorders (Tables 14.3 and 14.4)

An important result of the DSM developmental process is its increased reliability. Field studies have shown that interrater agreement for Axis I disorders is very high (between .73 and 1.00). DSM-IV has repeatedly been

Table 14.3 The multiaxial classificatory systems in ICD-10 and DSM-IV

DSM-IV	
Axis I	Clinical disorders
Axis II	Personality disorders Mental retardation
Axis III	General medical conditions
Axis IV	Psychosocial and environment problems
Axis V	Global assessment of functioning
ICD-10	
Axis I	Clinical diagnoses
Axis II	Disablements
Axis III	Contextual factors

Table 14.4 DSM-IV and ICD-10 classification of mental disorders

DSM-IV (Axis I)	*ICD-10*
Disorders first diagnosed in infancy, childhood or adolescence	Organic disorders
Delirium, dementia, amnestic and other cognitive disorders	Schizophrenia, schizotypal and delusional disorders
Mental disorders due to general medical conditions	Mood (affective) disorders
Substance-related disorders	Neurotic, stress-related and somatoform disorders
Schizophrenia and other psychotic disorders	Behavioural syndromes associated with physical factors, e.g. eating disorders
Mood disorders	Disorders of adult personality and behaviour
Anxiety disorders	Mental retardation
Somatoform disorders	Disorders of psychological development
Factitious disorders	Behavioural and emotional disorders with onset in childhood and adolescence
Dissociative disorders	
Sexual and gender identity disorders	
Eating disorders	
Sleep disorders	
Impulse-control disorders	
Adjustment disorders	

demonstrated to show greater diagnostic stability over time and greater inter-clinician agreement than previous versions, especially for such diagnostic categories as schizophrenia, bipolar disorder, major depression and substance misuse. However, its reliability for other disorders, especially personality disorders has been less promising.

Critique of DSM-IV and ICD-10

The principal goal of DSM was to create an empirically based nomenclature and improve the reliability and validity of various diagnostic categories. It has achieved these aims to a moderate degree. It has generated a large body of research and, as a result, our knowledge of psychiatric disorders keeps improving and changing. Nevertheless, there are certain inherent disadvantages associated with any diagnostic system. An awareness of the limitations and potential dangers of the diagnostic systems is essential for any clinician involved in dealing with real people (Box 14.2).

The problem of 'comorbidity'. The cooccurrence of clinically independent conditions is referred to as comorbidity. The occurrence of more than one psychiatric disorder in the same patient is a fact of life in psychiatry. A typical finding is that of Zimmerman and Matia (1999). Using semi-structures

> **Box 14.2 Disadvantages of diagnosis and diagnosing**
>
> - Diagnosis often objectifies the person and sees him/her as the bearer of symptoms or disease
> - It encourages the tendency to believe that people are powerless to do any thing about their problem
> - It promotes the reification fallacy, the tendency to ignore the fact that diseases are man-made entities
> - The diagnosis, by itself, is usually inadequate to understand or manage the disorder

interviews in a clinical setting, they found that more than a third of the patients qualified for three or more Axis I disorders (DSM-IV and ICD-10 allow multiple diagnoses). This has lead to two responses from the psychiatric establishment. The 'lumpers', those who believe in broad diagnostic groupings such as 'the general neurotic syndrome' (Andrews et al., 1990) and the 'splitters' who argue that the spirit of the current diagnostic systems is to record the maximum amount of diagnostic information as a way of characterising the complexity of clinical presentations and hence encourage multiple diagnoses. Official classifications require that as many disorders as possible should be recorded to describe the complete state of the patient and they are, therefore, on the side of the splitters.

But the presence of comorbidity strains credibility and reflects adversely on the conceptual basis of current classifications. It has been argued that either the nature of psychiatric disorders is such that they always tend to occur in clusters, or the diagnostic classification fails to discriminate between true comorbidity and spurious comorbidity arising from shared clinical features.

Expansion of the concept of mental disorder. In general, there has been a recent tendency in Western countries to create new diseases and new treatments for normal life processes (e.g. child birth, ageing, sexuality, unhappiness, death) and a tendency to classify people's ordinary day-to-day problems (reactions to bereavement, trauma and losses) as diseases. In 2002, the *British Medical Journal* ran a vote on its website to identify the top ten 'non-diseases' (Table 14.5). The results showed that many doctors agreed that conditions like ageing and unhappiness were really 'non-diseases' that were being spuriously considered as diseases (Smith, 2002).

In the field of psychiatry there have been similar developments, resulting in blurring of the traditional boundaries of mental illness and extending the remit of psychiatry to include minor mental perturbations. There are concerns that the traditional distinction between major, long-lasting, severe disorders and minor, time-limited disturbances is being overridden. Many complain that common personal and social problems (e.g. loneliness, ageing, grief, criminality, and unhappiness) are being classified as mental disorders.

This wider definition of mental disorders is reflected in the massive expansion of the number of conditions within the official classificatory systems. For example, the number of diagnostic categories has increased from 106 in DSM-I (1952) to 357 in DSM-IV (1994). Many epidemiological studies using DSM

Table 14.5 'Top ten' physical non-diseases and six mental non-diseases as voted for on British Medical Journal website

Physical 'non-diseases'	*Mental 'non-diseases'*
Ageing	Unhappiness
Work	Road rage
Boredom	Loneliness
Bags under eyes	Bereavement
Ignorance	Alcohol misuse
Baldness	
Freckles	
Big ears	
Grey or white hairs	
Ugliness	

criteria for mental disorders have produced overall prevalence rates in the region of 25 to 30% in the general population. For example, the largest epidemiological study of psychiatric morbidity conducted in the UK produced prevalence rates of 12.3% and 19.5% for men and women respectively for neurotic disorders in a given week (Richman & Barry, 1985). The epidemiologic catchment area study (ECA), a household survey of 20000 people in five states across the USA, is reported to have found that the life-time prevalence of psychiatric disorders to be 32.2% and that 28% of Americans suffered from clinically significant and diagnosable mental disorder in the preceding year (Robins & Reiger, 1991).

These are huge numbers. Many have argued against the 'medicalisation of misery' and drawn attention to the broadening of the traditional boundaries of psychiatry resulting in mental health care being seen as the panacea for many different personal and social problems. They have pointed out, for instance, that normal shyness is being medicalised as social phobia and traumatic experiences as posttraumatic stress disorder. Pharmaceutical companies have actively promoted the extension of the boundaries of psychiatric care by proclaiming the success of various psychotropic drugs as the 'cure' for psychiatric condition (Double, 2002). Another adverse outcome is the massive demand for mental health care and the framing of many social problems as mental health issues. This has lead to the complaint that those with major mental illnesses are not receiving the care that they should get as resources get diverted towards the 'worried well'.

Reification fallacy. The disease concept has been misunderstood and misrepresented by many. Disorders are often referred to as quasi-disease 'entities' implying that they have a real existence. Often their origins in human imagination are forgotten and are assumed to have physical objective existence. The belief that the abstract or hypothetical are real and concrete is known as *reification* or, more correctly, *reification fallacy*. It needs to be emphasised that disorders, and similar concepts, are man-made constructions and what matters is their utility for the patient, the clinician and the research worker.

Tendency to pathologise. Although the ICD and DSM make it clear that the basis of their classification of mental disorders into types is based on syndromal descriptions and that no aetiology is presumed, it does create the spurious impression of precision and exactness. Many have come to believe that they are dealing with clear-cut disorders rather than arbitrary symptom clusters. The ICD and DSM diagnoses have become ends in themselves assuming the certainty of concrete givens. Given the bias that most medically trained doctors have toward pathology, blind adherence to diagnostic categories tends to frame the difficulties a person is experiencing as a pathology. It is easy for the eye trained in pathology to see one where none exists. Often this disempowers the patient, makes him view himself as defective, deficient, or even mad, leading to self-stigmatisation and disability.

The Rosenhan study, mentioned previously, is a valuable reminder of the tendency of doctors to commit type-two errors (the bias towards false positives) and see pathology where there is none. Trained in the medical tradition, doctors see their role primarily as identifying abnormal conditions (why should any normal person go to the doctor in the first place?). Indeed, the duty of the doctor is to identify the abnormality. By the mere process of selection, doctors see people with disorders rather than those without, therefore there is an inherent tendency for doctors to pathologise and commit the type-two error. In medical training, type-one error – missing the diagnosis – is considered to be a blunder. Trainers and teachers are scornful of trainees who fail to make correct diagnoses, candidates in examinations who misdiagnose are penalised and doctors get sued for negligence for not diagnosing a condition. Failure to identify a condition, even if it is a rare one, is thought of as professional incompetence. No wonder doctors are prone to make type-two errors, i.e. diagnose ill health rather than normality. Because the practice of psychiatry is reliant to a large extent on what patients tell their psychiatrists of their subjective experience and, moreover, because it lacks the benefit of radiological and laboratory data to verify clinical judgements, it is particularly liable to type-two errors.

Psychological distress is a common response to life's problems. Sometimes the distress may last for a period of time or result in transient psychological disturbance. When the disturbance is extreme and persistent it qualifies to be termed a disorder. Distinguishing between the various degrees of psychological difficulties is an essential part of good clinical practice (Figure 14.3).

Concept-driven perception. This is the tendency of clinicians to limit their thinking to those aspects of the clinical situation that are in accordance with

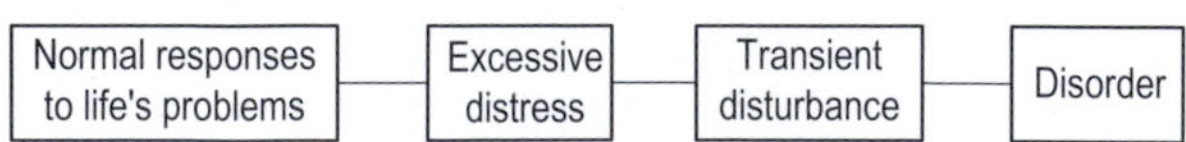

Fig.14.3 Spectrum of problems and difficulties people experience. Psychiatrists are most often presented with the extreme cases, i.e. mental disorders, and may fail to recognise or misdiagnose those at the other parts of the spectrum. The opposite is true of other mental health professionals.

their theoretical orientation and learning. In the case of psychiatrists steeped in the DSM and ICD tradition, the predilection to perceive primarily the diagnostic criteria in the manuals may take precedent over problems presented by the patient. A checklist approach to diagnosis encourages decontexualised formulations and can be misleading. This is especially true of trainee psychiatrists who want answers to the questions: What is the diagnosis? What is the drug of choice?

Limitations of DSM-IV

It is important to point out exactly what the DSM is, and also what it is not, for most of the criticisms of the DSM arise from a misunderstanding of its purpose. The DSM and ICD are *diagnostic and classificatory systems* – they are meant to provide reliable diagnoses. They do not aim to provide *assessments* and they are not intended to provide case formulations or treatment plans. DSM is a diagnostic manual that aspires to state succinctly how to identify the patient's disorder. Assessments, on the other hand, involve wider considerations of aetiological factors, impairments, meaning of symptoms, relational concomitants and so on. Moreover, assessments must be ideographic, i.e. unique to the individual. No two people with the same disorder show identical symptoms, the same level of suffering or similar aetiology. While all diagnostic systems take a nomothetic approach (see Chapter 3) emphasising the commonalities between diagnostic categories, clinical practice requires an idiographic perspective that emphasises the individuality, complexity and context of each person and his problems.

One of the unfortunate developments resulting from the use of DSM and ICD is the tendency among some clinicians, especially those with a biological orientation, to use the diagnostic process as a ritualistic, sterile exercise far removed from the experiences of the patient and the context in which these difficulties occur. This has lead some to complain that psychiatrists leave the human side of their patient to other practitioners and deal only with the 'being' side of the person.

Case example

A 24-year-old woman of Indian origin was involuntarily admitted to a psychiatric ward on a section of the Mental Health Act because of self-starvation and resulting weight loss. The consultant agreed with the social worker that she was endangering herself by severely restricting her eating, she had amenorrhoea and 'lacked insight'. A provisional diagnosis of anorexia nervosa was made. On admission she refused to eat the food provided by the ward on the pretext of 'not liking it'. She agreed that she wanted to lose weight and did not care whether she lived or died. She ran away from the ward and was brought back by the police.

At face value, the above case may be seen as fulfilling the criteria for an ICD/DSM diagnosis of anorexia nervosa. However, on closer examination, it would be evident that what we have is a decontexualised description of the problem. We know little about the circumstances of the eating problem, her relationships and the meaning of the 'symptoms' for her. As the story unfolded, a different picture emerged.

She came to the UK three years before, after marrying her husband who lived in the UK with his parents and two older brothers, who were already married. Her mother-in-law wanted her youngest son (the patient's husband) to be married to a young woman from her side of the family, but her husband (the patient's father-in-law) prevailed in his attempts to get him married to a girl from his side of the family. The mother-in-law and the two sisters-in-law were overtly hostile and got her (the patient) to do all the cleaning, washing and cooking. The situation became worse after she had a miscarriage 18 months previously. According to the female members of the family the patient was incapable of having children. The patient felt isolated and helpless and tried to persuade her husband to move to a house of their own, but he was financially dependent on his father and, though sympathetic to her request, found himself as helpless as her.

In this case it is clear that the patient's refusal to eat and the consequent loss of weight (and periods) were due to self-imposed starvation, which was a form of protest at her maltreatment at the hands of the family. A strictly biomedical approach made the situation worse by her being 'diagnosed' mentally ill because she appeared to almost fulfil the criteria for anorexia nervosa, an outcome that delighted the mother-in-law and restricted the patient's freedom until the family issues were identified.

Importance of diagnosis

Given these disadvantages of diagnoses, one might wonder, is there a role for diagnosis at all? The answer is a convincing 'yes' for the following reasons (Box 14.3):

1. Classification and categorisation, however imperfect, simplify complex data into manageable 'chunks' for information processing. Categorisation is a basic human cognitive process that helps us make sense of a complex world. The world of clinical medicine and psychiatry are no different.
2. Without diagnostic labels or similar classification system, epidemiological studies and research become almost impossible.
3. Diagnostic labels aid communication and act as shorthand ways of recording and understanding disorders, as long as there are agreed criteria.
4. Without proper ways of distinguishing between disorders, service planning and organisation, e.g. for early intervention in psychoses, becomes difficult.
5. There does not appear to be a viable alternative to classification and categorisation of mental health problems. The case formulation approach, which takes into account the unique features of the patient and his/her circumstances, is of great clinical value. But it is useless when it comes to epidemiological studies or studies of populations.

But, by itself, diagnosis can be limiting and, at times, can prove to be a hindrance to adequate patient care. The diagnosis alone is neither adequate for properly understanding the patient's experiences nor for formulating a

Box 14.3 Importance of making diagnoses in psychiatry

- Categorization is a normal cognitive process that helps identify and understand natural phenomena; it is used in other fields, e.g. biology, chemistry
- A short-hand way of communication
- Enables epidemiological studies to be carried out
- Assists the planning and organisation of services and helps research

management plan. In short, a diagnosis is a necessary but insufficient condition in clinical situations. No doubt it is a crucial piece of information, but it has to be supplemented by other data. One has to go beyond the diagnosis, enlarge the focus of enquiry to include other relevant personal, psychological and social domains. Both the zoom lens (for diagnostic assessment) and the wide-angled lens (for a comprehensive understanding of patients and their problems) are necessary. One way in which ICD-10 and DSM-IV have attempted to achieve all-inclusive formulations of the problems is by using a multiaxial classificatory system but it is not inclusive enough to provide most of the unique features of the patient and his/her illness.

Beyond DSM and ICD

The international systems of classification, ICD-10 and DSM-IV, have been major advances, but they provide only part of the information that we need in order to understand and manage patients and their problems. The psychosocial context in which the person's problems are embedded is as important as the disorder itself. In order to make sense of the patient's experiences and his/her narrative, clinicians need a framework around which all relevant information can be coherently and intelligibly organised. One such model is the *biopsychosocial* (BPS) *model* advocated by Engel (1980). However, before outlining the biopsychosocial model a short digression to describe the alternative model, the biomedical model, will help to provide the cultural background within which the BPS model has been developed.

The biomedical model

The prevailing dominant model in medicine and psychiatry today is the *biomedical model*. The biomedical model arose in the early nineteenth century with the discovery by microbiologists like Pasteur and others that certain germs caused diseases, such as smallpox and anthrax. Thus was born the 'germ theory' of disease. Certain bacteria were thought to 'cause' specific diseases. The introduction of antibacterial agents such as sulphanomides and penicillin lead to the 'cure' of many diseases. Following this huge breakthrough, researchers set out to discover the 'causes' of other major 'diseases', including mental disorders, so that a 'cure' could be discovered for them.

The main assumptions that underpin the biomedical model (Figure 14.4) are that: (1) disorders or diseases arise from one or more identifiable

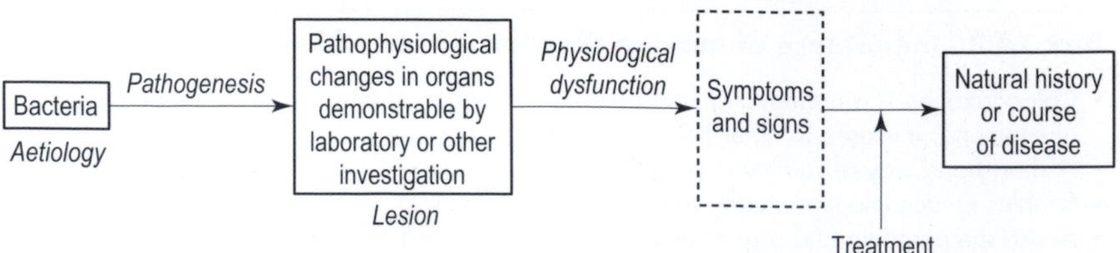

Fig. 14.4 The 'bacterial theory' of disease. Current psychiatric diagnoses are based on symptoms and signs and sometimes on the course of the disorder. Thus far no laboratory or radiological tests are available to confirm them.

aetiological causes (e.g. bacteria); (2) the aetiological agent produces a structural (lesion) or physiological dysfunction, called pathology (e.g. inflammation) and pathophysiology (e.g. reduced cardiac output); (3) the pathology leads to a recognisable pattern of symptoms and signs (syndromes); (4) the disease follows a certain temporal course (natural history); and (5) the course of the disease may be interrupted by some form of intervention (usually through drug treatment). Even a cursory examination of the model would indicate that it could not be applied even to the majority of physical illnesses. For example, diseases such as diabetes, ischaemic heart disease, cancer and hypertension, are not aetiological categories, as the 'bacterial hypothesis' would lead us to believe.

Following its initial success in physical medicine, there were similar attempts to apply the model to mental disorders. Emil Kraepelin, considered to be the father of modern psychiatry, was one of the first to apply the biomedical model to psychiatry. He believed that psychiatric disorders were mental equivalents of physical diseases and that future research would establish the causes of mental disorders (Box 14.4). Unfortunately, no such direct 'causes' of mental disorders have yet been discovered. Despite extensive research over more than a hundred years, psychiatry is nowhere near achieving the idealised biomedical model described above. Except for a very few conditions, like Alzheimer's disease, no structural pathology has been described and, despite all the research, no pathophysiology has been demonstrated for most psychiatric disorders. Moreover, there are no external criteria such as objective laboratory, radiological and histological findings against which the diagnoses can be validated. Extensive research carried out into the aetiology of disorders has singularly failed to identify the 'cause' of most disorders, including physical diseases (e.g. cancers, ischaemic heart disease). Now it is believed that all disorders, including most physical disorders, are the result of interaction between different types of social, psychological and

Box 14.4 Assumptions of the neo-Kraepelinian approach to psychiatry

- Psychiatry is a branch of medicine
- A boundary exists between the normal and the abnormal
- Mental illnesses exist
- It is the task of psychiatry to investigate the causes of mental illnesses
- Diagnostic criteria should be codified and validated

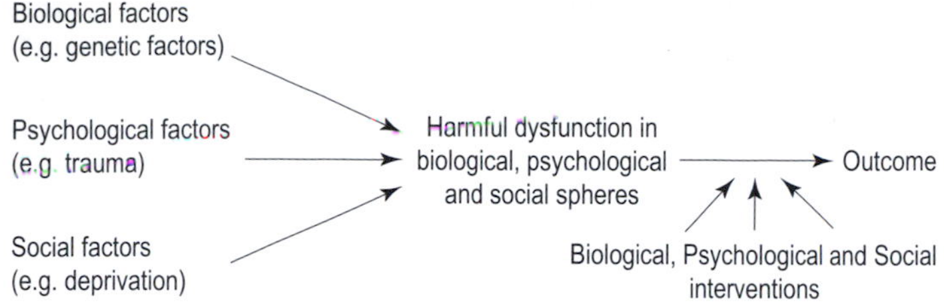

Fig. 14.5 Current understanding of physical (e.g. diabetes) and mental (psychiatric) disorders.

biological factors, i.e. they are multifactorial in origin (Figure 14.5). In contrast to the biomedical model of disease, the biopsychosocial model takes a multidimensional and multifaceted view of disorders.

The biopsychosocial (BPS) model

The origins of the biopsychosocial model can be traced back to Adolf Meyer. Meyer was critical of the Kraepelinian approach to psychiatry. He insisted that the assessment of patients' problem must be in relation to their personal history and not merely their current mental state. He argued against the mechanistic, rule-following Kraepelinian approach to diagnosis (the philosophy behind DSM-IV). For Meyer, the careful understanding of particular cases in their biographical context was more important than attempting to fit the patient's symptoms into pre-existing diagnostic categories. 'A diagnosis does justice to only one part of the facts and is merely a convenience of nomenclature', he wrote (Meyer, 1957). He argued that biological susceptibility due to inheritance or neurological abnormalities might be important but was not sufficient to explain why that person was mentally ill, in that way, at that time in their life. His model came to be known as 'psychobiology'.

In recent times, the subject of the biopsychosocial model has been forcefully articulated by Engel (1980). According to Engel, most illnesses, whether physical or psychiatric, are influenced by biopsychosocial phenomena and the biopsychosocial factors are central to the predisposition, onset, course and outcome of most disorders. More importantly, they are of major importance in designing interventions and management plans.

The BPS model holds that the diagnosis need not be exclusively in terms of the biomedical model. Those favouring the biopsychosocial model have recently expressed concern that psychiatry is simply becoming a matter of ticking check-lists to satisfy DSM criteria, and that there is an unhealthy trend to 'return to medicine', by concentrating on drug therapy and devising more and more specialisms, tending to dominate the field (Tucker, 1998). The BPS model seeks to overcome the limitations of the biomedical model by embracing a number of theories and practices that are thought to represent a more inclusive approach to complex sciences, such as mental disorders.

The biopsychosocial approach is not prescriptive, rather it adopts a perspective that allows multifactorial causation and explores the biological, psychological and social ramifications of all disorders. The scope of the biopsychosocial model includes a person-centred approach (rather than a disease-centred one), integration of biopsychosocial domains and a strong commitment to a contextualised and systemic approach. Engel (1980) turned to the general systems theory as best suited to provide a conceptual framework within which both medical and psychiatric disorders can be understood. The general systems theory developed by the biologists Ludwig von Bertalanffy and Paul Weiss is fundamental to the biopsychosocial approach (see also Chapter 12, p. 316). The key characteristics of systems may be summarised as follows:

1. Mental (and physical) disorders emerge in individuals who are part of a *system*.
2. Systems are interconnected and operate together in an integrated and coordinated fashion to maintain stability. This coordination is achieved through interaction between component parts of the system such that they identify coherent patterns. The overall patterns are not simply reducible to the sum of the actions of the individual parts – a system is more than the sum of its component parts.
3. The systems are organised hierarchically with more-complex, larger units being superordinate to less-complex, smaller units. Each system is thus a subsystem of another and, at the same time, contains smaller systems within it. For example, tissues form organs but also contain cellar systems. The model conceptualises nature as arranged on a hierarchical continuum ranging from molecules, cells, tissues, and organs through individuals, to families and societies. (Figure 14.6). Indeed, an outstanding property of all life is the tendency to form multilevel structures of systems within systems.
4. Each level of the hierarchy represents an organised dynamic. A system has distinctive properties such that it can be identified and named. The names cells, organs, person, and family each indicate a level of complex integrated organisation. The methods and rules appropriate for one level, such as the cell, cannot be applied to the study of another level, such as the person. While each system level interacts with those levels above and below it, each level also represents a 'dynamic whole' in its own right. A logical extension of this idea is that each system level can have its own type of dysfunction and that dysfunction at one system level will impact on the other system levels.
5. Lower-level organisations are *necessary* for higher ones to exist but they are not *sufficient* to describe or explain their nature. Central to systems theory is the idea that a system has characteristics that are *emergent*. At each level of complexity, the observed phenomena exhibit properties that do not exist at the lower level. Taking an example from biology, the taste of sugar is not present in carbon, hydrogen or oxygen atoms (Capra, 1997).

Although not without faults, the biopsychosocial model has achieved general acceptance in medicine and psychiatry. The implication of the model for nosology is that classification of disorders specific to each level are needed. Because current classifications are based on dysfunction at the *individual* level and neglect descriptions at other levels. DSM and ICD have, therefore, been

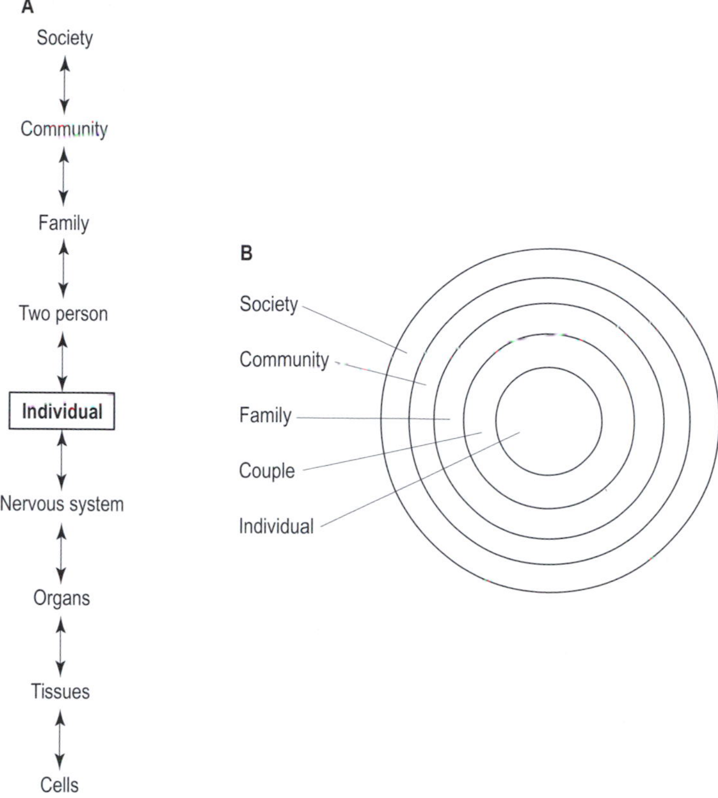

Fig. 14.6 Levels of organisation and systems hierarchy: A, the clinician is usually presented with problems that manifest at the level of the *individual*, but for an adequate understanding of the issues one has to study each component part of that system (individual) as well as other systems in the hierarchy (adapted from Engel, 1980); B, the ecological approach is another way of representing the same systems

found to be restricting. The BPS model helps overcome the limitations of the DSM and ICD to some degree.

The merit of the model is that it compels one to consider that a human is both a biological organism and a person who lives in the context of a family and a community. In contrast to the biomedical approach, which is disease centred, the biopsychosocial model is patient centred because it assesses the person with the disorder within the context of both support and the stresses affecting his daily life. The BPS model has important implications for the aetiology of disorders because it includes biological, psychological and social factors in their causation and continuation. The model also provides a framework for the management of patients' problems through biological, psychological and social interventions (Figure 14.7).

In recent years many psychiatrists have started emphasising the necessity for a high degree of psychological sensitivity when dealing with patients' mental disorders, including those patients with psychoses. It is important to adopt both humanistic and biological perspectives in understanding and

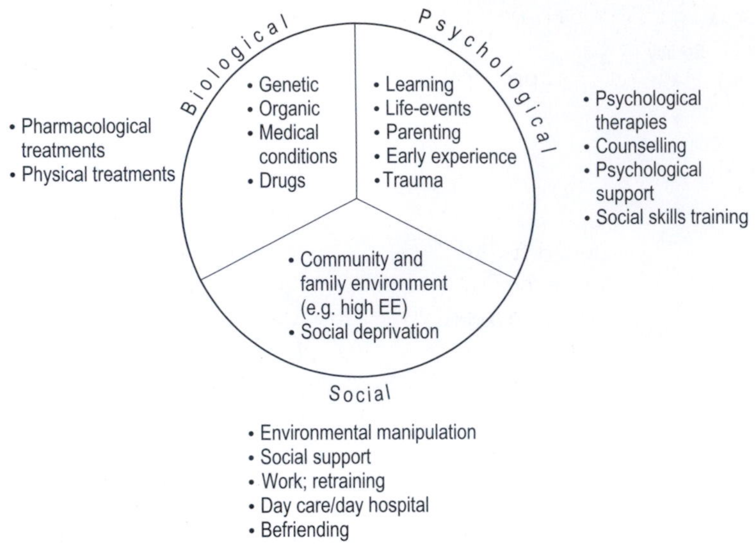

Fig. 14.7 Biopsychosocial factors in aetiology and management of disorders

working with persons with mental disorders. The overly optimistic expectation that neuroscience will find a pharmacological solution to the numerous and multifaceted problems presented by persons with mental disorders has lead to the loss of psychological skills of many psychiatrists. Our ability to understand mental disorders depends to a large extent on both the sciences and the humanities; science provides the insight into the causes of the problems and enables us to provide explanations while the humanities provide insight into their meanings. Psychiatry, if it is to establish itself as a mature science, must draw from both these sources. Of late, there has been a welcome resurgence of interest in psychological approaches to the assessment and treatment of those with mental disorders, especially those with psychoses. In general, psychiatry has been slow to embrace new developments in thinking and practice or has not been open to new ways of working. However, if a profession is to reach maturity there must be recognition that practice continuously exposes the limitations of a purely scientific approach, and ways need to be developed to help practitioners deal with the uncertainties and complexities of the everyday reality of psychiatric practice. The following are some of the psychological methods and/or frameworks that can make a significant contribution to the care of our patients. Some of these have already received brief mention elsewhere in the book, and only a few of the approaches are outlined here.

- Systemic approaches.
- Patient-centred care.
- Ecological approaches.
- Lifespan/developmental approaches.
- Narrative approaches.

- Integrating biopsychosocial domains.
- Reflective practice.
- Social constructivist approaches.

Narrative approach

The traditional emphasis in psychiatry about 'listening to patients' has recently been developed further by the introduction of what has been called the 'narrative' in mental health care. Narrative is one of the three fundamental modes of human understanding (the other two are the hypothetico-deductive mode and the categorical mode). Stories are fundamental features of all cultures and are universal mechanisms for transmitting meaning. We think, dream and tell our concerns in narrative form. Stories are also used to interpret and give coherence to past episodes in our lives and shape our future activities. Often individuals revise and rewrite their personal histories to support a current self-view. The concept of 'narrative' refers to what had happened to the subject, and 'narration' refers to how the narrative is presented to the clinician. So, narrative refers to events, relationships, experiences, whereas 'narration' describes what is communicated to the clinician and how the information is conveyed.

A narrative does not consist of random series of events, but a series of events related to one another in terms of cause and effect. The causal link implied by the narrator is often the way he or she makes sense of the events and reflects the underlying belief about the presenting problem. Patients present narratives of their illnesses, experiences and concerns to us. Every episode of illness is a milestone in the patient's narrative. Narrative provides the meaning and context to the patient's predicament. According to Bruner (1990), narratives are important because they:

- Give meaning to human action.
- Mediate between the culture and beliefs, desires and hopes of persons.
- Allow us to make sense of unusual or threatening events.
- Tell us what to expect.
- Allow us to explore how things might be different.

What makes stories so powerful? First, the brains of human beings are built to process stories better than other forms of information. Second, the process of storytelling itself provides a connection between the teller and listener. Third, stories are more powerful than statistics. Stories are recalled and imagined more readily and vividly in detail than mere numbers.

In the biomedical model the sole authorised narrative of illness is the physician's account of it and it occupies a privileged position. The common saying that 'illness is what the person has on the way to the doctor and disease is what he has on the way home' neatly summarises both the narrative of the patient and that of the doctor. Every time the person presenting with the problem and a health professional interact there is the potential for new stories to emerge. Since such stories (such as giving a diagnosis or an alternative explanation) have a powerful influence on the life of the help seeker, it is incumbent on practitioners to be aware of the powerful effects the stories create in the person. Alternative stories such as one of resilience, resourcefulness and recovery may create very different effects. In the case discussed above, the initial narrative of eating disorder requiring treatment was later replaced by one of protest by going on 'hunger strike', which proved to be more useful than the disorder story. Narrative approaches encourage 'richer' narratives to emerge from disparate descriptions of experience. Greenhalgh and Hurwitz (1998) have provided a fascinating account of narrative approaches to medicine.

Patient-centred approach

Medical students and doctors are now routinely taught and trained in patient-centred methods of interviewing and communication. In addition to active listening, establishing rapport and being culturally sensitive, a patient-orientated approach demands that the physician be aware of and take pains to elicit, the patient's explanatory model of the illness. This means that the practitioner has to sensitively explore the hypotheses patients may have for their difficulties.

Reflective practice

Reflection is a central process for learning about the world and ourselves. Experimental psychology has given us a variety of learning theories (conditioning, social learning, etc.) but neglected learning by reflection – the capacity to reanalyse, re-evaluate and find new meaning for past, present and future events. Although current psychiatric practice claims to be based on scientific theory and evidence-based practice, and while there is safety in the certainty of the scientific model, many, if not most, clinical situations are characterised by uniqueness, unexpectedness and value conflicts. A reflective paradigm gives us the opportunity to examine our practice with a critical eye. Whereas the scientific-practitioner model offers one method for discovering truths, the reflective position provides a framework for evaluating the status of these so-called truths. Thus, reflective practice leads us to take a critical and evaluative position in relation to our understanding of the practice of psychiatry and the perceived wisdoms of our profession.

The foundation for reflective practice in professions was laid down by Donald Schön (1983). He described the processes involved in reflective practice as follows:

- *Reflection in action*. This refers to the process where, while you are acting, you reflect cognitively and emotionally about what you are doing and what you should do next. This type of reflection occurs (or should occur) when faced with the unexpected or when theory-driven actions have reached their limits.
- *Reflection on action*. This happens after the event and may take place in clinical supervision or as a result of reflection by the professional about one's practice.

- *Reflection upon impact on others.* Since most of the time our professional lives are spent in interpersonal contexts, we need to reflect on the effect of our actions on others through feedback or by other means. This is particularly significant when working in teams and with other colleagues.
- *Reflection upon self.* This refers to the personal use of self-awareness about what we bring and take from clinical encounters. It compels the practitioners to question constructively all aspects of theory and practice and gets them to question themselves: What is the model I am using? What role(s) am I playing or am I made to play (e.g. expert, advocate, providing support, satisfying the managers) in a particular clinical situation? What are the core values that underpin my practice and when am I pressured to override them? In what other ways can I frame the problem in the best interest of the patient? Such reflective practice promotes self-awareness and professional development.

Reflective practice forms an important part of adult learning and continuous professional development. It has been considered as the critical factor that distinguishes expert practitioners from average practitioners. According to Skovholt and colleagues: 'A therapist and a counsellor can have 20 years of experience or one year of experience 20 times. What makes the difference? A key component is reflection' (Skovholt, Rønnestad, & Jennings, 1997). The power of reflection becomes clear if one recalls that Freud's reflections on no more than a few dozen of his patients formed the basis of his theoretical and practical formulations.

Thus, reflective practice forms an important part of personal and professional development and requires to be acknowledged as such in both the training of competent practitioners and the support of established clinicians. This is all the more important in the case of psychiatrists, who, by definition, are confronted with the most complex of cases and have to make difficult decisions.

Epistemology

Discussions on what constitutes a disorder, the appropriateness of classificatory systems and how we understand abnormality inevitably lead on to the philosophic question: what is the nature and source of knowledge and how do we make sense of our world? The branch of philosophy that is concerned with the origin and nature of knowledge is known as *epistemology*. It attempts to answer the basic question: what distinguishes true (adequate) knowledge from false (inadequate) knowledge? In practical terms the question that it raises for the clinician is: how can we develop models and theories that are better than existing ones?

Rational knowledge derived from experience and experimentation constructs a map of reality in which things are reduced to abstract concepts and symbols characterised by categorisation, measurement and linear sequential structures. But the natural world is complex, multidimensional and consists of infinite varieties occurring randomly. Modern physics tells us that even empty space is curved and that there are four dimensions in the natural world. It is evident that our abstract system of reality can never describe or understand this reality completely and we have to admit to the limitations of our understanding of the world (Capra, 1982). Based on findings from modern physics, Capra (1982) has called for a 'new paradigm thinking' in science, which includes the following:

- Knowledge of structure does not predict function.
- Knowledge is constructed.
- Process is primary and predicts structure.
- The observer is part of the whole system and observations are not independent of the observer.
- There are no fundamental equations.
- All rules, descriptions and equations are approximations.

Albert Einstein, who strove all his life to understand the forces of nature and capture them in scientific laws and equations, acknowledged the limitations of science and 'scientific thinking' when he said:

> *Imagination is more important than science.*
> Albert Einstein, *On Science*

REFERENCES

Andrews G, Stewart G, Morris-Yates A, Holt P, Henderson S (1990) Evidence for a general neurotic syndrome. British Journal of Psychiatry, 157, 6–12.

APA (1994) Diagnostic and Statistical Manual of Mental Disorders (4th ed.). Washington, DC: American Psychiatric Association.

Bruner J (1990) Acts of Meaning. Cambridge, MA: Harvard University Press.

Capra F (1982) The Tao of Physics. London, UK: Flamingo.

Capra F (1997) The Web of Life. London, UK: Flamingo

Double D (2002) The limits of psychiatry. British Medical Journal, 324, 900–904.

Engel GL (1980) The clinical application of the biopsychosocial model. American Journal of Psychiatry, 137, 535–544.

Greenhalgh T, Hurwitz B (1998) Narrative-based Medicine: dialogue and discourse in clinical practice. London, UK: BMJ Books.

Kendell RE (1975) The role of diagnosis in psychiatry. Oxford: Blackwell Scientific Publications.

Meyer A (1957) Psychobiology: a science of man. Springfield, IL: Charles C Thomas.

Richman A, Barry A (1985) More and more is less and less, the myth of massive psychiatric need. British Journal of Psychiatry, 146, 164–168.

Robins L, Reiger D (eds) (1991) The Epidemiologic Catchment Area Study. New York: Free Press.

Rosenhan DL (1973) On being sane in insane places. Science, 179, 250–258.

Schön DA (1983) The Reflective Practitioner. New York: Basic Books.

Skovholt TM, Rønnestad MH, Jennings I (1997) The search for expertise in counselling, psychotherapy and professional psychology. Educational Psychology Review, 9, 361–369.

Smith R (2002) In search of 'non-disease'. British Medical Journal, 324, 883–885.

Tucker GJ (1998) Putting DSM-IV in perspective. American Journal of Psychiatry, 155, 457–469.

Tyrer P (2003) Defining personality difficulties and personality disorders. Progress in Neurology and Psychiatry, 7(4), 11–16.

Tyrer P, Johnson T (1996) Establishing the severity of personality disorders. American Journal of Psychiatry, 153, 1593–1597.

WHO (1992) The ICD-10 Classification of Mental and Behavioural Disorders: clinical descriptions and diagnostic guidelines. Geneva: World Health Organization.
Zimmerman M, Matia JI (1999) Psychiatric diagnoses in clinical practice: is comorbidity being missed? Comprehensive Psychiatry, 40, 182–191.

FURTHER READING

Barron JW (ed.) (1998) Making Diagnosis Meaningful: enhancing evaluation and treatment of psychological disorders. Washington, DC: American Psychological Association.
- A thoughtful critique of DSM-IV by various authorities, mostly psychologists and psychotherapists.

Kendell RE (1975) The Role of Diagnosis in Psychiatry. Oxford: Blackwell Scientific Publications.
- An in-depth account of disease concept in psychiatry, somewhat dated. Updated by the author in subsequent articles in the *British Journal of Psychiatry*.

Wakefield JC (1992) The concept of mental disorder: on the boundary between biological facts and social values. American Psychologist, 47(3), 373–388.
- An influential paper outlining the 'harmful' dysfunction' view of mental disorders.

Index

Note: Page numbers suffixed with 'f' refer to figures; those suffixed with 't' refer to tables or boxes.

C

E

F

G

J

K

M

U

V

W